Measurement of Cardiac Deformations from MRI: Physical and Mathematical Models

Computational Imaging and Vision

Volume 23

Measurement of Cardiac Deformations from MRI: Physical and Mathematical Models

Edited by

Amir A. Amini

Washington University St. Louis, U.S.A.

and

Jerry L. Prince

Johns Hopkins University, Baltimore, U.S.A.

KLUWER ACADEMIC PUBLISHERS

DORDRECHT / BOSTON / LONDON

A C.I.P. Catalogue record for this book is available from the Library of Congress.

ISBN 1-4020-0222-X

Published by Kluwer Academic Publishers,
P.O. Box 17, 3300 AA Dordrecht, The Netherlands.

Sold and distributed in North, Central and South America
by Kluwer Academic Publishers,
101 Philip Drive, Norwell, MA 02061, U.S.A.

In all other countries, sold and distributed
by Kluwer Academic Publishers,
P.O. Box 322, 3300 AH Dordrecht, The Netherlands.

Printed on acid-free paper

Printed in the Netherlands.

Contents

Contributors xi
Preface xiii

1 Regional Stress and Strain in Healthy and Diseased Ventricular Myocardium
1.1 Introduction 1
1.2 Ventricular Geometry and Structure 2
1.3 Regional Myocardial Mechanics 3
1.4 Engineering Models of Wall Stress 7
1.5 Analyzing Wall Strain Distributions 8
1.6 Regional Strain Distributions in Disease 9
1.7 Future Directions 10
Acknowledgments 11
References for Chapter 1 11

2 Clinical Applications of Cardiac Tagging
2.1 Introduction 17
2.2 Imaging Techniques 18
2.3 Tagged Image Data Analysis 19
2.4 MR Tagging in Normal Human Heart 22
2.5 MR Tagging in Ischemic Heart Disease 24
2.6 MR Tagging in Left Ventricular Hypertrophy 28
2.7 Cardiomyopathies 29
2.8 Right Ventricular Mechanics 30
2.9 Pericardial Constriction 30
2.10 Summary 30
Acknowledgments 31
References for Chapter 2 31

3 Finite Element Modeling for Three-Dimensional Motion Reconstruction and Analysis
3.1 Introduction 37
3.2 The Finite Element Model 38
3.2.1 Basis Functions 39

3.2.2 Global Parameters 40
3.2.3 Coordinate Systems 40
3.2.4 Kinematics 42
3.3 Model Tags: 3D Formulation 43
3.3.1 Geometric Fits 43
3.3.2 Model Tag 3D Fitting 44
3.3.3 Image Analysis 45
3.3.4 Minimization 46
3.4 Reconstruction of RV Surface Deformation 48
3.4.1 RV Free wall geometry 49
3.4.2 Model Tags: Surface Formulation 49
3.5 Principal Component Analysis 51
3.5.1 Generating the Data Set 53
3.6 PCA of Normal Geometry and Deformation 53
3.7 Future Work 55
References for Chapter 3 56

4 Modeling and analysis of the RV and LV from MRI-SPAMM
4.1 Introduction 59
4.2 Biventricular Model Geometry 61
4.2.1 RV Contour Segmentation 62
4.2.2 Processing Contour Data 62
4.2.3 Finite element mesh generation 64
4.3 3D RV and LV motion reconstruction 64
4.3.1 MRI Input Data 65
4.3.2 Model Dynamics 65
4.3.3 External Forces from SPAMM data 67
4.3.4 External forces From Contour Data 69
4.3.5 Internal Forces Due To Stiffness 70
4.4 Motion and Deformation Analysis 72
4.4.1 Motion Parameters 72
4.4.2 Data Analysis 73
4.5 Results 74
4.5.1 Model fitting behavior 75
4.5.2 Validation studies 75
4.5.3 Clinical Data 79
4.6 Discussion 84
4.7 Conclusions and Future Work 85
Acknowledgments 85
Appendix 85
Finite Element Shape Functions 85
Strain Calculation Using Finite Elements 86
References for Chapter 4 89

5 Motion Analysis of the Whole Heart
5.1 Motivation and Background 91
5.2 Introduction and Background 92
5.2.1 Anatomy and Physiology 93
5.2.2 Studying Right Ventricular and Atrial Dynamics 94
5.2.3 MR Imaging of Right Ventricular and Atrial Function . . . 95
5.2.4 B-Spline based Motion Tracking 97
5.3 Methods 98
5.3.1 MR Imaging 98
5.3.2 Ventricular Motion Analysis 100
5.3.3 Atrial Surface Fitting 101
5.3.4 Calculation of the Atrial Motion Field 103
5.4 Results 106
5.4.1 Motion Analysis of Right and Left Ventricles 106
5.4.2 Motion Analysis of Atria 108
5.5 Discussion 109
5.6 Conclusion 112
Acknowledgments 113
References for Chapter 5 113

6 Harmonic Phase MRI
6.1 Introduction 119
6.2 A Harmonic Model of Tagged MR Images 120
6.3 HARP Motion Measurement Principles 123
6.3.1 Apparent Motion 125
6.3.2 Spatial and Temporal Derivatives 126
6.4 CINE-HARP (CHARP) Methods 127
6.4.1 Tracking Motion 127
6.4.2 Lagrangian Strain 130
6.4.3 Velocity Fields 134
6.4.4 Strain-rate Maps 137
6.5 Single-shot HARP (SHARP) Methods 139
6.5.1 Tagline Synthesis 139
6.5.2 Radial and Circumferential Eulerian Strain 140
6.5.3 Minimum and Maximum Eulerian Strain 142
6.5.4 Contraction Angle 145
6.6 Combining CHARP and SHARP Methods 146
6.7 Summary and Conclusion 146
Acknowledgments 148
References for Chapter 6 149

7 Automated Tag Detection
7.1 Introduction 151
7.2 Signal Models 152

7.2.1 Tagged Myocardium 153
7.2.2 Untagged Tissue 155
7.3 Tag Center Estimation 156
7.3.1 Single Tag Center Estimation 156
7.3.2 Tag Line Estimation 158
7.4 Hypothesis Testing 160
7.4.1 Myocardium Detection 161
7.4.2 Tag Line Detection 161
7.4.3 Removal of False Tag Points 162
7.5 Algorithm Implementation 163
7.5.1 Black Blood Images 163
7.5.2 White Blood Images 166
7.6 In Vivo Experiments 169
7.6.1 Imaging Protocol 169
7.6.2 Black Blood Images 169
7.6.3 White Blood Images 171
7.7 Discussion 171
Acknowledgments 177
Appendix 178
Likelihood Function Derivative 178
References for Chapter 7 179

8 Analysis of Tagged MR Cardiac Images with B-spline Models
8.1 Introduction 183
8.2 B-spline basics 186
8.2.1 Definitions and Notations 186
8.2.2 Properties 187
8.3 Coupled B-snake Grids 188
8.4 Constrained Thin-Plate Spline Reconstruction 190
8.4.1 Solution Using Subspace Approximations 193
8.4.2 Validations 196
8.4.3 Myocardial Strains 203
8.5 Measurement of 3D Motion of Myocardial Beads 204
8.5.1 Imaging Protocol 205
8.5.2 Reconstruction of Tag Planes 206
8.5.3 Computing 3D Coordinates of Myocardial Beads 207
8.5.4 Validations 213
8.6 Conclusions 214
8.7 Acknowledgments 215
References for Chapter 8 215

9 MR Physics and Imaging of Phase Contrast MRI
9.1 Introduction 219
9.2 Basic Principles of Phase Contrast MRI 220

9.2.1 Flow and Motion Compensation . . . 221
9.2.2 Velocity Encoding . . . 221
9.3 Implementation issues . . . 223
9.3.1 Gradient Echo imaging . . . 223
9.3.2 Respiratory Motion . . . 224
9.3.3 Segmented Scans . . . 225
9.3.4 Black Blood Preparation . . . 225
9.3.5 Measurement Timing and Pulse Sequence Design . . . 226
9.3.6 Multi Echo Approaches . . . 228
9.3.7 Measurement Timing . . . 230
9.3.8 View Sharing Approaches . . . 231
9.4 Data Processing . . . 232
9.5 Results . . . 237
9.5.1 Volunteers . . . 237
9.5.2 Patients . . . 238
9.6 Discussion . . . 243
Appendix . . . 245
Signal Phase . . . 245
References for Chapter 9 . . . 246

10 Myocardial Spatiotemporal Tracking
10.1 Introduction . . . 257
10.1.1 Imaging Cardiac Motion . . . 258
10.1.2 Mapping Velocity With Phase Contrast MRI . . . 259
10.1.3 Analyzing Motion . . . 262
10.2 DMESH Motion/Strain Mapping . . . 264
10.2.1 The Spatiotemporal Finite Element Model . . . 265
10.2.2 The DMESH Tracking Algorithm . . . 267
10.2.3 Reproducibility Analysis . . . 268
10.2.4 Lagrangian Strain Field Computation . . . 269
10.2.5 Extended Use of DMESH Tracking . . . 270
10.3 Experiments . . . 271
10.3.1 Computer simulation studies . . . 271
10.3.2 *In vitro* and *in vivo* studies . . . 275
10.3.3 Combined use of displacement and velocity data . . . 277
10.4 Discussion . . . 280
Acknowledgments . . . 282
References for Chapter 10 . . . 283

11 Computational Platforms for Integrated Cardiac Image Analysis
11.1 Introduction . . . 289
11.2 Obtaining Estimates of Cardiac Displacements . . . 290
11.2.1 Methods Relying on Magnetic Resonance Tagging . . . 290
11.2.2 Methods Relying on Phase Contrast MRI . . . 291

11.2.3 Computer-Vision Based Methods 292
11.2.4 The Shape-Based Tracking Approach 293
11.3 Modeling used for Interpolation and Smoothing 296
11.3.1 The Strain Tensor 297
11.3.2 Material Models 300
11.3.3 A Bayesian Estimation Framework 303
11.4 Experimental Results 305
11.4.1 Pre and post-occlusion comparison 306
11.4.2 Shape-Based Estimates vs MR Tagging 308
11.5 Future Research Directions 309
Acknowledgments 310
References for Chapter 11 310
Index 315

Contributors

Amir A. Amini
CVIA Laboratory, Box 8086, 660 S. Euclid Ave., Washington University School of Medicine, St. Louis, MO 63110

Kevin F. Augenstein
Department of Engineering Science, School of Engineering, University of Auckland, New Zealand

Leon Axel
Department of Radiology, University of Pennsylvania, Philadelphia, PA

Yasheng Chen
CVIA Laboratory, Box 8086, 660 S. Euclid Ave., Washington University School of Medicine, St. Louis, MO 63110

Thomas S. Denney Jr.
Department of Electrical and Computer Engineering, Auburn University, Auburn, AL

James S. Duncan
Department of Diagnostic Radiology, Department of Electrical Engineering, Yale University School of Medicine, New Haven, CT 06520-8042

Idith Haber
Cardiovascular Research Division, Children's Hospital and Harvard Medical School, Boston, MA

Jürgen Hennig
Uniklinik Freiburg, Abt. Rontgendiagnostik, Sect. of Medical Physics, Hugstetter Str. 55, D 79106 Freiburg, Germany

Michael Markl
Uniklinik Freiburg, Abt. Rontgendiagnostik, Sect. of Medical Physics, Hugstetter Str. 55, D 79106 Freiburg, Germany

Andrew D. McCulloch
Department of Bioengineering and The Whitaker Institute of Biomedical Engineering, University of California San Diego, 9500 Gilman Drive, La Jolla, CA 92093-0412, USA

Elliot R. McVeigh
Laboratory of Cardiac Energetics, NHLBI, Building 10, Room B1D416, Bethesda, MD 20892-1061

Dimitris Metaxas
Department of Computer and Information Science, University of Pennsylvania, Philadelphia, PA

Nael F. Osman
Department of Radiology, Johns Hopkins University, 3400 N. Charles St., Baltimore, MD 21218

Cengizhan Ozturk
Bogazici University, Institute of Biomedical Engineering, 80815 Bebek, Istanbul, Turkey

Xenophon Papademetris
Department of Diagnostic Radiology, Yale University School of Medicine, New Haven, CT 06520-8042

Norbert J. Pelc
Department of Radiology
Stanford University, Palo Alto, CA

Jerry L. Prince
Electrical and Computer Engineering, Johns Hopkins University, 3400 N. Charles St., Baltimore, MD 21218

Nathaniel Reichek
Research and Education Foundation, DeMatteis Center, St. Francis Hospital, 100 Port Washington Blvd., Roslyn, NY 11576

Britta Schneider
Uniklinik Freiburg, Abt. Rontgendiagnostik, Sect. of Medical Physics, Hugstetter Str. 55, D 79106 Freiburg, Germany

Albert J. Sinusas
Section of Cardiovascular Medicine, Department of Internal Medicine, Yale University School of Medicine, New Haven, CT 06520-8042

Alistair A. Young
Department of Anatomy with Radiology, School of Medicine, University of Auckland, New Zealand

Yu-Ping Wang
The Advanced Digital Imaging Research, LLC., 2525 South Shore Blvd., #100, League City, TX 77573

Yudong Zhu
GE Corporate Research and Development, Schenectady, New York

Preface

This book describes the latest imaging and image analysis techniques that have been developed at leading centers for the visualization, analysis, and understanding of normal and abnormal cardiac motion with magnetic resonance imaging (MRI). The use of MRI in measuring cardiac motion is particularly important because MRI is non-invasive, and it is the only modality capable of imaging detailed intramural motion *within* the myocardium. Other imaging modalities must infer the motion of the myocardium from the motion of just the endocardium and epicardium. In addition to its novel capabilities for imaging the intramural myocardial motion in 3D, first-pass contrast perfusion imaging, delayed contrast-enhanced imaging of myocardial viability, and MR imaging of the coronary arteries are experiencing rapid progress as well, making the one-stop-shop goal of cardiovascular MRI a reality in the near future.

There have been many significant advances in the field of cardiovascular MRI over the past several years. This book brings together many of the key advances in the imaging of cardiac motion — the data acquisition, image processing, and image analysis — in one bound volume. The book is organized to provide fundamentals about the mechanical properties of the heart, acquisition technologies including MR tagging and phase-contrast, and image processing and analysis methods that are used to reveal detailed myocardial velocity, displacement, and strain patterns in the heart muscle. While primary emphasis is on the left ventricle, new emerging applications to the right ventricle and atria are presented here as well. Information about the use of cardiac MR imaging of function for the scientific purpose of understanding heart motion and for the clinical need to diagnose heart disease is also represented herein.

We have collected chapters for inclusion in this book which should serve a variety of purposes. Biomedical engineers, medical physicists, computer scientists, and physicians interested in learning about the latest advances in cardiovascular MRI should find this book to be a valuable educational resource. In particular, it is more tutorial in nature than most of the technical papers where the research was originally published. Practitioners and researchers working in the field of cardiovascular MRI will find the book to be filled with practical technical details and references to other work, enabling the implementation of existing methods and serving as a basis for further research in the area. Non-specialists may find the reading to be technically challenging, but will certainly be inspired by the successful interplay between medical and engineering challenges, a key aspect of research developments described herein.

We now give a brief overview of the chapters contained within the book.

In Chapter 1, Andrew McCulloch gives an overview of the relationship between stress and strain in the myocardium. Stress is the force per unit area which acts on surfaces between adjacent regions of the muscle, whereas strain is a measure of the resulting deformation; often reported as a percent change in length. Measurement of these quantities, especially the strain of myocardial deformation, is a recurring theme in the book. This chapter provides the foundations for understanding the importance of this concept.

In Chapter 2, Nathaniel Reichek gives an overview of clinical application of cardiac tagging. Applications of MR tagging for assessment of strain and fiber shortening in normal physiology, and the changes in left-ventricular hypertrophy, ischemic heart disease, cardiomyopathies, and pericardial constriction are discussed. Additionally, a discussion of stress-testing with MRI using inotropic stimulation is provided.

In Chapter 3, Kevin Augenstein and Alistair Young discuss their latest Finite Element Modeling (FEM) approaches to analysis of tagged MRI data of the intact left and right ventricles. Using principal component analysis (PCA) in a normal population, Augenstein and Young report on the principal statistical modes of deformation of the left-ventricle from fitted FEM models.

In Chapter 4, Idith Haber, Dimitris Metaxas, and Leon Axel describe physics-based FEM deformable models for analysis of left and right ventricles. The approach fits a biventricular FE model to tag data based on the Lagrangian equations of motion. Application of methods to tagged MRI data collected in normal and hypertrophic hearts are reported.

In Chapter 5, Cengizhan Ozturk and Elliot McVeigh, describe methods for motion analysis of the whole heart, concentrating on atrial motion. Since the atria are thin and tagged MR methods do not lend themselves to atrial motion analysis, they describe a surface-based registration method for determining atrial deformations from MRI. For left and right ventricular motion analysis, circumferential strains are reported as a function of time.

In Chapter 6, Nael Osman and Jerry Prince describe HARmonic Phase (HARP) MRI, a new method based on tagged MRI for fast assessment of myocardial kinematics. Due to the relatively little post-processing which is involved, HARP may be used in the future within a cardiac monitoring or MRI stress testing setting.

In Chapter 7, Thomas Denney Jr. describes Bayesian methods for localization of tag lines in short-axis and long-axis tagged MRI slices. For carrying out comprehensive analysis of cardiac deformations over time, tag lines need to be localized on all acquired image data. The approach automatically estimates location of tag lines on tagged MRI slices of the left-ventricle.

In Chapter 8, Yasheng Chen, Yu-Ping Wang, and Amir Amini describe B-spline methods for analysis of tagged MRI data. They develop a fast approach to reconstruction of 2D tissue deformations from tagged MR images using a shifted B-spline bases representation of the deformation field. Additionally, they use deformable B-spline surface representations for triplets of intersecting tag planes to compute and track 3D location of myocardial beads.

In Chapter 9, Michael Markl, Britta Schneider, and Jürgen Hennig discuss MRI phase velocity encoding for assessment of ventricular function. The chapter provides a thorough description of phase-contrast MRI and describes an approach to analysis of acquired velocity data which involves decomposing the myocardial motion into radial (thickening) and tangential (angular and torsional) components.

In Chapter 10, Yudong Zhu and Norbert Pelc describe a dynamic FEM-based approach called DMESH for analysis of phase-velocity data. The approach which involves fitting velocity samples over an extended region at all time frames, analytically constructs the displacement and strains from the collected velocity data.

In Chapter 11, Xenophon Papademetris, Albert Sinusas, and James Duncan use biomechanically inspired models to measure displacements and strain from Cine MRI. The approach uses expected fiber directions in normal volunteers across the myocardial wall in a Bayesian framework to interpolate initial endocardial and epicardial surface displacements. Initial surface displacements are measured by tracking curvature landmarks.

We are thankful for the help of many people during the development of this book. We would first like to thank all the contributors for spending time to write the excellent chapters that comprise this volume. The product is primarily a result of their expertise and hard work. We are also grateful for the help of two of our students, whose efforts were truly indispensable in the preparation of this book. Jordan Woerndle (Washington University in St. Louis) set up and maintained a highly professional web site for the authors' use in the development of the book and Aaron Carass (Johns Hopkins University) painstakingly solved all the LaTeX 2_ε problems, edited and re-edited all of the chapters, and compiled the final product before you. We would like to thank Paul Roos and James Finlay of Kluwer Academic Publishers, who guided us through the details of book publishing (and who tolerated numerous delays in getting the final book to press). Finally, we would also like to thank Max Viergever, Editor of the Kluwer's Computational Imaging and Vision book series. Max first suggested the idea for this book to us in the summer of 1999 and has patiently urged and guided us to its completion.

Amir A. Amini	and	Jerry L. Prince
Washington University in St. Louis		Johns Hopkins University

Chapter 1

Regional Stress and Strain in Healthy and Diseased Ventricular Myocardium

Andrew D. McCulloch

Department of Bioengineering and
The Whitaker Institute of Biomedical Engineering,
University of California San Diego,
9500 Gilman Drive, La Jolla, CA 92093-0412, USA
amcculloch@ucsd.edu

1.1 Introduction

The primary function of the heart is fundamentally mechanical. The basic measures of myocardial mechanics are the three-dimensional stresses and strains, which depend on position and orientation in the myocardium, and vary in time through the cardiac cycle. A host of physiological and pathophysiological processes are directly or indirectly regulated by regional myocardial stress and strain. Most of these factors – such as coronary flow and myocyte energetics, excitation and arrhythmia, hypertrophy and development, remodeling and repair – themselves affect stress and strain in the ventricular wall. For example, increased wall stress due to altered hemodynamic load can cause ventricular hypertrophy, which in turn alters wall stress by changing chamber geometry and material properties. If this feedback loop establishes a new equilibrium, hypertrophy can be compensated. But if stress continues to increase, a transition to decompensated hypertrophy and pump failure can ensue. As treatments for myocardial infarction and ischemia have improved, the incidence of congestive heart failure has risen alarmingly. Some important load-induced responses are now known to be regulated by stress and strain directly at the level of the myocyte, endothelial cell and fibroblast. For these advances in basic cardiac biology to be applied in the clinical setting, a better understanding of the biomechanics of ventricular remodeling *in-vivo* will surely be needed.

From the perspective of biomechanics, there are three key determinants of ventricular wall stresses and strains: the three-dimensional geometry and structure of

A.A. Amini and J.L. Prince (eds.),
Measurement of Cardiac Deformations from MRI: Physical and Mathematical Models, 1–15.

the ventricular walls; the pressure boundary conditions and physical constraints imposed by the blood and surrounding tissues such as the pericardium, atria and great vessels; and the nonlinear material properties of the resting and contracting myocardium. Given this information, a continuum mechanics model based on the conservation laws of physics can be formulated to estimate wall stress and strain distributions. The capability of cardiac MRI to provide high-resolution three-dimensional information on ventricular geometry and structure, noninvasively and without the need for ionizing radiation, is therefore a valuable tool in the development of such theoretical and computational models.

Suitable three-dimensional measurements are also needed to validate and refine the model analysis of wall stress and strain. At present, it remains much more practical to measure regional strain distributions than stresses. The advent of cardiac MRI "tagging" and other techniques for identifying regional wall strains and strain-rates was thus a major milestone in myocardial biomechanics. In this chapter, I briefly introduce the engineering concepts of stress and strain and discuss the roles of cardiac MRI in improving our knowledge and understanding of ventricular biomechanics. I will discuss how the modeling methods for simulating ventricular wall mechanics and analyzing functional cardiac MRI data are starting to coalesce. Finally, I point to some challenges for the future.

1.2 Ventricular Geometry and Structure

Since three-dimensional geometry and structure are fundamental determinants of myocardial stress and strain, it is not surprising that MRI has been a useful modality for generating geometric models of ventricular anatomy for engineering analysis. Parametric image modeling techniques such as deformable contours [22] have also become popular tools for segmenting the image volumes. A variety of geometric approximations have been used to parameterize left and right ventricular geometries obtained from MR or other three-dimensional image sets. A natural extension to the popular use of prolate spheroidal geometric models, has been the fitting of polynomials or other interpolation functions to segmented ventricular boundaries using a prolate spheroidal (elliptic-hyperbolic-polar) coordinate system. Investigators have also recognized that the task of segmenting the tagged MRI images can even be combined into the model-fitting analysis [42].

The use of tomographic imaging to reconstruct ventricular geometric models is neither new nor limited to MRI. On the other hand, an application of MR phase-sensitive imaging is finding a novel use for measuring myocardial fiber architecture, a crucial determinant of regional ventricular mechanics. MR diffusion-sensitive imaging uses phase dispersion mapping to measure diffusion coefficients in six non-parallel directions allowing the local three-dimensional diffusion tensor to be reconstructed [4].

The heart has a complex three-dimensional anatomy which plays a significant role in the generation of regional wall deformation. The predominant myofiber direction is almost parallel to the plane of the epicardial and endocardial surfaces, but has a pitch angle that varies 120° or more across the wall from that of a left-handed helix on the epicardium to a steep right-handed helix on the endocardium with circumferential fibers near the ventricular midwall [34]. The more recent dissections and histological findings of LeGrice et al. [16] also suggest a higher level of organization of myofibers into a sheet structure with loose perimysial collagen connections between tightly coupled laminae 4-8 myocytes thick.

Initial studies using magnetic resonance diffusion tensor imaging in myocardium [9] showed that the diffusion of water in isolated perfused rat hearts is anisotropic with a well defined principal axis of the greatest diffusion coefficient. Studies by Hsu et al. [12] in dog hearts and Scollan et al. [33] in rabbit hearts used histology to confirm that the principal axis of maximal diffusion coincides with the local myocardial fiber direction, with a 12° uncertainty, (which also happens to be the degree of local dispersion of myocyte orientation within a typical histological section of myocardium [14]). The eigenvalues of the diffusion tensor may also be informative. The greater the ratio of largest to smallest, the stronger the anisotropy. Pathological disarray of muscle fibers should be associated with decreased anisotropy. In patients with familial hypertrophic cardiomyopathy, this promises to be a useful way to detect focal lesions that occur randomly in the ventricular wall, most commonly in the interventricular septum [38].

Scollan et al. [33] took myocardial diffusion tensor imaging a step further by describing a qualitative alignment between the orientation of laminar myofiber sheets in the ventricular wall and the second eigenvector of the diffusion tensor (the minor eigenvector appeared to be transverse to the laminar sheet plane). Unfortunately, this finding has yet to be confirmed conclusively by histological studies. Part of the difficulty in this may be explained by a recent study by Arts and colleagues [1], who proposed that there may be two principal sheet planes about 45° apart in many parts of the ventricular wall, rather than a single unique sheet orientation.

Reese et al. [32] have adapted the MR diffusion technique to *in-vivo* imaging of canine and human subjects. With this technology it recently became possible to measure three-dimensional fiber architecture non-invasively simultaneously with functional imaging of strain distributions in man [35]. This will be especially helpful in experimental models of disease where the effects of individual variation in anatomy can be unpredictable.

1.3 Regional Myocardial Mechanics

In cardiology, the terms "stress" and "strain" are often used almost interchangeably. While one invariably affects the other, they are actually distinct physical quantities. Stresses are interaction forces acting across surfaces between adjacent regions of muscle. Thus, stress has units of force/area. Since a vector is needed to denote a force, and another to indicate the orientation of a surface, the stress is defined by two vectors: Like the diffusion, it is a tensor, that can be represented by a symmetric 3×3 matrix for a given reference system of coordinates, as shown in Figure 1.1.

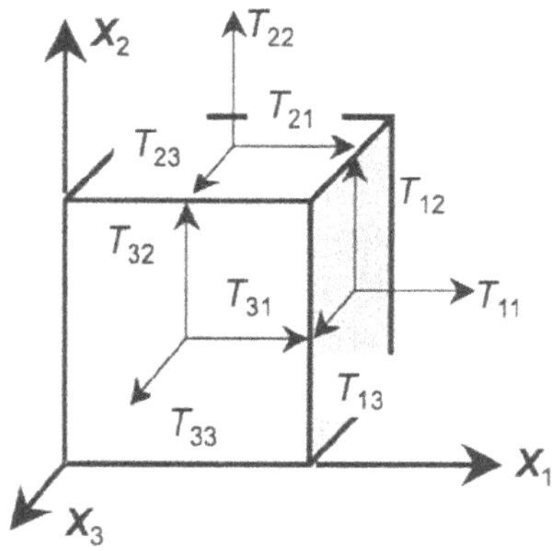

Figure 1.1: The nine components of the stress tensor. By conservation of angular momentum, the tensor is symmetric.

Strain is also a symmetric 3×3 tensor. It represents the change of shape at any point in the wall between the original reference state and the subsequent deformed state, as seen in Figure 1.2 .

For measuring systolic function, end-diastole is a conventional unstrained reference state for strain. However, for analyzing myocardial stress, the appropriate reference state is the stress-free state. Unfortunately, this state can not be observed *in-vivo* [30]. The closest approximation is during diastasis at a low ventricular diastolic pressure.

The matrix components of the stress and strain tensors depend on the chosen frame of reference. It is conventional to choose an orthogonal system, such as the local circumferential, longitudinal, and radial axes, or perhaps one defined by local myofiber architecture (e.g., fiber, cross-fiber and radial axes) as shown in Figure 1.2.

The three diagonals of the stress and strain tensors are the normal components, representing tensile or compressive loading along each of the three coordinate axis directions. Positive normal stresses and strains are associated with tension and stretch, while negative values describe compression and shortening.

The off-diagonals are the shear stress and strain components, associated with off-axis distortions of the wall such as torsion due to rotation of the apex relative to the base. Shear is always a consequence of the chosen reference frame. There is always a set of orthogonal axes (corresponding to the eigenvectors of the strain tensor) that make the shear stress or strain components vanish. These principal axes can change from place to place and are not necessarily the same for stress and strain. Referred to the principal axes, the three principal stresses or strains are

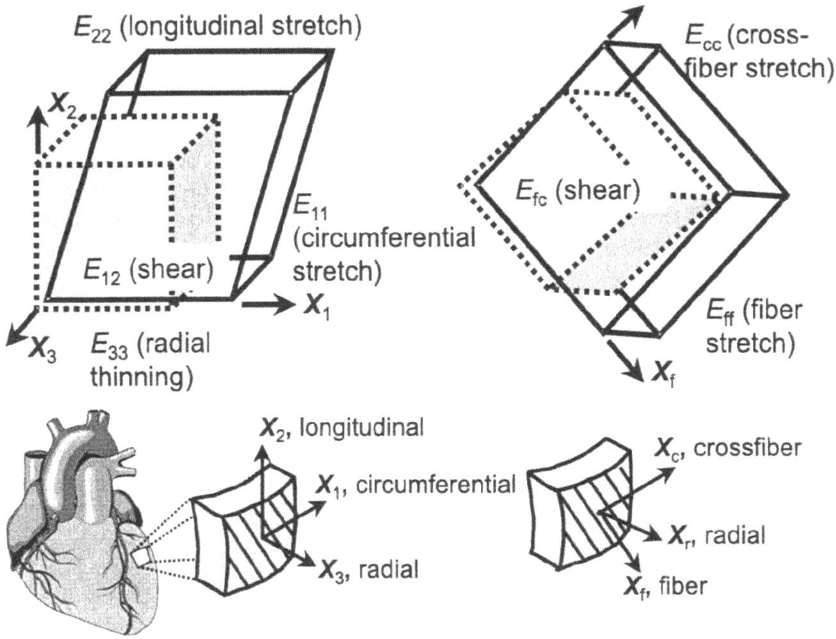

Figure 1.2: Components of the strain tensor resolved with respect to anatomic circumferential, longitudinal and radial coordinates (left) or local fiber, cross-fiber , crossfiber and radial coordinates (right).

purely extensional and they always include the greatest tensile and compressive components. Knowing the orientations of the three principal axes of strain and the length changes along each of them, one has complete information on the shape change at that location. But with only the normal strains along the three axes of an arbitrary reference system, one would not generally have complete information; the three shear strains would be needed too.

The principal axes of stress or strain do not usually coincide with global anatomic axes. Therefore, we typically observe significant shearing in the myocardium [37]. Positive torsional shear strain during ejection reflects the fact that greatest shortening does not occur in the short-axis plane. Nor is it necessarily found along the myofiber direction. In the healthy heart, greatest systolic shortening typically has a principal axis that is 30-45° clockwise from circumferential [37]. That is the orientation of subepicardial muscle fibers, but it is perpendicular to that of subendocardial fibers (Figure 1.3).

Hence, the fiber direction is the axis of greatest shortening near the epicardium, but the axis of least shortening near the endocardium. This is the main mechanism by which systolic fiber shortening during systole can be uniform across the wall [3] even though circumferential, longitudinal and radial strains are all largest on the subendocardium to accommodate wall thickening [11]. This uniform fiber

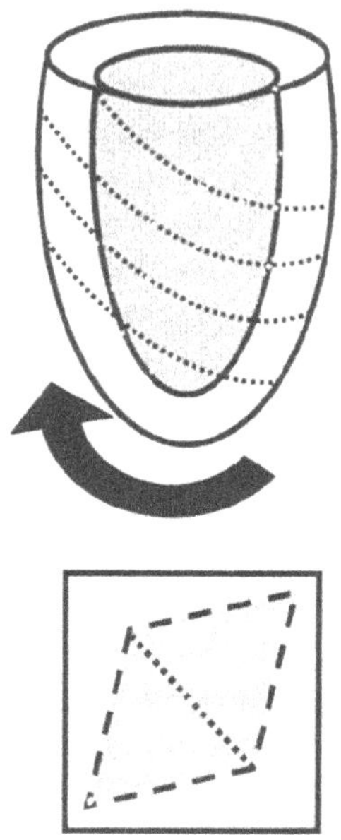

Figure 1.3: Left-handed torsion during systole augments subepicardial fiber shortening and reduces subendocardial fiber shortening. This compensates for larger subendocardial shortening, associated with the greater decrease in subendocardial diameter that must occur as the wall thickens, with the result that sarcomere lengths can remain transmurally uniform during ejection.

shortening has been proposed as a mechanism that maximizes myocardial energy efficiency [6] and minimizes the risk of myofiber injury.

The same mechanism maintains transmural uniformity of fiber lengthening during filling, when the ventricle experiences a small negative torsional shear [31]. Thus, the helical ventricular muscle fiber architecture appears to be optimized to minimize gradients of sarcomere length across the thickness of the ventricular wall in the healthy heart [10]. This property may be regulated by mechanical stimuli during development. In a recent study [39], type I collagen deficiency in the osteogenesis imperfecta murine was associated with significantly altered ventricular myofiber orientations. The difference was enough to help maintain ventricular torsional shear strain during passive filling despite lower stiffness and anisotropy in the absence of large perimysial collagen fibers.

Ventricular wall stress and strain are nonhomogeneous. Their components can change significantly from place to place in the myocardium. Compressive radial stress must, for example, match the ventricular pressure on the endocardium and the pericardial pressure on the epicardium. This heterogeneity makes understanding ventricular mechanics a significant challenge. Fortunately, invasive and non-invasive techniques have been developed for measuring regional distributions of three-dimensional strain in intact myocardium. They rely on tracking three-dimensional displacements of closely spaced material points within the myocardium; for example, by MRI tagging [45]. It is also possible to measure myocardial strain rates from velocity encoded images of the heart walls such as phase-contrast MRI [38, 46].

1.4 Engineering Models of Wall Stress

Because there are no reliable experimental methods for measuring the components of the three dimensional stress tensor, clinicians and scientists have long relied instead on engineering models to compute myocardial stresses [41]. The best known is the Law of *LaPlace*, in which "wall stress" is equal to pressure times radius divided by twice the wall thickness. This simple and instructive formula derives from the highly simplified assumption that the ventricle is a thin, spherical pressurized membrane; like a balloon. When the radius is constant and the wall is very thin, radial stresses can be ignored and the tangent stresses are the same everywhere. If the sphere remains circular under loading, the shear stress is always zero and the circumferential and meridional components of stress are equal by symmetry. By thus reducing the unknowns in the analysis to a single constant stress, *LaPlace's* formula is derived simply from the equilibrium of global forces.

However, the ventricles are not thin-walled and spherical; they are thick, three-dimensional structures. Without the aid of *LaPlace's* assumptions, more information is needed to complete the analysis. In addition to ventricular geometry and hemodynamics, a three-dimensional model of myocardial stress requires the material properties of the resting and active muscle. The constitutive relation describes these properties as a relationship between stress and strain under various loading conditions. Most available experimental data are one-dimensional tests in isolated cells, papillary muscles or trabeculae, but biaxial properties have also been measured in isolated muscle sheets [17].

With the nonlinear and dynamic material properties of myocardium measured, detailed structural data on three-dimensional ventricular wall geometry and myofiber architecture [27], and accurate measurements of hemodynamic loading conditions, we are ready to formulate the analysis. Solving the conservation equations of mechanics usually requires computational engineering techniques — notably the finite element method — that must be adapted for many of the special features of ventricular mechanics [13, 40]. Early models gave valuable insight into basic mechanisms such as the roles of myofiber orientation and ventricular torsion [2]. However, only recently have these analyses begun to reproduce the degree of detail in regional wall strains that three-dimensional imaging techniques have revealed, especially in heterogeneous pathologies such as ischemic disease [20]. Now, the objective is to extend these simulations to include more structural and physiological detail, such as anatomic structures like valves and papillary muscles, the biophysics of excitation-contraction coupling, the mechano-energetics of crossbridge interactions, or the interactions between coronary vessels and myocytes [18].

1.5 Analyzing Wall Strain Distributions

To validate and optimize computational models of cardiac mechanics, measurements of regional strain distributions are needed for comparison with model predictions. By modifying material parameters to improve the agreement between model and experiment, new insight into the three dimensional structural properties of the intact myocardium during health and disease can be obtained.

Cardiac MRI tagging is the only non-invasive modality for tracking the large displacements of material points in the ventricular myocardium through the cardiac cycle. And compared with other more invasive strain analysis techniques, such as biplane radiography of implanted radiopaque markers, MRI tagging also allows three-dimensional myocardial displacements to be imaged throughout the ventricular walls, rather than in a limited number of locations.

Using these image sets to compute three-dimensional strain distributions requires considerable analysis. The simplest three-dimensional strain analysis, is a homogeneous strain analysis, in which the displacement of four non-coplanar material points can be used to estimate identically the six components of the symmetric strain tensor in the neighborhood of the points [36]. Why four points? They form a tetrahedron with four sides whose linearly independent length changes are then sufficient to compute the six strains. However, homogeneous strain analysis has limitations: it assumes that strains within the region of the tetrahedron are constant, when they are invariably nonhomogeneous. To minimize the influence of this approximation, the material points must be close together, but this compromises the accuracy of the computed lengths and strains.

A more general approach is nonhomogeneous strain analysis. In this case, functions are fitted by least squares to the three-dimensional displacements throughout the wall. From the gradients of these displacement functions the strain can be estimated as a continuous tensor field throughout the wall. Various basis functions have been used for nonhomogeneous analysis, the most popular being piecewise linear and cubic polynomials (i.e., finite elements) [43] and spherical harmonic expansions [29]. Thus, three-dimensional methods for nonhomogeneous myocardial kinematic analysis are inherently model-based. Investigators have recognized that the task of segmenting the tagged MRI images can also be combined into the model fitting analysis [42].

The critical trade-off in model-based nonhomogeneous kinematic analysis is between allowing sufficient degrees of freedom in the model to accommodate the greatest degree of myocardial inhomogeneity without over-parameterizing and fitting noise. The spatial resolution of cardiac MRI is still limiting the density of material points that can be reconstructed and the accuracy with which they can be localized. Thus, methods have been developed to regularize the calculation and compensate for the relative sparsity of material tag lines [45].

A successful approach to regularization is to incorporate constraints based on physical prior knowledge, such as the mechanical properties of the myocardium [7]. For computational efficiency, these regularization techniques tend to model cardiac physical properties using heuristic rules.

At the same time, predictive finite element models based on mechanical first principles are improving [20], and it is feasible to use them in semi-inverse analyses together with measured ventricular strain fields to identify myocardial material parameters from experimental or clinical recordings [24, 28]. Thus, we are at the threshold of a convergence of stress and strain models for ventricular mechanics. As computational power continues to increase, it is feasible that heuristic parametric models could be replaced by physically detailed finite element models, and used to identify regional strains, stresses and material properties directly from MRI tagging or velocity-encoded recordings of regional ventricular function. There are still limitations to overcome, most crucially the need for accurate hemodynamic recordings simultaneously with cardiac imaging, and the need for optimization algorithms that reduce bias in the inverse analysis resulting from the strong mechanical nonlinearity of the myocardium.

1.6 Regional Strain Distributions in Disease

The ultimate clinical goal of regional cardiac mechanical analysis is to quantify and characterize regions of altered mechanical function and correlate this with alterations in perfusion, structure, or metabolism. These data are valuable, not only for acute diagnosis but for identifying the risk of long term remodeling and disease progression. Numerous cardiac pathologies are associated with altered regional ventricular wall mechanics, many of which have been studied by MRI tagging, including acute ischemia and myocardial infarction [26], hypertrophic [45] and dilated [44] cardiomyopathies, and arrhythmias [23].

For clinical application, one primary concern is whether the tissue is viable or not. If the tissue is necrotic, then an aggressive and expensive treatment such as coronary bypass graft surgery, may not be beneficial. However, if it can be shown that significant dysfunctional myocardium remains viable then restoration of normal circulation can help to restore normal function. A related issue is to quantify the degree of dysfunction. A patient exhibiting only a 20% loss of contractile function can perhaps be treated with a less aggressive, less expensive pharmacologic regimen, while a patient with a 80% loss of regional function will perhaps need more immediate aggressive therapy, such as balloon angioplasty, to restore vascular patency.

Dobutamine or adenosine stress testing has been suggested for non-invasive detection of hibernating myocardium in conjunction with MRI motion tracking. Croisille et al. [5] found improved function in response to inotropic stimulation in at-risk regions of canine hearts subject to left anterior descending coronary artery occlusion and reperfusion. Regions of unchanged function after dobutamine infusion were shown to be correlated with areas of infarction as evidenced by triphenol tetrazolium chloride staining.

In acute ischemia and infarction, a similar clinical problem arises in distinguishing stunned versus hibernating myocardium. In the latter, regional flow and function are concomitantly impaired, whereas in the former contractile function remains temporarily decreased while flow has returned to normal. Indeed, even in acute ischemia, there is no one-to-one relationship between regions of altered perfusion and wall strain. For example, normally perfused myocardium adjacent to an ischemic region can display decreased systolic strain [20], and subendocardial ischemia can lead to subepicardial dysfunction [21]. Hence, the potential for regional perfusion and strain to be imaged in a single MRI study is particularly appealing [15].

1.7 Future Directions

The mechanics of the beating heart depend on three-dimensional ventricular geometry, regional myocardial strain, myocardial fiber architecture and local wall stresses. We have shown examples of promising techniques to independently assess anatomy, strain and fiber architecture. At present, integrative computational models are the only way to synthesize this information and predict regional stress distributions [19].

Although, it is not yet possible to directly measure myocardial stresses *in-vivo* without damaging the tissue or significantly altering the measurement, there is a promising non-invasive MRI method for measuring soft tissue elastic stiffness, at least in the linear limit of infinitesimal strains. Magnetic resonance elastography [8,25] combines acoustic or ultrasonic excitation with MR phase-sensitive imaging to monitor the propagation of transverse acoustic shear waves through soft tissue with high sensitivity. However, obstacles must still be overcome before these techniques can be applied successfully to the heart *in-vivo*.

We can expect continued progress on several fronts in the use of MRI as an integral tool for the analysis of myocardial mechanics and structure function relations in health and disease. As work with diffusion tensor imaging progresses, it should be possible to image myocardial fiber structure with greater detail and efficiency. As our understanding of the laminar architecture of myofiber sheets improves, more structural detail will be available form the diffusion tensor. As motion correction techniques improve, more structural detail can be anticipated from *in-vivo* studies. Because MRI is non-invasive, the prospect for serial studies in animals and man should improve as the cost effectiveness of scanner time improves. As the speed of imaging protocols increases, the practicality of more comprehensive studies that combine anatomy, mechanical function, perfusion and metabolism will increase. In order for these studies to be tightly integrated with computational models, better estimates of hemodynamics and the unloaded reference state of the ventricular and atrial walls will be needed.

Finally, beyond more detailed descriptions of regional mechanics in animals and man during health and disease and their relationship to ventricular structure and physiology, a central goal is to identify the molecular and genetic determinants of regional myocardial mechanical function and dysfunction. Here, the prospects for *in-vivo* imaging of regional gene expression and high-field imaging in gene-targeted mice during development, growth and the progression of disease are particularly promising.

Acknowledgments

The author's laboratory is supported by the NIH, NSF, American Heart Association, UC Life Science Informatics program, and the National Space Biomedical Research Institute.

References

[1] Arts, T., K. D. Costa, J. W. Covell, and A. D. McCulloch. Relating myocardial laminar architecture to shear strain and muscle fiber orientation. Am J Physiol: Heart Circ Physiol (in press):, 2001.

[2] Arts, T., R. S. Reneman, and P. C. Veenstra. A model of the mechanics of the left ventricle. Ann Biomed Eng 7: 299-318, 1979.

[3] Arts, T., P. C. Veenstra, and R. S. Reneman. Epicardial deformation and left ventricular wall mechanics during ejection in the dog. Am J Physiol 243: H379-H390, 1982.

[4] Basser, P. J., J. Mattiello, and D. LeBihan. MR diffusion tensor spectroscopy and imaging. Biophys J 66: 259-67., 1994.

[5] Croisille, P., C. C. Moore, R. M. Judd, J. A. Lima, M. Arai, E. R. McVeigh, L. C. Becker, and E. A. Zerhouni. Differentiation of viable and nonviable myocardium by the use of three dimensional tagged MRI in 2-day-old reperfused canine infarcts. Circulation 99: 284-91, 1999.

[6] Delhaas, T., T. Arts, F. W. Prinzen, and R. S. Reneman. Estimates of regional work in the canine left ventricle. Prog Biophys Mol Biol 69: 273-87, 1998.

[7] Duncan, J., P. Shi, T. Constable, and A. Sinusas. Physical and geometrical modeling for image- based recovery of left ventricular deformation. Prog Biophys Mol Biol 69: 333-51, 1998.

[8] Dutt, V., R. R. Kinnick, R. Muthupillai, T. E. Oliphant, R. L. Ehman, and J. F. Greenleaf. Acoustic shear-wave imaging using echo ultrasound compared to magnetic resonance elastography. Ultrasound Med Biol 26: 397-403., 2000.

[9] Garrido, L., V. J. Wedeen, K. K. Kwong, U. M. Spencer, and H. L. Kantor. Anisotropy of water diffusion in the myocardium of the rat. Circ Res 74: 789-93, 1994.

[10] Guccione, J. M., A. D. McCulloch, and L. K. Waldman. Passive material properties of intact ventricular myocardium determined from a cylindrical model. J Biomech Eng 113: 42-55, 1991.

[11] Hexeberg, E., D. C. Homans, and R. J. Bache. Interpretation of systolic wall thickening. Can thickening of a discrete layer reflect fiber performance? Cardiovasc Res 29: 16-21, 1995.

[12] Hsu, E. W., A. L. Muzikant, S. A. Matulevicius, R. C. Penland, and C. S. Henriquez. Magnetic resonance myocardial fiber-orientation mapping with direct histological correlation. Am J Physiol 274: H1627-34, 1998.

[13] Hunter, P. J., and B. H. Smaill. The analysis of cardiac function: a continuum approach. Prog Biophys Mol Biol 52: 101-164, 1989.

[14] Karlon, W. J., J. W. Covell, A. D. McCulloch, J. J. Hunter, and J. H. Omens. Automated measurement of myofiber disarray in transgenic mice with ventricular expression of ras. Anatomical Record 252: 612-625, 1998.

[15] Kraitchman, D. L., N. Wilke, E. Hexeberg, M. Jerosch-Herold, Y. Wang, T. B. Parrish, C. N. Chang, Y. Zhang, R. J. Bache, and L. Axel. Myocardial perfusion and function in dogs with moderate coronary stenosis. Magn Reson Med 35: 771-80, 1996.

[16] LeGrice, I. J., B. H. Smaill, L. Z. Chai, S. G. Edgar, J. B. Gavin, and P. J. Hunter. Laminar structure of the heart: ventricular myocyte arrangement and connective tissue architecture in the dog. Am J Physiol 269: H571-82, 1995.

[17] Lin, D. H. S., and F. C. P. Yin. A multiaxial constitutive law for mammalian left ventricular myocardium in steady-state barium contracture or tetanus. J Biomech Eng 120: 504-517, 1998.

[18] May-Newman, K., and A. D. McCulloch. Homogenization modeling for the mechanics of perfused myocardium. Progress in Biophysics and Molecular Biology 69: 463-482, 1998.

[19] Mazhari, R., and A. D. McCulloch. Integrative models for understanding the structural basis of regional mechanical dysfunction in ischemic myocardium. Ann Biomed Eng 28: 979-990, 2000.

[20] Mazhari, R., J. H. Omens, J. W. Covell, and A. D. McCulloch. Structural basis of regional dysfunction in acutely ischemic myocardium. Cardiovasc Res 47: 284-293, 2000.

[21] McCulloch, A. D., D. Sung, J. M. Wilson, R. S. Pavelec, and J. H. Omens. Flow-function relations during graded coronary occlusions in the dog: effects of transmural location and segment orientation. Cardiovasc Res 37, 1998.

[22] McInerney, T., and D. Terzopoulos. Deformable models in medical image analysis: a survey. Med Image Anal 1: 91-108., 1996.

[23] McVeigh, E. R., F. W. Prinzen, B. T. Wyman, J. E. Tsitlik, H. R. Halperin, and W. C. Hunter. Imaging asynchronous mechanical activation of the paced heart with tagged MRI. Magnetic Resonance in Medicine 39: 507-13, 1998.

[24] Moulton, M. J., L. L. Creswell, S. W. Downing, R. L. Actis, B. A. Szabo, and M. K. Pasque. Myocardial material property determination in the *in-vivo* heart using magnetic resonance imaging. Int J Card Imaging 12: 153-67, 1996.

[25] Muthupillai, R., and R. L. Ehman. Magnetic resonance elastography. Nat Med 2: 601-3., 1996.

[26] Nagel, E., M. Stuber, M. Lakatos, M. B. Scheidegger, P. Boesiger, and O. M. Hess. Cardiac rotation and relaxation after anterolateral myocardial infarction. Coron Artery Dis 11: 261-7., 2000.

[27] Nielsen, P. M. F., I. J. Le Grice, B. H. Smaill, and P. J. Hunter. Mathematical model of geometry and fibrous structure of the heart. Am J Physiol 260: H1365-H1378, 1991.

[28] O'Dell, W., W. Hunter, E. McVeigh, and A. McCulloch. Determination of material properties for the passively filling canine left ventricle. Ann Biomed Eng 25: S-27, 1997.

[29] O'Dell, W. G., C. C. Moore, W. C. Hunter, E. A. Zerhouni, and E. R. McVeigh. Displacement field fitting approach to calculate 3-D deformations from parallel-tagged MR images. Radiology 195: 829–835, 1995.

[30] Omens, J. H., and Y. C. Fung. Residual strain in rat left ventricle. Circ Res 66: 37-45, 1990.

[31] Omens, J. H., K. D. May, and A. D. McCulloch. Transmural distribution of three-dimensional strain in isolated arrested canine left ventricle. Am J Physiol 261: H918-H928, 1991.

[32] Reese, T. G., V. J. Wedeen, and R. M. Weisskoff. Measuring diffusion in the presence of material strain. J Magn Reson B 112: 253-8, 1996.

[33] Scollan, D. F., A. Holmes, R. Winslow, and J. Forder. Histological validation of myocardial microstructure obtained from diffusion tensor magnetic resonance imaging. Am J Physiol 275: H2308-18, 1998.

[34] Streeter, D. D., Jr, and D. L. Bassett. An engineering analysis of myocardial fiber orientation in pig's left ventricle in systole. Anat Rec 155: 503-511, 1966.

[35] Tseng, W. Y., T. G. Reese, R. M. Weisskoff, T. J. Brady, and V. J. Wedeen. Myocardial fiber shortening in humans: initial results of MR imaging. Radiology 216: 128-39., 2000.

[36] Waldman, L. K. Multidimensional measurements of regional strains in the intact heart. In: Theory of Heart; Biomechanic, Biophysics, and Non-Linear Dynamics of Cardiac Function, edited by L. Glass, P. Hunter and A. D. McCulloch. New York: Springer-Verlag, 1991, p. 145-174.

[37] Waldman, L. K., D. Nossan, F. Villarreal, and J. W. Covell. Relation between transmural deformation and local myofiber direction in canine left ventricle. Circ Res 63: 550-562, 1988.

[38] Wedeen, V. J., W.-Y. I. Tseng, T. G. Reese, H. Kantor, and R. M. Weisskoff. Magnetic resonance imaging finds normal myocardial fiber shortening and reduced crossfiber shortening in hypertrophic cardiomyopathy. Circulation 98: I-514, 1998.

[39] Weis, S. M., J. L. Emery, D. Becker, D. J. McBride, J. H. Omens, and A. McCulloch. Myocardial mechanics and collagen structure in the osteogenesis imperfecta murine. Circulation Research 87: 663-669, 2000.

[40] Yin, F. C. P. Applications of the finite-element method to ventricular mechanics. CRC Crit Rev Biomed Eng 12: 311-342, 1985.

[41] Yin, F. C. P. Ventricular wall stress. Circ Res 49: 829-842, 1981.

[42] Young, A. A. Model tags: direct three-dimensional tracking of heart wall motion from tagged magnetic resonance images. Med Image Anal 3: 361-72., 1999.

[43] Young, A. A., and L. Axel. Three-dimensional motion and deformation in the heart wall: estimation from spatial modulation of magnetization - a model-based approach. Radiology 185: 241-247, 1992.

[44] Young, A. A., S. Dokos, K. A. Powell, B. Sturm, A. D. McCulloch, R. C. Starling, P. M. McCarthy, and R. D. White. Regional heterogeneity of function in nonischemic dilated cardiomyopathy. Cardiovasc Res 49: 308-318., 2001.

[45] Young, A. A., C. M. Kramer, V. A. Ferrari, L. Axel, and N. Reichek. Three-dimensional left ventricular deformation in hypertrophic cardiomyopathy. Circulation 90: 854-67, 1994.

[46] Zhu, Y., M. Drangova, and N. J. Pelc. Estimation of deformation gradient and strain from cine- PC velocity data. IEEE Trans Med Imaging 16: 840-51., 1997.

Chapter 2

Clinical Applications of Cardiac Tagging

Nathaniel Reichek
Research and Education Foundation,
DeMatteis Center, St. Francis Hospital,
100 Port Washington Blvd.,
Roslyn, NY 11576
reichek@wpahs.org

2.1 Introduction

In vitro assessment of myocardial contraction is possible in experimental models at many levels, from the classical papillary muscle model down to video tracking of deformation of individual loaded or unloaded myocytes. However, *in vivo* assessment of myocardial contraction remains critically important for understanding disease pathophysiology and responses to potential therapeutic interventions. Invasive methods using implanted markers at discrete material points in the myocardium to depict local myocardial deformation that are suitable for use in experimental models have long been available for cardiovascular investigation [1,2]. Such methods include pulse transit time recordings between pairs or arrays of sonomicrometry crystals as well as cineangiographic imaging of arrays of tantalum markers. However, such methods are too invasive to be used commonly in man, although a few studies in patients undergoing cardiac surgery, particularly cardiac transplantation, have been performed [3]. For research in humans and for clinical applications, many cardiac imaging methods now permit projection, tomographic or 3D assessment of cardiac chamber, epicardial, endocardial and valvular motion. These include roentgenographic contrast ventriculography, transthoracic or transesophageal echocardiography, electron beam CT with intravenous contrast injection, radionuclide SPECT and PET and conventional magnetic resonance (MR) imaging. However, the heart translates through and rotates within any imaging plane during the cardiac cycle. Thus, apparent motion of endocardial and epicardial borders has a complex relationship to local myocardial deformation. Therefore, none of these conventional imaging methods permit assessment of myocardial

A.A. Amini and J.L. Prince (eds.),
Measurement of Cardiac Deformations from MRI: Physical and Mathematical Models, 17–36.

deformation. The practical result until recently was that inferences about human myocardial mechanical function was inherently compromised in disorders in which the relationship between chamber dynamics and actual intramural myocardial contraction is altered, including ischemic heart disease and pressure overload hypertrophy, in particular. MR tagging was the first widely applied noninvasive method for assessment of actual local myocardial deformation in human beings [4, 5]. It has provided the opportunity to assess local myocardial deformation and motion in man as well as to assess it comprehensively and serially in experimental models of disease. Other methods, such as MR phase contrast imaging [6] and MR strain imaging [7] have also emerged, but as of this writing have not seen extensive application in clinical disease states.

2.2 Imaging Techniques

Myocardial tagging methods have been thoroughly reviewed in other chapters of this book. However, there are a number of considerations particularly relevant to research or clinical applications in human beings. To obtain volumetric studies in conscious humans, particularly those with symptomatic heart disease, combining data in orthogonal imaging planes requires fast imaging. The most common practical approach at present is to use breath-hold segmented k space Cine MR [8] which is fast, typically requiring only 16-18 heartbeats per slice. Generally imaging is performed with a field of view between 24 and 32 cm in adults with a 128×256 matrix interpolated to 256×256. Tagging applications in humans have most commonly used the 3D cubic grid approach often referred to as SPAMM, for spatial modulation of magnetization [5]. Some centers have used interleaved image pairs, each of which contains a set of parallel tag lines [9]. The orientation of the tag lines is orthogonal in plane in the two members of the image pair. Thus the same data is obtained as is available with the SPAMM method. Using this approach can improve image quality sufficiently to offset the loss in temporal resolution for some applications. A third approach that provides somewhat different data is use of a set of radially distributed tagging planes oriented orthogonal to the image plane and centered in the center of the left ventricle [10].

Tagged image data can be obtained with sufficient speed to make it possible for myocardial tagging to be suitable for stress testing applications such as dobutamine tagged MR [11, 12]. The breath-hold is used to eliminate respiratory motion effects over the cardiac cycles required for data acquisition. Breath-hold duration is thus a function of cardiac cycle length and typically ranges from 12–20 seconds at heart rates from 100 to 60 beats per minute. Newer MR imaging approaches applicable to tagged imaging include "true FISP" sequences, which provide better contrast between blood and myocardium, breath-hold 3D tagged imaging and a variety of hybrid real-time or near realtime imaging strategies [13]. Extensive further development of 3D and real-time approaches will be required to obtain sufficient SNR, spatial and temporal resolution. Using a 3D square grid of tag lines, tag plane separations currently practical for application in humans range from 5–7 mm. Using the segmented k space methods, variation in the number of segments acquired per cardiac cycle can be used to vary the number of cardiac cycles during which data must be taken and, at high heart rates, to increase temporal resolution. Such breath-holds are feasible in cardiac patients even early after acute myocardial infarction, or in stable patients with relatively advanced congestive heart failure, provided that dyspnea due to severe pulmonary congestion or concomitant disease such as severe obstructive airways disease are not present and the patient is oriented and cooperative. However, it is essential to create a high level "safety net" for patients with advanced heart disease in the scanner. This is especially true when pharmacologic stress testing using progressive infusion of dobutamine is planned because of the potential risks of arrhythmia, myocardial ischemia and pulmonary congestion. Typical monitoring includes noninvasive blood pressure, EKG with multiple channel selection, pulse oximetry and two-way audio combined with video observation of the patient in the scanner. During dobutamine infusion it is desirable to have a nurse with cardiac care training in the scanner room. In addition, cardiac arrest is, inevitably, a small but potentially devastating risk in patients with advanced cardiac disease. Thus, full provisions for cardiopulmonary resuscitation must be made immediately adjacent to the scanner, time to removal of the patient from the scanner room must be sufficiently short (<60 sec) to permit timely resuscitation, cardiac arrest practice drills must be held for the MR group and at least one member of the group in attendance at each study should be qualified in advanced cardiac life support. Supplemental oxygen is commonly administered in patients with heart failure or myocardial ischemia and monitoring of blood pressure, EKG, pulse oximetry and respiratory motion are desirable in many patients. For dobutamine stress, where 3–5 minute stages at each dose infusion level are required, coordination and very fluent performance of imaging by a team including the scanner operator, a skilled cardiovascular nurse and a cardiologist are required. With the advent of new fast gradient systems optimized for fast cardiac imaging including interactive plane-steering and real-time imaging, development of rapid myocardial tagging methods, particularly for use with pharmacologic or exercise stress is likely to advance considerably further.

2.3 Tagged Image Data Analysis

Tagged cardiac images can be informative about local myocardial function even when simple qualitative visual interpretation of cine loops is performed by an experienced observer. However, the strength of tagged imaging lies in the utility and rigor of the quantitative analysis methods that have been developed. The major problem facing efforts at widespread application of quantitative analysis of tagged imaging in human beings continues to be the time cost and tediousness of image analysis and data reduction. In early applications, skilled observers laboriously performed completely manual analysis of images [14]. This has been replaced by semi-automated analyses based on snakes algorithms in a number of centers in recent years, but the work is still very slow. More automated approaches may be practical with improved image SNR using newer sequences or with methods such as HARP in which deformation information is extracted without conventional postprocessing approaches [15, 16]. Quantitative analysis of tagged images can be performed at a variety of levels of complexity. The simplest is to track changes in the side-to-side separation of tag lines or tag line intersections in a single image plane over the cardiac cycle along a single spatial axis. This is often done using side-to-side distances between pairs of tag lines and the center of each line is typically defined as the pixel showing the nadir of signal amplitude within the dark saturation stripe. The change in distance between such line pairs at end-diastole and end-systole represents unidimensional shortening or elongation of the myocardium in that direction. Ordinarily, such measurements are normalized to the end-diastolic distance between tag lines. When pairs of tag lines oriented perpendicularly to the endocardium are analyzed in this manner, the resultant measurement is equivalent to circumferential segment shortening (%S) [10]. Advantages of this approach include its extreme simplicity, familiarity to cardiologists based on an extensive experimental literature on human disease states using implanted sonomicrometry crystal pairs to obtain analogous measurements and the ability to measure at multiple levels across the wall thickness (subendocardial, midwall, subepicardial). Tagged MRI %S data and radial thickening data generally agree well with sonomicrometry data when compared directly [17, 18]. Comparison of deformation at subendocardial and subepicardial sites may be of great potential value given the normal gradient in deformation across the myocardium from endo- to epicardium [10] and the fact that ischemic dysfunction tends to begin at the subendocardium. Even when %S determination is done by an operator without automation of the analysis, inter and intraobserver reproducibility is excellent. Disadvantages of unidimensional tag analyses such as circumferential %S include the fact that rotation, translation and the other components of strain tensor available in the images are not extracted. In addition, the number of sites on a given image plane where measurements can be made with this method is limited. Finally, through plane motion is not accounted for using either 1D or 2D in-plane analysis of tagged images. However, this last issue might be relatively unimportant in clinical studies of the left ventricle in conditions in which longitudinal deformation is not uniquely affected if the imaging plane is normal to long axis shortening. Since the tag separation at end- diastole is known throughout 3D space and is identical on every image plane, so long as the analysis is done on true short axis tagged images and myocardium moves in a direction perpendicular to the imaging plane as the left ventricle empties, in plane strains will be correctly depicted. Limited data in normal humans (E. Hoffman, personal communication) indicates that these conditions are roughly met with short-axis LV imaging. These considerations may explain the good agreement with sonomicrometry results that can be obtained in experimental models.

A more informative approach to tagging analysis than 1D %S is to perform a two-dimensional in-plane analysis [19]. The analysis separates components of rigid body motion, such as in-plane rotation and translation of points within the myocardium, from the actual deformation within the tissue, or strains, reflecting motion of points within the myocardium relative to each other. Two dimensional strain analyses are typically determined using triangular elements of myocardium bounded by intersections of 3 tag lines. Each strain vector has a magnitude of lengthening or shortening and an angular orientation within the plane. Typically, the maximal strain (magnitude and direction of maximal lengthening of tissue, often termed λ_1) and the minimal strain (magnitude and direction of maximal shortening of tissue within the triangular element, often termed λ_2) are derived. However, radial and circumferential strains can also be derived from the data. Further, if the orientation of myocardial fibers across the ventricular wall is known, shortening in the fiber direction and in the direction orthogonal to the fiber length-so-called cross-fiber shortening, can be derived [21]. This is generally possible only in experimental models of disease where extensive histologic studies can be performed. In normal human myocardium, λ_1 is oriented relatively close (typically $\leq 10°$) to the direction of wall thickening and λ_2 is oriented close to the direction of circumferential segment shortening. However, the direction or orientation of these strains may be altered in disease. For example, in the extreme case, in acute severe transmural myocardial ischemia, there may be actual systolic wall thinning, so that the direction of the two strains will be reversed. Two dimensional strain analysis has a number of limitations. These include weighting of the data toward the ventricular midwall, with underrepresentation of the subendocardial and subepicardial fibers. This occurs due to the fact that tag intersections at endocardial and epicardial edges as well as those occurring in the blood pool or mediastinum just beyond the myocardium are lost so that adjacent myocardium is not assessed. In human studies, tag spacing cannot be made close enough to provide triangular myocardial elements completely located within subendocardium or subepicardium. Furthermore, the array of parameters derived, including rigid body translation and rotation, as well as strain magnitudes and orientations is not familiar to clinicians.

Full 3D analyses of myocardial strains and motion are of course optimal in principle and obviate many limitations of simpler approaches. Such analyses have long been possible and have been applied to small populations in a number of disease states. [20, 27] However, while analytic tools have progressively improved, full 3D analyses remain complex, relatively slow, somewhat difficult to interpret and generally available only to relatively few investigators using research software developed locally. In general, 3D analyses have tended to improve understanding of the regional heterogeneity of deformation and motion of the myocardium in selected disease states but have not resulted in fundamental qualitative differences in interpretation of cardiac mechanics in human disease as yet.

Using radial tagging approaches, other analytic approaches have been emphasized in a limited number of human studies . One is analysis of so-called "twist", or rotation of the apex of the left ventricle relative to its base during systole [28,29].

This parameter reflects the effects of the 3D spiral orientation of sheets of myocardial fibers. Twist increases in parallel with myocardial contractile state. Systolic twist is largely an ejection index, like other strain parameters, wall thickening and chamber emptying. Therefore twist is sensitive to both afterload and preload. However, some data suggest that diastolic untwisting occurs in large part during isovolumic relaxation, generating much of the ventricular pressure fall during isovolumic relaxation- so-called "ventricular suction" that generates mitral valve opening [28]. Thus isovolumic untwisting may behave like isovolumic LV pressure decay and could therefore serve as a noninvasive index of Tau, the time constant of isovolumic pressure decay, a very useful index of active myocardial relaxation that cannot otherwise be readily measured noninvasively in humans.

Radial tag data analysis has also been used in animal models to calculate strains on the endocardial and epicardial surfaces of the myocardium. Since fiber orientation on these surfaces is simple to determine using pathologic specimens, fiber and cross-fiber strains are readily determined [21, 30]. This sort of analysis is hard to apply in humans since it depends on either direct determination of or assumptions about fiber orientation. Such assumptions would be tenuous in diseased hearts, particularly ischemic heart disease with regional inhomogeneity of myocardial function. It is possible to directly determine fiber orientation with diffusion MRI [31], which might help increase applicability of this approach to human hearts. However, the diffusion methods have been challenging to apply.

Analysis of tagged image data is complex and generates a great deal of data. Thus development and wide availability of improved, commercially available software with automated data reduction and improved parametric displays is badly needed. Without it there is little possibility that the great promise of tagged imaging applications to human physiology and disease can be fully realized.

2.4 MR Tagging in Normal Human Heart

Investigators using myocardial tagging have made valuable contributions to our understanding of normal human cardiac mechanics and physiology, see Figure 2.1. Tagged imaging made it possible early on to demonstrate that the normal human left ventricle shows a transmural gradient in circumferential segment shortening, as previously demonstrated using sonomicrometry in animal models [14]. This finding is somewhat counterintuitive since spiral sheets of myocardial fibers in the subepicardium and subendocardium have a more longitudinal orientation while fiber sheets in the midwall show more circumferential fiber orientation. One might assume that segment shortening would be maximal in the direction of myocardial fiber orientation, but this is not the case. Rademakers and co-workers provided an informative analysis in an animal model, by comparing strains and fiber orientation to permit determination of fiber strain and so-called cross-fiber strain [21]. Thus it has emerged that fiber strain is fairly uniform across the wall of the left ventricle. However, cross-fiber strain is maximal at the subendocardium and mini-

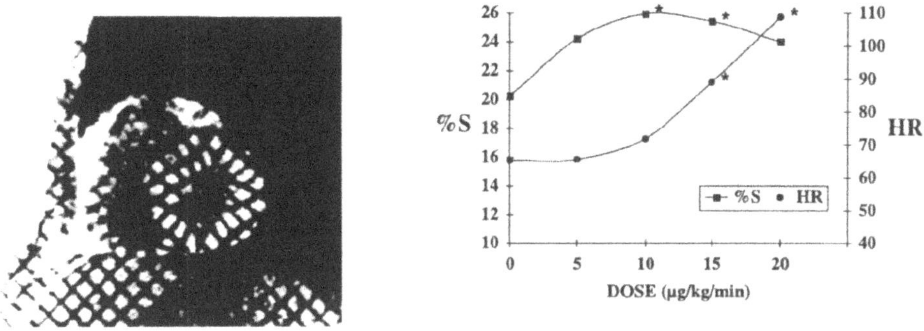

Figure 2.1: **Left:** Tagged end-systolic short axis image of a mid-ventricular slice through normal human LV. Diaphragm and liver shown below heart. In the liver, the original square 7mm × 7mm tag grid pattern is shown which was deposited at end-diastole. Within the myocardium, the grid has been deformed by the systolic contraction of the myocardium. The differences in grid line and intersection separations between the original grid and the end-systolic myocardial grid can be used to calculate local deformation within small elements of myocardium, including differences between subendocardial and subepicardial deformation.
Right: Response of normal human LV circumferential segment shortening (%S) to dobutamine infusion by MRI tagging. *Left axis:* %S. *Right axis:* Heart rate. *Horizontal axis:* dobutamine dose. %S reaches maximum values at 10 mcg/kg/min, before HR rises, showing dissociation of inotropic state and heart rate (reprinted with permission from [11]).

mal at the subepicardium. Therefore high circumferential %S and wall thickening in the subendocardium is attributable largely to cross-fiber strain, which must be transmitted across the wall from the midwall and subepicardium. Indeed, subepicardial injury can markedly diminish strains in the subendocardium. The ways in which the orientation of myocardial fiber sheets and the suspension of myocytes within a complex interstitium contribute to these complex mechanical events remain poorly understood and the foci of very active investigation. Tagging methods have also made it possible to assess the regional heterogeneity of myocardial deformation and rigid body motion in normal left ventricle, using one, two and three-dimensional techniques [14, 21, 22, 30, 32].

Tagging analysis has resulted in improved understanding of the effects of adrenergic stimulation of the myocardium, which can result in both an inotropic stimulus and alterations in heart rate and loading conditions, see Figures 2.1, 2.2. Dobutamine is commonly used for inotropic support of patients with markedly impaired myocardial function and for pharmacologic stress to detect regional ischemia in combination with a variety of imaging methods. Tagging studies during dobutamine infusion have shown that in normal myocardium, maximal absolute regional deformation is achieved at relatively low doses, 10 g/kg/min or less, well before heart rate begins to accelerate, see Figure 2.1 [11, 12]. During infusion of higher doses of dobutamine, tachycardia occurs and absolute deformation does not increase further. However, the strain rate continues to increase, reflecting in-

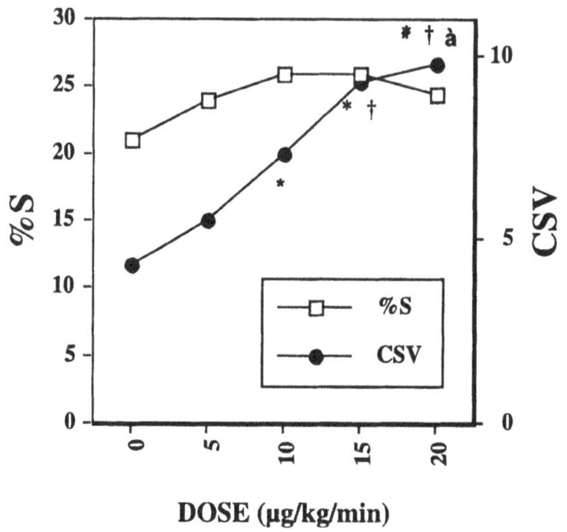

Figure 2.2: Tagged %S during dobutamine infusion in normals (left Y axis) versus circumferential shortening velocity (CSV, right Y axis), over increasing doses of dobutamine (X axis). Although %S in normals reaches maximum at 10 micrograms/kg/min, the velocity of shortening (CSV) continues to increase linearly with dobutamine dose after maximum with permission from [11]).

creasing inotropic effect. Presumably, despite the increased rate of myocardial relaxation at higher heart rate and during inotropic stimulation, the shortening of diastole has an overriding effect on preload so that absolute deformation cannot increase further. Much of untwisting occurs during isovolumic relaxation and it appears that untwisting may account for "ventricular suction", the normal fall in left ventricular early diastolic pressure that permits the mitral valve to open and ventricular filling to begin [28].

2.5 MR Tagging in Ischemic Heart Disease

Regional heterogeneity of myocardial contraction in ischemic heart disease is a hallmark of the disorder. Such heterogeneity is found in six different clinical scenarios central to the natural history and treatment of the disorder: acute ischemia, acute myocardial infarction, chronic myocardial infarction, myocardial stunning after an episode of acute ischemia, myocardial hibernation in the setting of chronic or recurrent ischemia and as part of the process of post-infarction left ventricular remodeling. Thus assessment of such heterogeneity is central to the problem. In order to make a clinical decision about pharmacologic management or revascularization with catheter-based intervention or bypass surgery it is often necessary to determine how much dysfunctional myocardium exists and how much of it is viable and capable of recovery of normal or near-normal function. Revascularization in patients who have a lot of viable but dysfunctional myocardium improves clinical outcomes, but revascularization in the absence of viable myocardium does not. A variety of common clinical noninvasive methods are available for assessment of viability, but none of them are entirely satisfactory. In general there are two classes: assessment of contractile reserve by imaging regional wall motion and assessment of perfusion and metabolism by radionuclide methods. Clinical wall motion imaging methods tend to underestimate the extent of myocardial viability and potential for recovery of regional deformation, while perfusion and metabolism imaging methods tend to identify viability in many regions which do not recover contractile function. Common clinical methods for assessment of regional wall motion also have important fundamental limitations, outlined above (see Section 2.1).

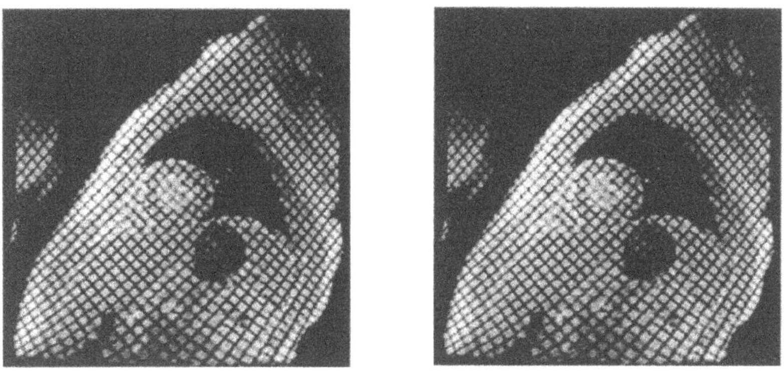

Figure 2.3: End-diastolic (left) and end-systolic (right) short axis left ventricular tagged images in a patient with recent reperfused inferior myocardial infarction. The culprit artery (the right coronary artery) had been reopened with primary stenting and there was no residual stenosis. The end-systolic image shows relatively normal tag deformation in the anteroseptal, anterior and anterolateral walls from eleven o'clock to four o'clock on the image. In contrast, the infarct region from five o'clock to nine o'clock shows markedly reduced or absent deformation. Delayed enhancement imaging demonstrated that most of the dysfunctional region was not necrotic, with necrosis limited to the subendocardium from five to 7 o'clock. The remainder of the dysfunctional myocardium was therefore stunned.

Used at rest or with dobutamine inotropic stimulation, tagged MR imaging or analogous methods such as phase contrast MR imaging or strain rate imaging offer important advantages for assessment of regional heterogeneity of myocardial deformation in ischemic heart disease, whether the problem is acute ischemia, effects of acute or chronic infarction, presence of stunned or hibernating but viable myocardium or effects of postinfarction remodeling, see Figures 2.3, 2.4. Similar information can currently be obtained only by highly invasive studies unsuitable for widespread clinical use, based on three-dimensional arrays of sonomicrometry crystals or intramyocardial tantalum markers. Such techniques are suitable for use in experimental large animal models, but not in man.

Only a fraction of the potential clinical applications of tagged MR imaging in

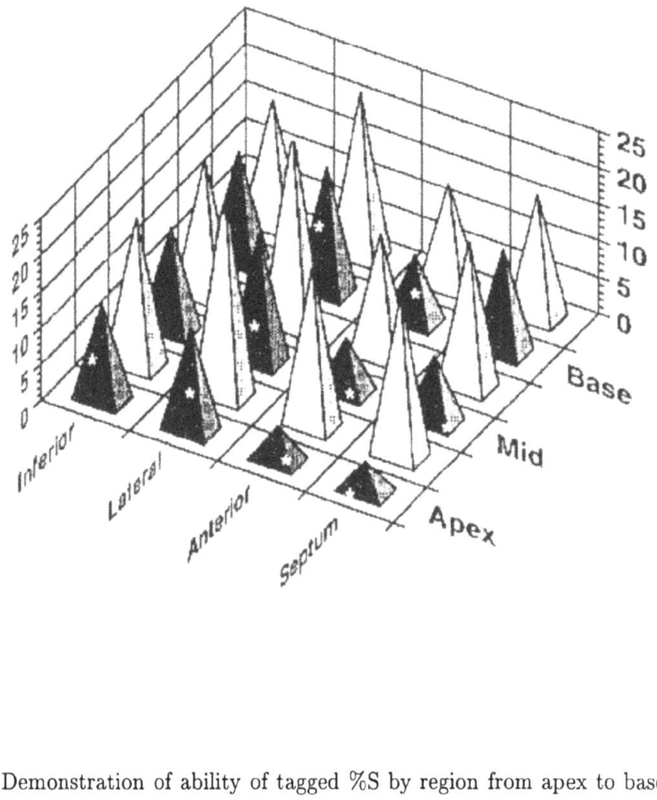

Figure 2.4: Demonstration of ability of tagged %S by region from apex to base and over inferior, septal, anterior and lateral walls in patients with recent anteroapical MI (dark pyramids) and normal controls (white pyramids). In addition to the anticipated reduction of function in the infarct zone at the apex, significant reductions of %S extend beyond the infarct region (From [38], with permission).

human ischemic heart disease have even been initially explored at present. The best studied thus far have been recent acute myocardial infarction, post-infarction stunning and post-infarction remodeling. In acute infarction, myocardial deformation may be diminished, abolished or altered to systolic stretching in the infarct region-which is itself quite heterogeneous [17, 18, 33–36]. Systolic stretching is generally found only in the necrotic center of unreperfused infarcts or in regions of acute transmural ischemia. Stretching is expressed as negative circumferential %S in a 1D analysis, while lesser degrees of contractile abnormality result in reduced or absent circumferential %S. In contrast, findings on 2D strain analysis are less intuitively obvious to clinicians. The strain vectors often remain large in magnitude, but shift in direction so that maximal lengthening no longer lies close to the radial direction with maximal shortening close to the circumferential plane in the left ventricular short axis plane. Rather, maximal strain is oriented at a larger angle to the radial direction with stretching expressed as an angle of 90° to the radial [33]. Further, the orientation of deformation is dynamic and dependent on load and contractile state. Thus, in experimental models, reduction in afterload and/or preload shift strain vectors toward the normal orientation, as myocardium deforms more normally with reduced afterload or augmented contractile state. Several studies have been published examining regional tagging data in patients with recent acute infarction-typically treated with reperfusion therapy by either thrombolysis or primary angioplasty. In such patients, the early post-infarction dysfunction is more extensive than necrosis and extends beyond the so-called risk region of the culprit artery to affect remote myocardium, even in the absence of local perfusion abnormalities [37–40] Several mechanisms appear to be at work. First, myocardial stunning may be present within the risk region in myocardium that was transiently ischemic but did not become necrotic and is left with transiently reduced contractile function but relatively normal perfusion and preserved metabolic function. In addition, physical tethering of adjacent and remote myocardium to the necrotic region may result in increased regional afterload even in regions remote from the infarct. This has not been proven by empirical data to date given our inability to directly measure or reliably estimate wall stress in regionally heterogeneous myocardium. Nonetheless, this mechanism best explains the continuous gradient of increasing deformation found in infarcted left ventricle from the edge of the infarct to remote normal myocardium [41]. Experimental data suggests that other contributors include, sympathetic denervation due to transient ischemia in noninfarcted portions of the risk region as well as multiple other functional and compositional changes in the myocyte and interstitium in the non-infarcted risk region. These may include reversible damage to the myocytes contractile apparatus, impaired calcium handling, depressed energetics, and reduced β-receptor function and downstream coupling of the receptor.

In reperfused infarction some residual active myocardial deformation is often found even in central infarct regions [38–40]. This could be due to survival of small islands of viable myocardium or to effects of cross-fiber shortening resulting from contraction in an epicardial rim of surviving myocardium. After reperfused infarction, viable but stunned myocardium generally returns to normal or near normal function a few months after infarction. Viability can be demonstrated early after infarction using either low dose dobutamine administration with MR tagging or demonstrating absence of delayed myocardial enhancement 20 minutes after gadolinium contrast injection [42–44]. Combining the two methods further improves recognition of viable myocardium in this setting [45]. Augmented contraction with dobutamine generally occurs in regions that have some very low level residual normally oriented deformation in the basal state. The better the basal state deformation, the greater the dobutamine response and the greater the probability that marked improvement will occur over time [42, 45].

After infarction with an extensive region of necrosis and depressed left ventricular ejection fraction, progressive adverse left ventricular remodeling often occurs over a period of years resulting in further left ventricular dilation and further reduction of left ventricular pump function [46, 47]. Remodeling is associated with persistent impaired regional deformation adjacent to and remote from the original infarct. The remodeling process may be blunted by administration of angiotensin converting enzyme inhibitors (ACEI) and this blunting is associated in experimental models with improved recovery of deformation in adjacent and remote myocardium. Recently, in an animal model, combination of ACEI with an angiotensin receptor blocker has been shown to further reduce adverse remodeling and its effects on regional function [48].

MR imaging techniques are progressing rapidly in speed, improved SNR, resolution and volumetric coverage of the heart. Thus it has become increasingly feasible to perform complex multifaceted imaging protocols in patients with recent myocardial infarction, who typically tolerate no more than an hour in the MR scanner. Volumetric coverage of the left ventricle with tagged or untagged images is now routine in 15 minutes or so and real-time techniques will soon reduce that time by two-thirds. This makes it quite practical to combine tagged imaging with global volumetric assessment of ventricular chamber volume, ejection fraction and myocardial mass, first pass and delayed contrast imaging and low dose dobutamine stress in the post-infarction patient or the patient with chronic coronary artery disease and left ventricular dysfunction. Use of tagged imaging in such "multiparametric" imaging studies in patients can be expected to grow rapidly in the future for both research and clinical use, particularly if tagged image post-processing can be sufficiently automated to make data reduction timely and inexpensive.

2.6 MR Tagging in Left Ventricular Hypertrophy

In experimental models of left ventricular pressure overload hypertrophy (LVH) myocardial function becomes abnormal at the myocardial segment and myocyte levels, with associated changes in myocardial calcium handling, energetics and contractile proteins, long before ventricular pump function is impaired. MRI tagging methods have made it possible to examine intramural myocardial function in man. Results demonstrate reduced myocardial deformation even in mild pressure-overload hypertrophy with normal left ventricular ejection fraction [32]. Reductions in deformation of over 40% may be found even in mild hypertrophy. In addition, patterns of regional heterogeneity of deformation and rigid body motion are also altered. However, transmural gradients in deformation are preserved. These results have stimulated the clinical cardiac imaging community to more widely examine the distinction between chamber function and myocardial function and the potential significance of altered intramural function in pressure overload hypertrophy. Such studies have been made more feasible by the development and application of simple echocardiographic methods for estimation of left ventricular midwall shortening that have been extensively applied in large-scale studies of hypertension and, in smaller studies, to pressure overload due to aortic stenosis [49]. The methods used are somewhat indirect and require simplified assumptions about the distribution of intramural deformation across the wall and the constancy of myocardial volume over the cardiac cycle. Nonetheless, they have been quite useful and results are generally concordant with those obtained more directly from tagging studies. Early reports suggest that reduced midwall shortening may be another marker for increased risk of adverse events and that midwall shortening abnormalities reverse with regression of left ventricular pressure overload hypertrophy induced by effective pharmacologic management of hypertension with at least some antihypertensive agents. In contrast to pressure overload LVH, limited data indicates that the physiologic hypertrophy produced by high level athletic conditioning, which is known to be fully reversible, does not result in abnormal intramural myocardial function.

2.7 Cardiomyopathies

Tagged imaging has been applied in man to non-ischemic cardiomyopathies to a limited degree. In dilated cardiomyopathy, depressed left ventricular ejection fraction is due to depressed fiber and cross-fiber strain, the severity of which parallels depressed chamber function, but the transmural gradients in these strain components are preserved [30]. Hypertrophic cardiomyopathy, a genetic disorder of one of several contractile proteins, has been studied somewhat more extensively. In this disorder, left ventricular ejection fraction is often normal or supernormal, but circumferential segment shortening is depressed in the septum and inferior wall [50]. When 3D deformation is assessed, reduced strain in the septum is most striking, but left ventricular torsion is preserved [22, 23]. The relationship of preserved torsion and of reduced strains in thicker myocardium to preserved chamber function in this disorder remain to be clarified. Some investigators have noted similar findings in ordinary pressure overload LVH.

2.8 Right Ventricular Mechanics

Tagging studies of the right ventricle have been relatively few in number. Tagged imaging and data reduction in thin-walled right ventricles is difficult, but application of the method to hypertrophied right ventricles is considerably easier [51]. Three-dimensional analysis can also be performed and are particularly promising because of the complex shape and patterns of motion of the right ventricle [52]. Early studies suggest that application of tagging methods will be particularly fruitful in congenital heart disease with right ventricular overload and in congenital heart disease with univentricular heart [53].

2.9 Pericardial Constriction

A relatively common non-myocardial application of tagged imaging merits mention. Constrictive pericarditis is a disorder in which biventricular filling in diastole is impaired by thickened, scarred pericardium adherent to the epicardium that greatly increases diastolic cardiac stiffness. Conventional noninvasive and invasive imaging methods have important limitations in assessment of this disorder. Transthoracic echocardiography does not image the pericardium very well and relies on other indirect evidence of constrictive physiology. Even invasive hemodynamics may be confusing if coexistent myocardial disease is present. MR imaging is an excellent method for assessment of myocardial thickness around the entire cardiac perimeter. However, constriction may occur with relatively thin myocardium, so thickness measurement alone does not suffice. Tagged imaging can directly demonstrate adhesion of the parietal pericardium to the epicardium of the cardiac chambers. In normal heart, sliding of epicardium against pericardium results in loss of registration of tag lines over systole. In constrictive pericarditis, registration of pericardial tag lines with epicardial ends of tag lines is preserved. Thus the combination of untagged MR imaging of pericardial thickness and tagged imaging of pericardial adhesion has become a powerful approach for assessment of this disorder. Instances of partial constriction limited to all or part of the epicardium of a single chamber can be identified despite often atypical clinical and hemodynamic findings [54, 55]. The literature has been limited by the small number of such patients seen at any one center and a report of a large series of such patients is badly needed.

2.10 Summary

MR tagging of the myocardium is a powerful method for assessment of regional myocardial deformation. It has permitted important new insights with regard to normal physiology, myocardial disease and pericardial disease in man. In particular, applications to ischemic heart disease have great value and are likely to become more commonplace. Application of tagging methods in patients has been limited in the past by relatively slow MR imaging methods and the cost and time requirements of data reduction. Further increases in imaging speed and automation of analysis of tagged images, as well as incorporation of tagging sequences and analytic tools into commercial MRI software for imaging and postprocessing are badly needed. With solution of these problems, tagged imaging is likely to become a very important technique for clinical assessment of myocardial function.

Acknowledgments

I would like to thank many colleagues and trainees, past and present, for their valuable contributions to development of MR tagging and its application in patients: Leon Axel, Walter Rogers, Joao Lima, Neil Clark, Christopher M. Kramer, Alistair Young, Eric Hoffman, Victor Ferrari, Linda Palmon Calhoun, Susan Yeon, Thomas Power and Genady Geskin. Jan Meister's careful editing and production of this chapter is very gratefully acknowledged.

References

[1] Vatner SF; Millard RW; Patrick TA; Heyndrickx GR: Effects of isoproterenol on regional myocardial function, electrocardiogram, and blood flow in conscious dogs with myocardial ischemia. J Clin Invest. 1976 May;57(5):1261-71.

[2] Gallagher KP; Kumada T; Koziol JA; McKown MD; Kemper WS; Ross J Jr. : Significance of regional wall thickening abnormalities relative to transmural myocardial perfusion in anesthetized dogs. Circulation 1980 Dec;62(6):1266-74

[3] Hansen DE; Daughters GT 2nd; Alderman EL; Ingels NB Jr; Miller DC : Torsional deformation of the left ventricular midwall in human hearts with intramyocardial markers: regional heterogeneity and sensitivity to the inotropic effects of abrupt rate changes. Circ Res 1988 May;62(5):941-52

[4] Zerhouni EA; Parish DM; Rogers WJ; Yang A; Shapiro EP : Human heart: Tagging with MR imaging - a method for noninvasive assessment of myocardial motion. Radiology 1988;169:59-63

[5] Axel L; Dougherty L: MR imaging of motion with spatial modulation of magnetization. Radiology 1989;171:841-45

[6] Pelc NJ; Drangova M; Pelc LR; Zhu Y; Noll DC; Bowman BS; and Herfkens RJ: Tracking of cyclic motion with phase-contrast cine MR velocity data. J Magn Reson Imaging 1995 May-Jun;5(3):339-45

[7] Wedeen VJ; Weisskoff RM; Reese TG; Beache GM; Poncelet BP; and Rosen BR: Dinsmore RE: Motionless movies of myocardial strain-rates using stimulated echoes Magn Reson Med 1995 Mar;33(3):401-8

[8] McVeigh ER; Atalar E: Cardiac tagging with breath-hold cine MRI. Magn Reson Med 1992 Dec;28(2):318-27

[9] Denney TS; McVeigh ER: Model-free reconstruction of three-dimensional myocardial strain from planar tagged MR images. J Magn Reson Imaging 1997 Sep-Oct;7(5):799-810.

[10] Bolster BD; McVeigh ER; Zerhouni EA: Myocardial tagging in polar coordinates with use of striped tags. Radiology 1990 Dec;177(3):769-72.

[11] Power TP; Kramer CM; Shaffer AL; Theobald TM; Petruolo S; Reichek N; Rogers WJ Jr: Breath-hold dobutamine magnetic resonance myocardial tagging: normal left ventricular response. Am J Cardiol 1997 Nov 1;80(9):1203-7

[12] Scott CH; Sutton MS; Gusani N; Fayad Z; Kraitchman D; Keane MG; Axel L; Ferrari VA: Effect of dobutamine on regional left ventricular function measured by tagged magnetic resonance imaging in normal subjects. Am J Cardiol 1999 Feb 1;83(3):412-7

[13] Tang C; McVeigh ER; Zerhouni EA: Multi-shot EPI for improvement of myocardial tag contrast: comparison with segmented SPGR. Magn Reson Med 1995 Mar;33(3):443-7

[14] Clark NR; Reichek N; Bergey P; Hoffman EA; Brownson D; Palmon L; Axel L.: Circumferential Myocardial Shortening in the Normal Human Left Ventricle. Assessment by Magnetic Resonance Imaging Using Spatial Modulation of Magnetization. Circulation 84(1): 67-74, 1991.

[15] Osman NF; McVeigh ER; Prince JL: Imaging heart motion using harmonic phase MR IEEE Trans Med Imaging 2000 Mar;19(3):186-202

[16] Garot J; Bluemke DA; Osman NF; Rochitte CE; McVeigh ER; Zerhouni EA; Prince JL; Lima JA: Fast determination of regional myocardial strain fields from tagged cardiac images using harmonic phase MRI. Circulation 2000 Mar 7;101(9):981-8.

[17] Yeon S; Reichek N; Palmon LC; Tallant B; Brownson D; Hoffman E; Axel L: Segmental Shortening by Magnetic Resonance Tagging in Experimental Myocardial Infarction. Circulation 82(IV):763, 1990(Abstr).

[18] Lima JA; Jeremy R; Guier W; Bouton S; Zerhouni EA; McVeigh E; Buchalter MB; Weisfeldt ML; Shapiro EP; Weiss JL : Accurate systolic wall thickening by nuclear magnetic resonance imaging with tissue tagging: correlation with

sonomicrometers in normal and ischemic myocardium. J Am Coll Cardiol 1993 Jun;21(7):1741-51

[19] Young AA; Imai H; Chang CN; Axel L: Two-dimensional left ventricular deformation during systole using magnetic resonance imaging with spatial modulation of magnetization. Circulation 1994 Feb;89(2):740-52

[20] Young AA; Axel L: Three-dimensional motion and deformation of the heart wall: estimation with spatial modulation of magnetization–a model-based approach. Radiology 1992 Oct;185(1):241-7

[21] Rademakers FE; Rogers WJ; Guier WH; Hutchins GM; Siu CO; Weisfeldt ML; Weiss JL; Shapiro EP: Relation of regional cross-fiber shortening to wall thickening in the intact heart. Three-dimensional strain analysis by NMR tagging. Circulation. 1994 Mar;89(3):1174-82.

[22] Young AA; Kramer CM; Ferrari VA; Axel L; Reichek N: Three-dimensional left ventricular deformation in hypertrophic cardiomyopathy. Circulation 1994 Aug;90(2):854-67

[23] Dong SJ; MacGregor JH; Crawley AP; McVeigh E; Belenkie I; Smith ER; Tyberg JV; Beyar R: Left ventricular wall thickness and regional systolic function in patients with hypertrophic cardiomyopathy. A three-dimensional tagged magnetic resonance imaging study. Circulation 1994 Sep;90(3):1200-9

[24] Denney TS; McVeigh ER: Model-free reconstruction of three-dimensional myocardial strain from planar tagged MR images. J Magn Reson Imaging 1997 Sep-Oct;7(5):799-810.

[25] Kuijer JP; Marcus JT; Gotte MJ; van Rossum AC; Heethaar RM: Simultaneous MRI tagging and through-plane velocity quantification: a three-dimensional myocardial motion tracking algorithm. J Magn Reson Imaging 1999 Mar;9(3):409-19

[26] Moore CC; Lugo-Olivieri CH; McVeigh ER; Zerhouni EA: Three-dimensional systolic strain patterns in the normal human left ventricle: characterization with tagged MR imaging. Radiology 2000 Feb;214(2):453-66

[27] Ozturk C; McVeigh ER: Four-dimensional B-spline based motion analysis of tagged MR images: introduction and in vivo validation. Phys Med Biol 2000 Jun;45(6):1683-702.

[28] Rademakers FE; Buchalter MB; Rogers WJ; Zerhouni EA; Weisfeldt ML; Weiss JL; Shapiro EP: Dissociation between left ventricular untwisting and filling. Accentuation by catecholamines. Circulation 1992 Apr;85(4):1572-81

[29] MacGowan GA; Burkhoff D; Rogers WJ; Salvador D; Azhari H; Hees PS; Zweier JL; Halperin HR; Siu CO; Lima JA; Weiss JL; Shapiro EP: Effects of afterload on regional left ventricular torsion. Cardiovasc Res 1996 Jun;31(6):917-25

[30] MacGowan GA; Shapiro EP; Azhari H; Siu CO; Hees PS; Hutchins GM; Weiss JL; Rademakers FE: Noninvasive measurement of shortening in the fiber and cross-fiber directions in the normal human left ventricle and in idiopathic dilated cardiomyopathy. Circulation 1997 Jul 15;96(2):535-41

[31] Reese TG; Weisskoff RM; Smith RN; Rosen BR; Dinsmore RE; Wedeen VJ: Imaging myocardial fiber architecture in vivo with magnetic resonance. Magn Reson Med 1995 Dec;34(6):786-91

[32] Palmon LC; Reichek N; Yeon SB; Clark NR; Brownson D; Hoffman E; Axel L: Intramural myocardial shortening in hypertensive left ventricular hypertrophy with normal pump function. Circulation 1994 Jan;89(1):122-31

[33] Lima JA; Ferrari VA; Reichek N; Kramer CM; Palmon L; Llaneras MR; Tallant B; Young AA; Axel L: Segmental motion and deformation of transmurally infarcted myocardium in acute postinfarct period. Am J Physiol 1995 Mar;268(3 Pt 2):H1304-12

[34] Kraitchman DL; Young AA; Bloomgarden DC; Fayad ZA; Dougherty L; Ferrari VA; Boston RC; Axel L: Integrated MRI assessment of regional function and perfusion in canine myocardial infarction. Magn Reson Med 1998 Aug;40(2):311

[35] Aelen FW; Arts T; Sanders DG; Thelissen GR; Prinzen FW; Reneman RS: Kinematic analysis of left ventricular deformation in myocardial infarction using magnetic resonance cardiac tagging Int J Card Imaging 1999 Jun;15(3):241-51

[36] Bogaert J; Maes A; Van de Werf F; Bosmans H; Herregods MC; Nuyts J; Desmet W; Mortelmans L; Marchal G; Rademakers FE: Functional recovery of subepicardial myocardial tissue in transmural myocardial infarction after successful reperfusion: an important contribution to the improvement of regional and global left ventricular function. Circulation 1999 Jan 5-12;99(1):36-43

[37] Kramer CM; Lima JA; Reichek N; Ferrari VA; Llaneras MR; Palmon LC; Yeh IT; Tallant B; Axel L: Regional differences in function within noninfarcted myocardium during left ventricular remodeling. Circulation 1993 Sep;88(3):1279-88

[38] Kramer CM; Rogers WJ; Theobald TM; Power TP; Petruolo S; Reichek N: Remote noninfarcted region dysfunction soon after first anterior myocardial infarction a magnetic resonance tagging study. Circulation, 1996;94:660-666

[39] Kramer CM; Rogers WJ; Theobald TM; Power TP; Geskin G; Reichek N: Dissociation between changes in intramyocardial function and left ventricular volumes in the 8 weeks after first anterior myocardial infarction. J Am Coll Cardiol 1997;30:1625-1632.

[40] Bogaert J; Bosmans H; Maes A; Suetens P; Marchal G; Rademakers FE: Remote myocardial dysfunction after acute anterior myocardial infarction: impact of left ventricular shape on regional function: a magnetic resonance myocardial tagging study.J Am Coll Cardiol 2000 May;35(6):1525-34

[41] Kramer CK; Nicol PD; Rogers WJ; Suzuki MM; Shaffer A; Theobald TM; Reichek N: Reduced Sympathetic Innervation Underlies Adjacent Non-infarcted Region Dysfunction During Left Ventricular Remodeling.JACC 1997;30:1079-85

[42] Geskin G; Kramer CM; Rogers WJ; Theobald TM; Pakstis D; Hu YL; Reichek N: Quantitative assessment of myocardial viability after infarction by dobutamine magnetic resonance tagging. Circulation 1998 Jul 21;98(3):217-23

[43] Rogers WJ Jr; Kramer CM; Geskin G; Hu YL; Theobald TM; Vido DA; Petruolo S; Reichek N: Early contrast-enhanced MRI predicts late functional recovery after reperfused myocardial infarction Circulation 1999 Feb 16;99(6):744-50

[44] Kim RJ; Wu E; Rafael A; Chen EL; Parker MA; Simonetti O; Klocke FJ; Bonow RO; Judd RM: The use of contrast-enhanced magnetic resonance imaging to identify reversible myocardial dysfunction. N Engl J Med 2000 Nov 16;343(20):1445-53

[45] Kramer CM; Rogers WJ Jr; Mankad S; Theobald TM; Pakstis DL; Hu YL: Contractile reserve and contrast uptake pattern by magnetic resonance imaging and functional recovery after reperfused myocardial infarction. J Am Coll Cardiol 2000 Nov 15;36(6):1835-40

[46] Pfeffer MA; Pfeffer JM: Ventricular enlargement and reduced survival after myocardial infarction Circulation 1987 May;75(5 Pt 2):IV93-7

[47] Pfeffer MA; Lamas GA; Vaughan DE; Parisi AF; Braunwald E: Effect of captopril on progressive ventricular dilatation after anterior myocardial infarction. N Engl J Med 1988 Jul 14;319(2):80-6

[48] Mankad S; d'Amato TA; Reichek N; McGregor WE; Lin J; Singh D; Rogers WJ; Kramer CM: Combined angiotensin II receptor antagonism and angiotensin-converting enzyme inhibition further attenuates post-infarction left ventricular remodeling. Circulation, 2001 In Press

[49] Aurigemma GP; Silver KH; Priest MA; Gaasch WH: Geometric changes allow normal ejection fraction despite depressed myocardial shortening in hypertensive left ventricular hypertrophy. J Am Coll Cardiol 1995 Jul;26(1):195-202

[50] Kramer CM; Reichek N; Ferrari VA; Theobald T; Dawson J; Axel L: Regional Heterogeneity of function in hypertrophic cardiomyopathy. Circulation. 90:186-194, 1994.

[51] Young AA; Fayad ZA; Axel L: Right ventricular midwall surface motion and deformation using magnetic resonance tagging. Am J Physiol 1996 Dec;271(6 Pt 2):H2677-88

[52] Fayad ZA; Ferrari VA; Kraitchman DL; Young AA; Palevsky HI; Bloomgarden DC; Axel L: Right ventricular regional function using MR tagging: normals versus chronic pulmonary hypertension. Magn Reson Med 1998 Jan;39(1):116-23

[53] Fogel MA; Weinberg PM; Fellows KE; Hoffman EA: A study in ventricular-ventricular interaction. Single right ventricles compared with systemic right ventricles in a dual-chamber circulation. Circulation 1995 Jul 15;92(2):219-30

[54] Hasuda T; Satoh T; Yamada N; Sakamaki F; Kyotani S; Nakanishi N: A case of constrictive pericarditis with local thickening of the pericardium without manifest ventricular interdependence. Cardiology 1999;92(3):214-6

[55] Kojima S; Yamada N; Goto Y: Diagnosis of constrictive pericarditis by tagged cine magnetic resonance imaging. N Engl J Med 1999 Jul 29;341(5):373-4

Chapter 3

Finite Element Modeling for Three-Dimensional Motion Reconstruction and Analysis

Kevin F. Augenstein
Department of Engineering Science,
School of Engineering,
University of Auckland
k.augenstein@auckland.ac.nz

Alistair A. Young
Department of Anatomy with Radiology,
School of Medicine,
University of Auckland
a.young@auckland.ac.nz

3.1 Introduction

Magnetic resonance (MR) tissue tagging has become a useful tool for non-invasive analysis of heart wall motion (see Chapter 2). Typically, multiple parallel tagging planes are created orthogonal to the imaging plane in a short time interval (5–12 ms) on detection of the R wave of the ECG (end-diastole). Often a grid of tag planes is created, whose intersection with the image plane gives rise to dark bands ("image stripes") in the image, 1–2 mm in width and spaced 5–10 mm apart. With the advent of fast imaging techniques (segmented k-space, echo planar, SENSE and SMASH techniques), it is now possible to obtain a complete dataset suitable for 4D analysis in 5–15 minutes (a 4D dataset typically contains 5–8 short axis slices and 2–6 long axis slices in various orientations, each at 10–20 frames in the cardiac cycle).

The clinical utility of cardiac MR is currently limited by the prohibitively long time required for image analysis. Most analysis methods require the prior extraction of the inner and outer boundaries of the heart in each image, together with the localization of the image stripes in each frame [2, 13–17, 30]. The image inten-

A.A. Amini and J.L. Prince (eds.),
Measurement of Cardiac Deformations from MRI: Physical and Mathematical Models, 37–58.

sity information is however insufficient to completely characterize the boundary and tag locations in real clinical images, due in part to limited spatial and temporal resolution, lack of contrast between blood and muscle, and respiration and gating artifacts. User interaction with the tracking and segmentation processes is therefore fundamental, along with prior information on geometry and motion. FE models allow efficient incorporation of *a priori* information and lend themselves to intuitive user interaction.

Finite element (FE) modeling has been used extensively in cardiac mechanics to efficiently describe cardiac geometry and muscle micro-structure [8, 9, 12] and to solve the equations of equilibrium for material stress and strain [7]. It is the only computational method which allows incorporation of nonlinear material properties, finite deformations, material anisotropy and complex geometry into the stress estimation problem (See Chapter 1). FE analysis techniques for 3D motion reconstruction were developed initially for the reconstruction of epicardial surface geometry and motion from coronary cinéangiograms [19, 29]. A similar technique was used to estimate epicardial deformation from implanted beads [6]. A FE approach to reconstruction of 3D motion from tagged MRI was first presented in 1992 [22]. Variations of this approach have been developed subsequently, including RV motion analysis [28] and fast interactive modeling techniques [20]. An overview of these techniques is included in the first part of this chapter.

These methods have now been applied to a number of pathological cases and normal volunteers [5, 23, 27, 31]. Material strain in registered locations of the heart can be calculated directly from the model using standard continuum mechanics techniques [4]. While this has provided a wealth of information on regional deformation, it is unclear how the statistical analysis of these data should be performed. Collation of the results into meaningful physiological and pathological processes remains an open problem. Large numbers of models can be used to form a compact, efficient database of normal and abnormal geometry and motion. Such a database would allow systematic analysis of effects due to treatment or aging. Since each model is registered to the cardiac anatomy, the model parameters themselves can be used in multidimensional statistical analyses of motion and geometry. One powerful tool is principal component analysis (PCA). The second part of this chapter outlines one PCA approach and presents preliminary results from a group of normal volunteers. It is hoped that such an approach may lead to a sensitive research tool for the description and quantification of heart wall motion abnormalities.

3.2 The Finite Element Model

The finite element method (FEM) was developed to solve differential equations on a complex domain [32]. The solution domain is divided into small regions called *elements*, each of which is governed by a group of element parameters, normally defined at *nodes*. Over each element the field is defined by a weighted average of the element parameters, with the weights given by the element *basis functions*.

Low order polynomials are normally used to interpolate the element parameters between nodes. Similar basis functions can be used to define the model geometry as well as the solution field. Piecewise low order polynomials are commonly used in graphical modeling as their behavior is well understood. Low order polynomials have the advantages that high order oscillations are reduced and mathematical operations such as differentiation and integration can easily be applied. Continuity between elements is maintained by constraints between element parameters of neighboring elements. This continuity can be of any order, but is restricted by the basis functions and element connectivity.

3.2.1 Basis Functions

One-dimensional, linear Lagrange basis functions are given by

$$\begin{aligned} \varphi_1(\xi) &= 1-\xi, \\ \varphi_2(\xi) &= \xi. \end{aligned} \tag{3.1}$$

Given element parameters (nodal values) u_n, we can define the interpolated field with respect to the element coordinate, ξ.

$$u(\xi) = \sum_{n=1}^{N} \varphi_n(\xi)\, u_n, \tag{3.2}$$

where N is the number of element parameters (and basis functions).

Linear basis functions are limited in that they can only achieve C^0 continuity; to achieve higher levels of smoothness it is necessary to use higher order basis functions. Normally the highest order used is cubic basis functions. The cubic Hermite basis functions are defined as

$$\begin{aligned} \varphi_1(\xi) &= 1-3\xi^2+2\xi^3, \\ \varphi_2(\xi) &= \xi^2(3-2\xi), \\ \varphi_3(\xi) &= \xi(\xi-1)^2, \\ \varphi_4(\xi) &= \xi^2(\xi-1). \end{aligned} \tag{3.3}$$

In the linear case the element parameters were the field values at each node. In the cubic Hermite case we require the field derivatives as well.

It is easy to apply this method to multi-dimensional fields. To create 2D basis functions with two element coordinates we apply a tensor product between the two sets of basis functions. For example, to interpolate over a linear-cubic patch we would use the following basis functions

$$\begin{aligned}
\varphi_1(\xi_1,\xi_2) &= (1-\xi_1)\times\left(1-3{\xi_2}^2+2{\xi_2}^3\right)\,,\\
\varphi_2(\xi_1,\xi_2) &= \xi_1\times\left(1-3{\xi_2}^2+2{\xi_2}^3\right)\,,\\
\varphi_3(\xi_1,\xi_2) &= (1-\xi_1)\times{\xi_2}^2(3-2\xi_2)\,,\\
\varphi_4(\xi_1,\xi_2) &= \xi_1\times{\xi_2}^2(3-2\xi_2)\,,\\
\varphi_5(\xi_1,\xi_2) &= (1-\xi_1)\times\xi_2(\xi_2-1)^2\,,\\
\varphi_6(\xi_1,\xi_2) &= \xi_1\times\xi_2(\xi_2-1)^2\,,\\
\varphi_7(\xi_1,\xi_2) &= (1-\xi_1)\times{\xi_2}^2(\xi_2-1)\,,\\
\varphi_8(\xi_1,\xi_2) &= \xi_1\times{\xi_2}^2(\xi_2-1)\,.
\end{aligned} \tag{3.4}$$

3.2.2 Global Parameters

The individual elements are assembled into the model using a local-to-global parameter map. This map typically takes the form of a hash table. As the elements share nodes and borders, some field values must be conserved through these shared boundaries. After removing the duplicated nodes we end up with the global parameters. For example, if we consider two linear elements that abut one another, then the second node of the first element is the same as the first node of the second element, giving the following global parameters

$$\begin{aligned}
u_{11} &= U_1\,,\\
u_{21} &= U_2\,,\\
u_{12} &= U_2\,,\\
u_{22} &= U_3\,,
\end{aligned} \tag{3.5}$$

where u_{ij} is the nodal value at the ith node in the jth element and U_k is the kth global node.

3.2.3 Coordinate Systems

Left ventricle (LV) geometry is efficiently described in a prolate spheroidal coordinate system [12]. This is similar to a spherical coordinate system except the shape of a surface of constant radius is a regular ellipsoid, rather than a sphere. The conversion to Cartesian coordinates is

$$\begin{aligned}
x &= f\cosh\lambda\cos\mu\,,\\
y &= f\sinh\lambda\sin\mu\cos\theta\,,\\
z &= f\sinh\lambda\sin\mu\sin\theta\,.
\end{aligned} \tag{3.6}$$

Using the prolate coordinate system to fit the geometry of the LV simplifies the fitting problem to a linear least squares problem with data points projected along lines of constant μ and θ.

The deformation and motion of the heart is best modeled in a rectangular Cartesian coordinate system. A "cardiac" coordinate system is constructed as shown in Figure 3.1 to allow the comparison and registration of different cases in a consistent fashion. A central axis is defined to lie along the line between the LV apical and basal centroids. Fiducial markers placed at the LV apex and base are projected onto this central axis to give an estimate of LV length. The origin of the cardiac coordinate system is defined to be one-third the distance from the base towards the apex. The direction of the x-axis is aligned towards the apex. The y-axis is defined to be parallel to the line joining the right ventricle centroid to its projection on the central axis. The remaining z-axis is therefore oriented towards the LV posterior wall.

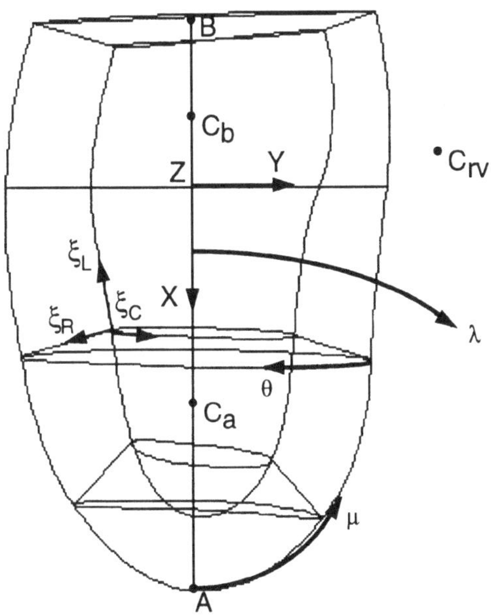

Figure 3.1: A wire frame mesh showing a model geometry fitted to the end-diastolic inner and outer contours in a normal heart. The model is defined in a "cardiac" coordinate system (X, Y, Z) with the X-axis joining the centroids of the most apical and basal contours (C_a and C_b respectively), and the Y-axis pointing toward the centroid of the RV contours (C_{RV}). Apex and base markers (A and B) define an overall scale for the model. Element coordinates are aligned in longitudinal (ξ_L), circumferential (ξ_C), and radial (ξ_R) directions. An initial prolate spheroidal system is also shown (λ, μ, θ). The overall view is from the posterior wall with the septum on the right.

3.2.4 Kinematics

Local material displacement, rotation, and strain can be calculated directly from the FE model using standard continuum mechanics methods [4]. Typically, strains are referenced to end-diastole (the "undeformed" state), although this is a convention only. For convenience, we use a local rectangular Cartesian coordinate system (Y_1, Y_2, Y_3) which is locally aligned along the circumferential (ξ_1), longitudinal (ξ_2), and radial (ξ_3) directions at each point in the undeformed model. The Y_M are known as material coordinates, whereas lower case symbols (y_1, y_2, y_3) are used to refer to the deformed state (e.g., end-systole).

A line segment in the undeformed material has components (dY_1, dY_2, dY_3). After the material deforms the line segment has the coordinates (dy_1, dy_2, dy_3). The deformation field expresses the deformed state, (y_i), as a function of the material coordinates, (Y_M). The deformation gradient tensor is given by $F = \frac{\partial y_i}{\partial Y_M}$. The deformation gradient tensor can be decomposed into RU, an orthogonal rotation matrix R and a symmetric strain matrix U.

Strain is a measurement of the relative length change undergone in deformation. The squared length of the deformed line segment is given by

$$\begin{aligned} ds^2 &= \sum_{k=1}^{3} dy_k dy_k\,, \\ &= \sum_{k=1}^{3} \left(\sum_{M=1}^{3} \frac{\partial y_k}{\partial Y_M} dY_M \sum_{N=1}^{3} \frac{\partial y_k}{\partial Y_N} dY_N \right), \\ &= \sum_{N=1}^{3} \sum_{M=1}^{3} C_{MN} dY_M dY_N\,, \end{aligned} \tag{3.7}$$

where $C_{MN} = \sum_{k=1}^{3} \frac{\partial y_k}{\partial Y_M} \frac{\partial y_k}{\partial Y_N} = F^T F$ is known as the right Cauchy-Green strain tensor. Note that F is referenced to the circumferential (C), longitudinal (L), and radial (R) directions and can be related to element coordinates by

$$F_{kN} = \frac{\partial y_k}{\partial Y_N} = \sum_{j=1}^{3} \frac{\partial y_k}{\partial \xi_j} \frac{\partial \xi_j}{\partial Y_N}\,. \tag{3.8}$$

Because $F = RU$ we can show that C is independent of rigid body rotations.

$$\begin{aligned} C &= F^T F\,, \\ &= (RU)^T RU\,, \\ &= U^T R^T RU\,, \\ &= U^2\,. \end{aligned} \tag{3.9}$$

The Lagrangian strain tensor can be calculated as

$$E = \frac{1}{2}\left(F^T F - I\right), \tag{3.10}$$

where I is the identity tensor. The diagonal components of E, (E_{CC}, E_{LL}, E_{RR}) are called normal strains and measure the contraction if negative or elongation if positive in the associated direction. The off-diagonal components (E_{CL}, E_{CR}, E_{LR}) are shear strains that measure the change in angle between planes that are initially orthogonal in the undeformed state. The eigenvalues of E, (E_1, E_2, E_3) are the principal strains, and the eigenvectors the direction in which they occur. The maximum and minimum principal strains are the maximum and minimum extension/contraction experienced by the tissue at that point. Typically, in a normal heart with end-diastole as the undeformed state, E_1 is positive and is associated with wall thickening, whereas E_3 is negative and is the maximum contraction [31].

It is sometimes convenient to express the normal strains as % shortening or % lengthening.

$$\%S_i = \frac{ds - ds_o}{ds} \times 100\% = (\sqrt{1 + 2E_{ii}} - 1) \times 100\%. \tag{3.11}$$

Shear angles (i.e., the change in angle between line segments which are initially perpendicular) can be calculated from [4]

$$\sin \alpha_{ij} = \frac{2E_{ij}}{\sqrt{1 + 2E_{ii}}\sqrt{1 + 2E_{jj}}}. \tag{3.12}$$

3.3 Model Tags: 3D Formulation

This section outlines a method for 3D LV motion estimation from multiplaner tagged images, without the need for separate 2D boundary and tag tracking [20]. It allows interactive reconstruction directly from the images under the guidance of the user.

A set of "model tags" were embedded into the finite element model, resulting in material surfaces which define the location of the tag planes within the model. Since the model tags deform with the finite element model, the intersections of the model tags with the images could be superimposed on the images as "model stripes". Image forces were then calculated in order to pull the model stripes towards the image stripes.

3.3.1 Geometric Fits

The initial geometry (at frame one or ED) of the LV was determined interactively using guide point fitting [26]. In this technique a small number of guide points are placed on the images and a 3D model is interactively fitted in real time. The epicardial and endocardial surfaces were defined in the prolate spheroidal coordinate system. The model was linear in μ and θ, which were held constant. The fitted λ field was bicubic in the circumferential and longitudinal directions. The scale factor f of the prolate system was chosen to allow a value of $\lambda = 1$ at the apex projection and $\mu = 120°$ at the aortic-mitral valve plane. The element coordinates, (ξ_1, ξ_2), for each data point were calculated by projecting the data point along radial λ lines onto an initial (constant λ) surface. A standard model has four elements in the circumferential direction and four in the longitudinal direction, giving sixteen elements.

The least squares fit minimized

$$E_{\text{contour}} = S(\lambda) + \sum_c \left(\lambda(\boldsymbol{\xi}_c) - \lambda_c\right)^2 , \tag{3.13}$$

where λ_c is the contour point and $\lambda(\boldsymbol{\xi}_c)$ is its projection onto the model. The smoothing term, $S(\lambda)$ is required because the sparse data distribution can allow wild oscillations in the fitted piecewise cubics in regions that are not well constrained by data. This ill-conditioning is a well-known problem in image modeling and has typically been solved by including a form of weighted Tikhonov regularization [18]. The most common form is "spline-type" smoothing which in this case takes the form,

$$\begin{aligned} S(\lambda) &= \int_{\xi_2}\int_{\xi_1} \alpha \left[\left(\frac{\partial \lambda^\star}{\partial \xi_1}\right)^2 + \left(\frac{\partial \lambda^\star}{\partial \xi_2}\right)^2 \right] \\ &\quad + \beta \left[\left(\frac{\partial^2 \lambda^\star}{\partial \xi_1^2}\right)^2 + 2\left(\frac{\partial^2 \lambda^\star}{\partial \xi_1 \partial \xi_2}\right)^2 + \left(\frac{\partial^2 \lambda^\star}{\partial \xi_2^2}\right)^2 \right] d\xi_1\, d\xi_2 . \end{aligned} \tag{3.14}$$

This type of smoothing is best imposed on the displacement field, $\lambda^\star = \lambda - \lambda_p$, from a target shape (or prior λ_p) to the fitted solution. The weight α then penalizes gradients in the displacement field, while β penalizes curvature in the displacement field.

Nodal values of the fitted surfaces were then converted into the rectangular Cartesian "cardiac" coordinate system. The two surfaces were joined by a linear interpolation in the radial direction. The resulting model was then defined in rectangular Cartesian space with three element coordinates, (ξ_1, ξ_2, ξ_3) aligned in the circumferential, longitudinal and transmural directions respectively (see Figure 3.1).

Real-time updates of the model-image intersection contours facilitated this interactive process. This method has since been developed to give fast, accurate volume and mass measurements in untagged ciné images [26].

3.3.2 Model Tag 3D Fitting

The location and orientation of the tag planes at the time of their creation were determined from the tagging pulse sequence parameters. The tag planes were intersected with the 3D LV model using a subdivision algorithm similar to marching

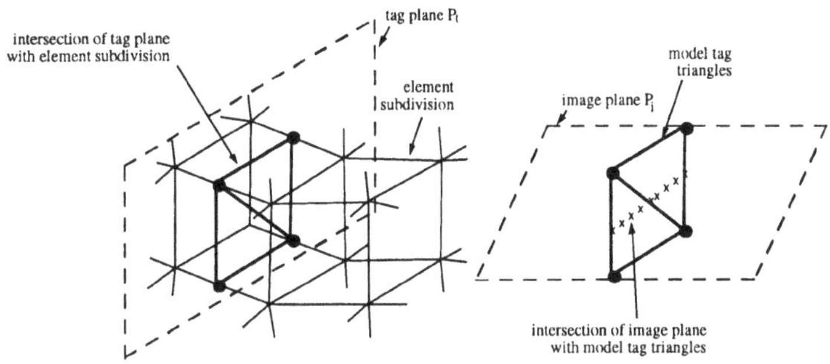

Figure 3.2: Calculation of model tags and model stripe points. Each model is subdivided into small linear elements, shown as the thin lines in the left figure. The tag plane, shown as the dashed lines, is intersected with the element subdivision using a marching cubes algorithm. This results in a set of triangles (dark lines). On the right, the triangles are intersected with the image plane (dashed lines) to give a set of model stripe points ($\times$).

cubes [10], resulting in a set of linked triangles describing the location of the tag plane within the model. These "model tags" define material surfaces within the model which deform as the model parameters change. At each stage in the minimization process, a set of "model stripe" points could be found by intersecting the model tags with the image planes. The intersecting line segments were sampled to give a 1–2 mm spacing between model stripe points. This process is outlined in Figure 3.2.

The ED geometry was deformed from frame to frame to minimize the following:

$$E(\boldsymbol{x}) = S(\boldsymbol{x}) + \sum_t w_t \left[\boldsymbol{n}_{T(t)} \cdot (\boldsymbol{x}(\boldsymbol{\xi}_t) - \boldsymbol{x}_t)\right]^2, \tag{3.15}$$

where $\boldsymbol{x}_t$ is the tth image stripe point, $\boldsymbol{n}_{T(t)}$ is the normal to the associated tag plane $T(t)$, and $\boldsymbol{x}(\boldsymbol{\xi}_t)$ is the corresponding model stripe point.

3.3.3 Image Analysis

Image stripe points $\boldsymbol{x}_t$ were found for each model stripe point $\boldsymbol{x}(\boldsymbol{\xi}_t)$ by searching the image in a small neighborhood about $\boldsymbol{x}(\boldsymbol{\xi}_t)$ for the most likely point on the image towards which the model stripe point should displace. For each pixel, a likelihood function in the form of a centerline detector was used to measure the probability of the pixel belonging to the center of an image stripe. Since image stripe orientations do not change substantially during the cardiac cycle (typically $< 20°$), the search direction and stripe normal $\boldsymbol{n}_T$ were kept constant throughout the tracking process (orthogonal to the original tag plane). This enabled the result of the search to be precalculated before the model fitting process. Displacement look-up images were generated which stored the displacement to the nearest image stripe point associated with each point on the image plane. Similarly, weighting images provided the associated weight, a measure of the strength or ambiguity of the image stripe point (see Figure 3.3).

3.3.4 Minimization

To minimize Equation (3.15) a Levenburg-Marquardt algorithm [11] was used. The smoothing term integrals were evaluated using Gaussian quadrature. Equation (3.15) can then be written as

$$E = \|\boldsymbol{Sq}\|_2{}^2 + \|\boldsymbol{Jq} - \boldsymbol{p}\|_2{}^2, \tag{3.16}$$

where $\boldsymbol{S}$ is a matrix containing derivatives of the deformation gradient tensor at the Gauss points (in the case of global deformation smoothing), $\boldsymbol{J}$ is a matrix containing model basis functions evaluated at $\boldsymbol{\xi}_t$ and weighted by the tag normals, $\boldsymbol{p}$ is a vector containing components of $\boldsymbol{x}_t$ weighted by the tag normals, and $\boldsymbol{q}$ is a vector of model parameters. Note that $\boldsymbol{J}$ varies with $\boldsymbol{q}$, but $\boldsymbol{S}$ does not.

The Newton method minimizes E by assuming the function is quadratic and neglecting the terms higher than second order in the Taylor series expansion, giving the following iteration which can be solved for $\boldsymbol{q}_{k+1}$:

$$\boldsymbol{H}_k \left(\boldsymbol{q}_{k+1} - \boldsymbol{q}_k\right) = - \left.\frac{\partial E}{\partial \boldsymbol{q}}\right|_k, \tag{3.17}$$

where $\boldsymbol{H}$ is the Hessian matrix of second derivatives of E. The right-hand side of Equation (3.17) has a component due to the change in $\boldsymbol{\xi}_t$ caused by $\boldsymbol{q}$. However, Equation (3.15) measures the squared distance from each data point to the model position $\boldsymbol{\xi}_t$ in a direction approximately perpendicular to the model surface. Since $\boldsymbol{\xi}_t$ can only change within the model tag, the contribution to the first derivative of the error function due to changes in model position will be small. We can therefore use the linear approximation

$$\frac{\partial E}{\partial \boldsymbol{q}} = \boldsymbol{S}^T\boldsymbol{Sq} + \boldsymbol{J}^T\boldsymbol{Jq} - \boldsymbol{J}^T\boldsymbol{p}. \tag{3.18}$$

Replacing the Hessian $\boldsymbol{H}$ with the linear approximation $\boldsymbol{S}^T\boldsymbol{S} + \boldsymbol{J}^T\boldsymbol{J}$, and adding a term $\Lambda\boldsymbol{I}$ ($\Lambda \geqslant 0$) to avoid non-positive definite $\boldsymbol{H}$, gives the iteration

$$\left(\boldsymbol{S}^T\boldsymbol{S} + \boldsymbol{J}_k^T\boldsymbol{J}_k + \Lambda\boldsymbol{I}\right)\boldsymbol{q}_{k+1} = \Lambda\boldsymbol{I} + \boldsymbol{J}_k^T\boldsymbol{p}. \tag{3.19}$$

If the value of Λ is large then the problem becomes one of steepest descent; if Λ is zero then we use a complete Gauss-Newton step.

Figure 3.4 shows the model tags at ED and ES.

Smoothing Term

Equation (3.15) contains a smoothing term $S(\boldsymbol{x})$ to regularize the problem. One problem with spline type smoothing is that large rigid body rotations are also penalized (rotations of approximately 20 degrees normally occur at the LV apex).

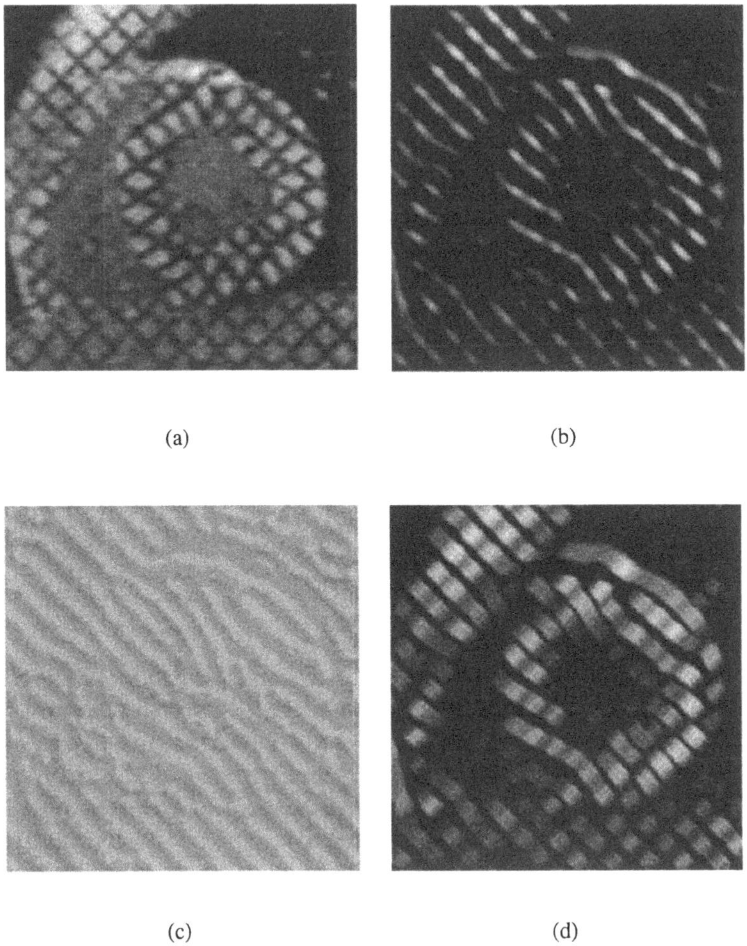

Figure 3.3: Precalculation of image displacement constraints as images. **(a)** the raw image. **(b)** image after the stripe detection filter in one orientation. **(c)** displacement image (lighter levels indicates displacement towards the top right.) **(d)** weight image (lighter levels indicate higher weighting.)

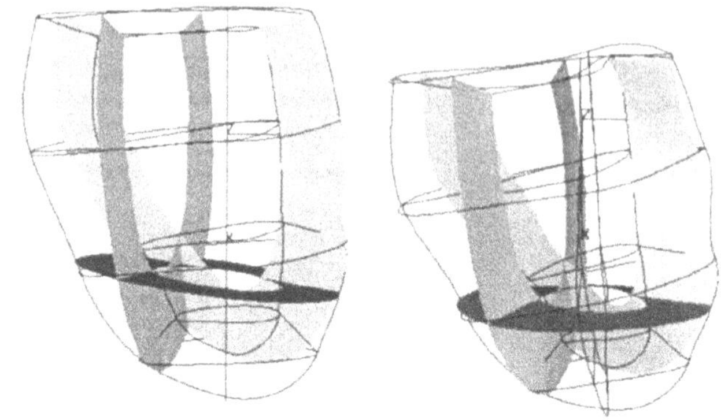

(a) (b)

Figure 3.4: Model tags at the time of creation **(a)** and at ES **(b)**. The lighter tags are from the short-axis images and the darker is from a long-axis image.

To solve this problem the following "global deformation" smoothing was proposed [21,22]

$$S(\boldsymbol{x}) = W \int_{\xi} \sum_{k,i,j} \left(\frac{\partial F_{ij}}{\partial \xi_k} \right)^2 d\xi \,, \tag{3.20}$$

where $\boldsymbol{F}$ is the deformation gradient tensor in fitting coordinates. This term penalizes the variation of the deformation with respect to the element (material) coordinates. The advantage of this measure is that it is minimized by any global affine transformation, including rigid rotations. Such deformations can be exactly recovered from the displacements of four or more linearly independent points. This results in a linear least squares problem giving deformation fields which are as near to homogeneous as the data will allow. Any variation in strain should therefore be entirely due to the data and not to the smoothing constraint.

3.4 Reconstruction of RV Surface Deformation

A variant of the model tags approach was used to reconstruct the motion of the right ventricular free wall [28]. Since the RV free wall is relatively thin, wall thickening and transmural shear deformations are not reliably measured using MR tagging. Rather, the mid-wall surface of the RV free wall was modeled as a 2D surface in 3D space. Firstly, RV mid-wall contours were drawn on each image. Secondly, the intersections between the tagging planes and the mid-wall contours (image stripe points) were tracked between frames. Fiducial markers were also determined as above and the cardiac coordinate system constructed with respect to the LV central axis.

3.4.1 RV Free wall geometry

The model contained three elements circumferentially and three elements longitudinally, giving sixteen nodes. Bicubic Hermite basis functions were used with nodal values shared between adjacent elements (C^1 continuity). The angular values for the boundary nodes were set using the extrema of the contours. The remaining nodes were equally spaced in the μ and θ directions. The contour data were projected along lines of constant μ and θ and a linear least squares fit was performed in the λ field as in Equation (3.13). The fitted nodal values were then transformed into rectangular Cartesian coordinates and the surface was then refitted by minimizing:

$$E_{\text{contour}} = \omega \sum_{c} \{\boldsymbol{n}_c \cdot [\boldsymbol{x}(\boldsymbol{\xi}_c) - \boldsymbol{x}_c]\}^2 , \tag{3.21}$$

where $\boldsymbol{x}_c$ is a contour (Cartesian) coordinate and $\boldsymbol{x}(\boldsymbol{\xi}_c)$ is the corresponding model point given by the projection of $\boldsymbol{x}_c$ onto the model in the direction of the contour normal $\boldsymbol{n}_c$. The minimization of this objective is nonlinear since the points were projected along lines of least distance to the Cartesian model, allowing the model projections to change with the nodal parameters.

3.4.2 Model Tags: Surface Formulation

The ED geometry was deformed to match the displacements of the tracked stripe data in each subsequent frame. The match between the model and the tracked stripe points is given by

$$E_{\text{tag}} = \sum_{t} \{\boldsymbol{n}_{T(t)} \cdot [\boldsymbol{x}(\boldsymbol{\xi}_t) - \boldsymbol{x}_t]\}^2 , \tag{3.22}$$

where $\boldsymbol{x}_t$ is the tth image stripe point, $\boldsymbol{n}_{T(t)}$ is the normal to the associated tagging plane $T(t)$, and $\boldsymbol{x}(\boldsymbol{\xi}_t)$ is the corresponding model stripe point. To establish correspondence between the model and the tags, a set of "model tags" L_T were constructed to define the material intersection between the tags and the model surface. The model tags were thus material line segments which deform with the surface and at all times should intersect the image planes at the tracked stripe points. Due to through plane motion, the model material point corresponding to the image tags (i.e., the model coordinates $\boldsymbol{\xi}_t$ above) may change during the minimization process, but must always lie on the associated model tag.

The model tag lines were found by intersecting the initial geometry with each tag plane P_T (see Figure 3.5) using a subdivision algorithm similar to that in Section 3.3.2. This results in a connected set of line segments describing the model tag location in model ($\boldsymbol{\xi}$) coordinates. At each iteration of the minimization process, the model tags were intersected with the image plane to give model stripe points. The distance between the model stripe points and the image stripe points in the direction of the tag normal was minimized in Equation (3.22).

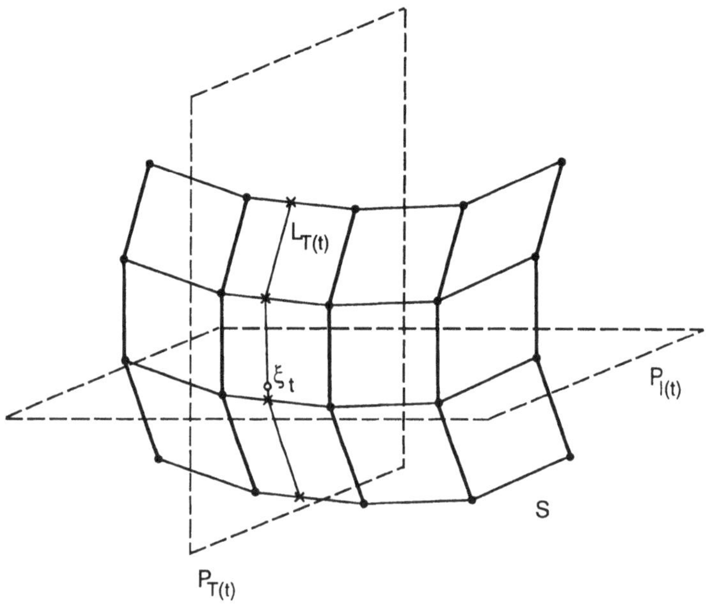

Figure 3.5: Calculation of element coordinates for tag data points. S, Surface Mesh subdivision; •, vertices of surface mesh subdivision; $P_{T(t)}$, tagging plane associated with image stripe point x_t; $P_{I(t)}$, image plane associated with image stripe point x_t; $L_{T(t)}$, line segments defining the intersection between S and $P_{T(t)}$; ×, vertices of line segments on the model tag; ○, intersection of $L_{T(t)}$ with the image plane $P_{I(t)}$. This locates the model stripe point ξ_t.

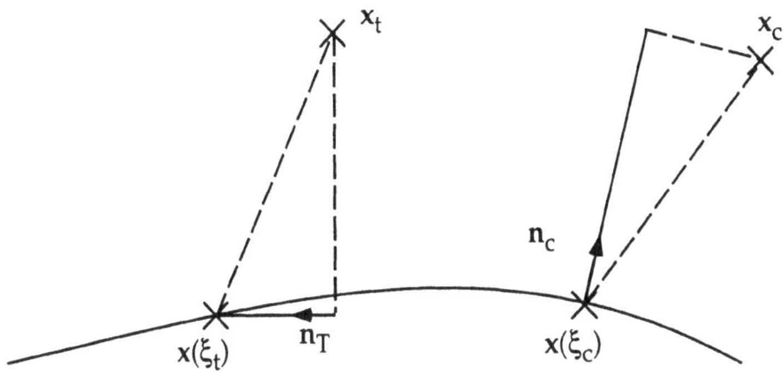

Figure 3.6: Tag and contour data constraints. Tag data imposes displacement constraints orthogonal to the tag stripes and approximately tangential to the surface. Contour data impose displacement constraints approximately orthogonal to surface. The solid lines represent the errors which are minimized in the fit.

Since Equation (3.22) constrains the deformation of the surface in the tag normal directions only, additional constraints were necessary to unambiguously determine surface motion. The constraint that the surface intersect the image plane at the RV mid-wall contour locations was imposed using Equation (3.21).

Note that since the image stripe points were only tracked if the tag was approximately normal to the mid-wall surface, the stripe and contour constraints (Equations (3.22) and (3.21) respectively) acted in approximately orthogonal directions (Figure 3.6).

The final objective function was made up of terms from the stripe, contour and smoothing constraints,

$$E_{\text{total}} = E_{\text{tag}} + E_{\text{contour}} + E_{\text{smooth}}, \tag{3.23}$$

and was minimized using the Levenburg-Marquardt algorithm outlined in Section 3.3.4.

3.5 Principal Component Analysis

We hope to characterize the healthy functioning heart using a set of orthogonal modes of deformation derived from principal component analysis (PCA). The PCA method describes the modes and their associated variance and can also remove the noise of insignificant modes. A new heart model it could be compared with the database distributions to see if statistical evidence of abnormal function exists.

One benefit of PCA is that it describes the heart with a small number of parameters (modes). Although the fitted FE models have hundreds of parameters, by using PCA on a training set we hope to distinguish the modes which truly differentiate the hearts, and remove the modes that are insignificant.

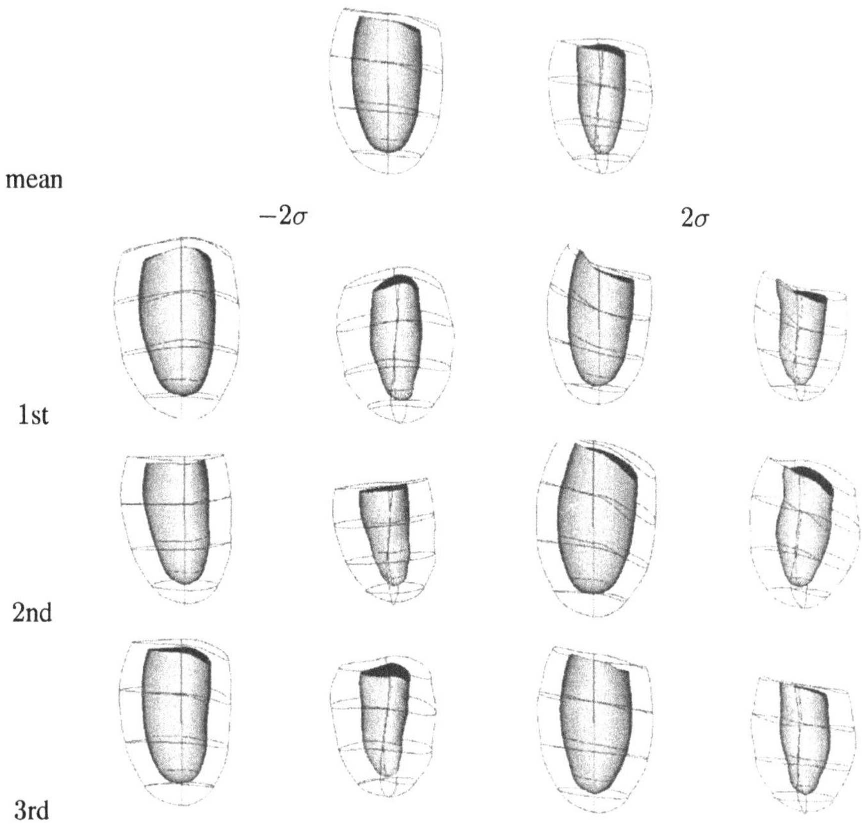

Figure 3.7: The geometry modes of the coupled ED and ES shapes. The top row shows the mean ED and ES shapes, and the three most significant modes are shown below at $+2\sigma$ and -2σ.

PCA has been used in many different fields. It has been used in the construction of point distribution models [1]. These models are used in the automatic segmentation of images. The principal component analysis is used to restrict the image guided model to modes which PCA has found in a training set of data.

PCA has also been used in the extrapolation of small data sets [3]. Using a set of densely sampled femurs, PCA was used to create a model of the bone with a small set of parameters, and remove the noise. The PCA provides a statistical model of the bone, which is used to fit a smaller sampling performed during surgery only on the exposed pieces of bone. This allows a full picture of the bone to be viewed in an interactive display, allowing correct placement of the graft in ligament reconstruction.

3.5.1 Generating the Data Set

Tagged MR images of fifteen normals were acquired. These were fitted with a four by four element mesh using the methods described in Section 3.3. The models are registered with respect to the cardiac coordinate system used in the fit, and can be completely described by the vector of parameters

$$\boldsymbol{U} = (U_{1s}, U_{2s}, \dots, U_{ms}, U_{1d}, U_{2d}, \dots, U_{md}) , \tag{3.24}$$

where U_i is the ith parameter of the model and s and d represent the ES and ED model respectively of a given case. Models were placed in a data matrix $\boldsymbol{X}$ describing the population. Each row $\boldsymbol{X}_i$ of the data matrix contains a separate case at ES and ED (i.e., $\boldsymbol{X}_i = \boldsymbol{U}$.)

The mean model was then calculated using

$$\overline{\boldsymbol{X}} = \frac{1}{n} \sum_{i=1}^{n} \boldsymbol{X}_i , \tag{3.25}$$

where n is the number of subjects in the database. The difference between each subject and the mean is then calculated as follows

$$\boldsymbol{\delta}_i = \boldsymbol{X}_i - \overline{\boldsymbol{X}} , \tag{3.26}$$

and the covariance matrix of the model parameters is given by

$$C_{ij} = \frac{1}{n} \boldsymbol{\delta}_i \cdot \boldsymbol{\delta}_j . \tag{3.27}$$

The modes of the variance are found using eigenvalue decomposition.

$$\boldsymbol{C} = \boldsymbol{P} \boldsymbol{\Lambda} \boldsymbol{P}^T , \tag{3.28}$$

where $\boldsymbol{P}$ is an orthogonal matrix which contains the modes of the variation and $\boldsymbol{\Lambda}$ is a diagonal matrix of eigenvalues (all ≥ 0). Each row of $\boldsymbol{P}$ contains the mode associated with the corresponding diagonal element of $\boldsymbol{\Lambda}$. Assuming the modes are normally distributed about zero, the variance of each mode is σ_i^2, the ith diagonal element of $\boldsymbol{\Lambda}$.

3.6 PCA of Normal Geometry and Deformation

The resulting modes show the statistical variation which would be expected in the motion of a normal heart. The modes are also orthogonal to each other and are independent in their distribution.

Figure 3.7 shows the relationship between the ED and the ES shape for the three most significant modes (largest eigenvalues of $\boldsymbol{C}$). The first two modes are clearly related to the position of the base plane. These modes are dominated ED shape

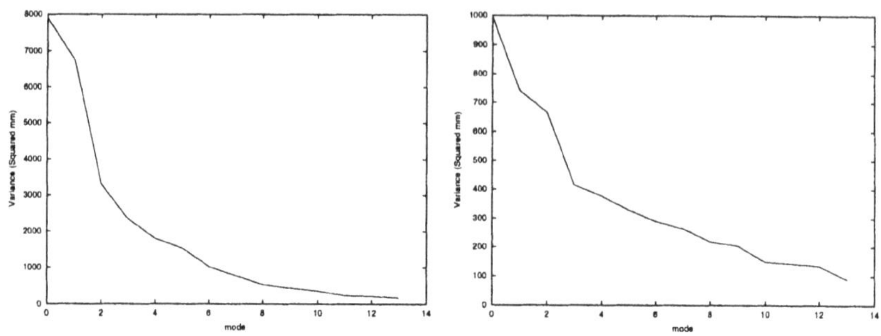

(a) (b)

Figure 3.8: The variance associated with each mode. (a) Shows the modes of the combined ED and ES model parameters, whereas (b) is the modes of the difference between ED and ES.

-2σ $+2\sigma$

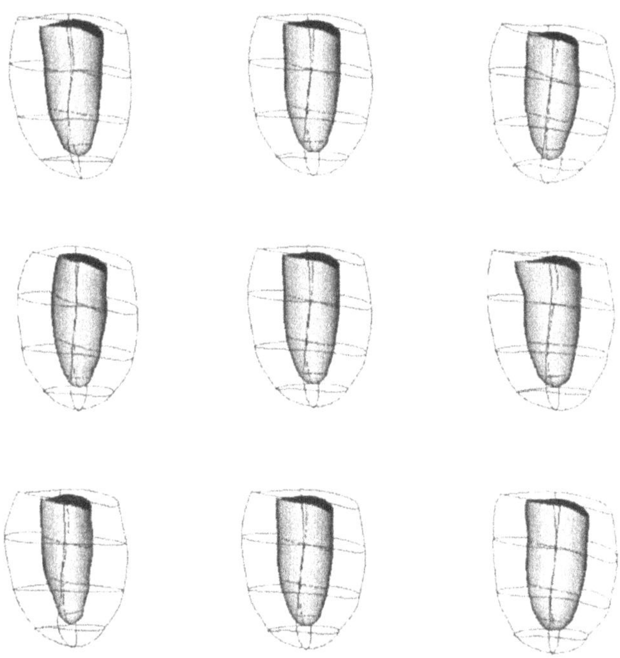

Figure 3.9: Shows the variance of the ES shape after performing a PCA on the displacement variables. The shapes have a common diastolic shape which is the mean diastolic shape illustrated in Figure 3.7. The middle column is the mean displacement (added to the mean ED shape).

rather than variation in deformation, the variances of the modes is shown in Figure 3.8.

To analyze the deformation rather than the geometry, the ES parameters were subtracted from the ED parameters to give a set of displacement parameters. This provides modes which illustrate how the systolic shape differs from the diastolic.

Figure 3.9 shows the first three displacement modes acquired from the data. This is done by varying the first three modes's weights between -2.0σ and 2.0σ. This range should accommodate most normal functioning of the heart. Because the modes represent the change from end-diastole to end-systole, the mean diastolic shape was added to each displacement mode to help in the visualization.

Since each of these modes has a known variance, it should be possible to see if a given subject lies within the normal range for this mode. The amount of each mode present in a particular fitted model, $\boldsymbol{u}$, is

$$b = \boldsymbol{P}^T \boldsymbol{U} . \tag{3.29}$$

A z-score can be written

$$z_i = \frac{b_i}{\sigma_i} , \tag{3.30}$$

which can then be used in a statistical test to determine the probability of the case arising from the population distribution. Equation (3.29) is the least squares representation of the model data, (i.e., $\boldsymbol{U}$ in the parameter space defined by $\boldsymbol{P}$.)

Figure 3.9 shows the extremes of the three largest modes. The first mode appears to vary the twist at the apex, the second the position of the base (i.e., longitudinal shortening) and the third mode appears to signify the size of the cavity (and therefore the ejection fraction and circumferential shortening).

3.7 Future Work

In addition to the deformation between ED and ES, temporal abnormalities in regional wall motion are important diagnostic indicators of disease. In particular, diastolic filling abnormalities often precede systolic dysfunction in many cardiac diseases. To quantify temporal behavior, two approaches have been taken. In the first, the smoothing constraint was extended to penalize temporal variation in the displacement field (velocity and acceleration) [24]. This adds viscosity and damping to the model formulation. The inclusion of temporal coherence in the model allows the influence of spatial smoothing to be reduced and enables a more accurate temporal description of LV motion. In the second approach, time basis functions are added to the model [25]. Fourier basis functions (sinusoidal functions) have the advantages that they are implicitly periodic and orthogonal. The number of terms can be increased until the desired accuracy is achieved. Many terms are however required to capture rapid filling in early diastole, and perhaps a time-varying temporal smoothing term should also be applied. Future work includes the testing of these approaches in the model tags formulation. As more data come to hand, the smoothing term can be replaced by a PCA of a group of suitable studies, allowing a statistical prior to be used in a Bayesian formulation of the model estimation problem.

Finite element models of stress and activation [7] may be directly applied to the model fitting or analysis problems. In the case of model fitting, a physical FE model of heart function may allow the definition of a few physiological parameters (material stiffness, regional blood volume, cross-bridge dynamics) which could be directly fitted to an image dataset. This approach would result in a more complete analysis of cardiac function based on biophysical parameter estimation rather than shape parameter estimation. We hope that this will provide more useful diagnostic information on disease and treatment processes than is currently available.

References

[1] Cootes, T. F., Hill, A., Taylor, C. J., and Haslam, J. (1994). The use of active shape models for locating structures in medical images. Image and Vision Computing, 12(6):355–66.

[2] Denney, Jr, T. S. and McVeigh, E. R. (1997). Model-free reconstruction of three-dimensional myocardial strain from planar tagged mr images. Journal of Magnetic Resonance Imaging, 7:799–810.

[3] Fleute, M. and Lavallée, S. (1998). Building a complete surface model from sparse data using statistical shape models: Applications to computer assisted knee surgery. Medical Image Computing and Computer-Assisted Intervention. First Internation Conference. , pages 879–87.

[4] Fung, Y. C. (1965). Foundations of Solid Mechanics. Prentice-Hall, New Jersey.

[5] Gentles, T., Cowan, B. R., Occleshaw, C., and Young, A. A. (1999). Normal left ventricular systolic function following repair of coarctation of the aorta. American Heart Association, Atlanta.

[6] Hashima, A. R., Young, A. A., McCulloch, A. D., and Waldman, L. K. (1993). Nonhomogeneous analysis of epicardial strain distributions during acute myocardial ischemia in the dog. Journal of Biomechanics, 26:19–35.

[7] Hunter, P. J. and Smaill, B. H. (1988). The analysis of cardiac function: A continuum approach. Progress in Biophysics and Molecular Biology, 52:101–64.

[8] Le Grice, I. J., Hunter, P. J., and Smaill, B. H. (1997). Laminar structure of the heart: a mathematical model. American Journal of Physiology, 272:H2466–76.

[9] Le Grice, I. J., Smaill, B. H., Chai, L. Z., Edgar, S. G., Gavin, J. B., and Hunter, P. J. (1995). Laminar structure of the heart: ventricular myocyte arrangement and connective tissue architecture in the dog. American Journal of Physiology, 269:H571–82.

[10] Lorensen, W. E. and Cline, H. E. (1987). Marching cubes: a high resolution 3d surface construction algorithm. Computer Graphics, 21:163–169.

[11] Marquardt, D. W. (1963). An algorithm for least squares estimation of non-linear parameters. J Soc Indust Appl Math, 11:431–41.

[12] Nielsen, P. M. F., Le Grice, I. J., Smaill, B. H., and Hunter, P. J. (1991). Mathematical model of the geometry and fibrous structure of the heart. American Journal of Physiology, 260:H1365–H1378.

[13] O'Dell, W. G., Moore, C. C., Hunter, W. C., Zerhouni, E. A., and McVeigh, E. R. (1995). Three-dimensional myocardial deformations: Calculation with displacement field fitting to tagged mr images. Radiology, 195(3):829–35.

[14] O'Donnell, T., Boult, T., and Gupta, A. (1996). Global models with parametric offsets as applied to cardiac motion recovery. Computer Vision and Pattern Recognition, pages 293–99, New York. IEEE Press.

[15] O'Donnell, T., Gupta, A., and Boult, T. (1995). The hybrid volumetric ventriculoid: New model for MR-SPAMM 3-D analysis. Computers in Cardiology, pages 5–8, New York. CRC Press.

[16] Park, J., Metaxas, D., and Axel, L. (1996a). Analysis of left ventricular wall motion based on volumetric deformable models and MRI-SPAMM. Medical Image Analysis, 1(1):53–71.

[17] Park, J., Metaxas, D., Young, A. A., and Axel, L. (1996b). Deformable models with parameter functions for cardiac motion analysis from tagged mri data. IEEE Trans. Medical Imaging, 15(3):278–89.

[18] Terzopoulos, D. (1988). The computation of visible-surface representations. IEEE Trans. Pattern Analysis and Machine Intelligence, 10:417–438.

[19] Young, A. A. (1989). Epicardial deformation from coronary cinéangiograms. Glass, L., Hunter, P. J., and McCulloch, A. D., editors, Theory of Heart, pages 175–208. Springer-Verlag.

[20] Young, A. A. (1999). Model tags: direct three-dimensional tracking of heart wall motion from tagged magnetic resonance images. Medical Image Analysis, 3(4):361–72.

[21] Young, A. A. and Axel, L. (1992a). Non-rigid heart wall motion using MR tagging. Proc Computer Vision and Pattern Recognition, pages 388–404.

[22] Young, A. A. and Axel, L. (1992b). Three-dimensional motion and deformation of the heart wall: Estimation with spatial modulation of magnetization–a model-based approach. Radiology, 185(1):241–7.

[23] Young, A. A., Biederman, R. W. W., Doyle, M., Thrupp, S., and Dell'Italia, L. J. (1998). Three dimensional left ventricular deformation in hypertensive LV hypertrophy. Proc. International Society of Magnetic Resonance in Medicine, 1, page 475.

[24] Young, A. A. and Cowan, B. R. (1997). Frame-based (3D) interactive modeling of heart motion. Proceedings IEEE Nonrigid and Articulated Motion Workshop,pages 128–35.

[25] Young, A. A. and Cowan, B. R. (1998). Four dimensional modeling of LV motion. Proceedings International Society of Magnetic Resonance in Medicine, volume 1, page 557.

[26] Young, A. A., Cowan, B. R., Thrupp, S. F., Hedley, W. J., and Dell'Italia, L. J. (2000). Left ventricular mass and volume: fast calculation with guide-point modeling on MR images. Radiology, 216(2):597–602.

[27] Young, A. A., Dokos, S., Powell, K. A., Strum, B., McCulloch, A. D., McCarthy, P. M., and White, R. D. (1999). Regional heterogeneity and recovery of septal function after successful (LV) volume reduction in nonischemic dilated cardiomyopathy. American Heart Association, Atlanta.

[28] Young, A. A., Fayad, Z. A., and Axel, L. (1996). Right ventricular midwall surface motion and deformation using magnetic resonance tagging. American Journal of Physiology, 271(6):H2677–88.

[29] Young, A. A., Hunter, P. J., and Smaill, B. H. (1989). Epicardial surface estimation from coronary cinéangiograms. Computer Vision and Graphics, 47:111–27.

[30] Young, A. A., Kraitchman, D. L., Dougherty, L., and Axel, L. (1995). Tracking and finite element analysis of stripe deformation in magnetic resonance tagging. IEEE Transactions on Medical Imaging, 14(3):413–21.

[31] Young, A. A., Kramer, C. M., Ferrari, V. A., Axel, L., and Reicheck, N. (1994). Three-dimensional left ventricular deformation in hypertrophic cardiomyopathy. Circulation, 90(2):854–67.

[32] Zienkiewicz, O. C. and Morgan, K. (1982). Finite elements and approximation. Wiley, New York.

Chapter 4

Modeling and analysis of the RV and LV from MRI-SPAMM

Idith Haber
Cardiovascular Research Division,
Children's Hospital and Harvard Medical School,
Boston, MA
Idith.Haber@tch.harvard.edu

Dimitris Metaxas
Department of Computer and Information Science,
University of Pennsylvania, Philadelphia, PA
dnm@graphics.cis.upenn.edu

Leon Axel
Department of Radiology,
University of Pennsylvania, Philadelphia, PA
axel@oasis.rad.upenn.edu

4.1 Introduction

In the past two decades, researchers have determined that the right ventricle (RV) plays an important role in normal and abnormal hemodynamics [2]. In addition, diseases that affect the right ventricle can adversely affect the left ventricle (LV), and may lead to heart failure. As in the LV, several types of RV disease, such as ischemia and hypertrophy, alter the normal motion and deformation of the RV free wall and septum. Furthermore, since the RV pumps blood into the pulmonary circulation, abnormalities of the lung can adversely affect the motion of the RV. As several diseases may adversely affect the motion of the RV, a method that quantifies abnormal RV kinematics may be useful in detecting the presence and severity of such diseases. In this chapter, we describe methods for modeling the RV geometry, extracting RV motion from MRI images using a computer vision/image analysis technique called deformable modeling, and analyzing these results using

A.A. Amini and J.L. Prince (eds.),
Measurement of Cardiac Deformations from MRI: Physical and Mathematical Models, 59–90.

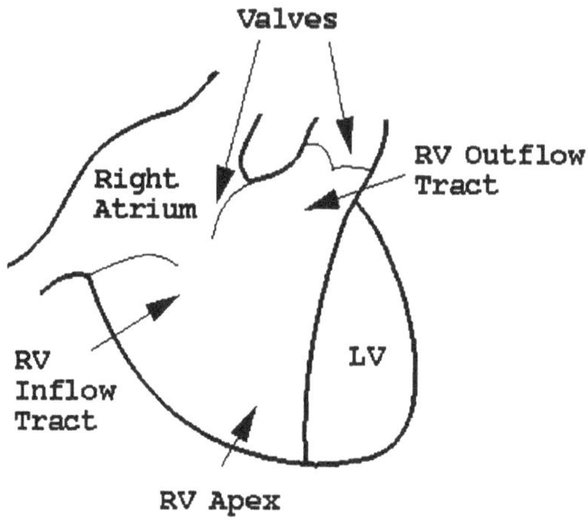

Figure 4.1: Schematic of partial heart anatomy. The RV can be separated into an inflow tract, outflow tract, and apex.

techniques from mechanics.

The RV receives deoxygenated blood from the right atrium and pumps it into the pulmonary artery, and then out to the lungs (Fig. 4.1). It appears crescent-like in a cross-sectional view and, unlike the LV, is difficult to approximate with any simple parameterized 3D shape. The RV shares a common wall with the LV (the septum), while its free (outer) wall is in mechanical contact with the pericardium and, through it, the lungs. The RV cavity can be conceptually separated into an inflow tract, a highly trabeculated apical portion, and a relatively smooth outflow tract [7]. The normally 3-5mm-thick RV free wall is thin relative to the 9-11mm-thick LV free wall [7].

Early studies of RV kinematics, which involved implanting radiopaque markers and following their motion, provided limited information about RV contraction [3]. In contrast, MRI tissue tagging techniques, such as SPAMM [1] (Chapter 2) provide a non-invasive means for studying RV wall motion in humans. Although MRI tagging has been shown to be a useful tool, the tomographic tagged MRI images cannot capture deformation and motion normal to the plane in which the image is acquired. Techniques for reconstructing the 3D motion from multiple image plane orientations (views) have primarily been developed for and applied to the LV (see Chapters 3,4,8). Some of these techniques have been extended to the RV (Chapter 3). The RV poses several challenging problems for 3D motion reconstruction: 1) with the current MR image resolution, tags are spaced approximately 6mm apart so that a limited number of tags fall on the RV wall; 2) the RV geometry cannot be described using any simple primitive; 3) RV wall motion varies temporally and regionally, thereby making it difficult to describe concisely; and 4) the RV exhibits significant motion through both short and long-axis image planes.

We describe an application of a deformable modeling technique to the task of capturing the full 3D motion of the RV wall. Previous work at the University of Pennsylvania involved fitting a generalized primitive deformable model of the LV to MRI tag intersections [15]. The current method retains the basic deformable modeling technique where *Lagrange's* equations of motion are used to deform the model under forces calculated from image data. However, the force calculation, geometric description of the deformable model, and model degrees of freedom differ in order to properly apply the technique to the RV.

The deformable modeling approach requires an accurate geometric model. Previous approaches to modeling the RV have been surface models of the free wall [23], a combination of quadratic surfaces [5], and biquadratic spline surface patches [18]. Volumetric RV models have usually included the LV, but excluded the outflow tract [12,16] [16] taken from ex-vivo wall contours. Another approach had been to fit a general RV-LV finite element mesh to digitized data from excised hearts [12]. We developed a new method for modeling the complex RV geometry. Instead of fitting a deformable geometric primitive to the initial contour data, a geometric model of the biventricular geometry is built *directly* from contours extracted from the initial time phases of the images. This approach allows us to account for the significant geometric variations which can occur in some RV diseases. Since the RV and LV are intricately connected, both are included in the model. A biventricular model opens the way for the quantitative study of inter-ventricular dependence and relative motion. However, the focus of this chapter is the analysis of RV free wall and septal systolic contraction.

Each reconstructed 3D model provides a dense and detailed set of motion data. The final phase of the methodology is to translate this data into both global and local motion variables. Principal strains and directions are used as indicators of contraction, since they are independent of any coordinate system. The motion quantities can be visualized in 3D using computer graphics techniques. In order to demonstrate the utility of the method, and to learn more about RV motion, we applied the reconstruction technique to both normal volunteers and patients with right ventricular hypertrophy (RVH). The results are consistent with previously documented knowledge of RV motion and provide a relatively detailed motion analysis of the normal RV motion. We also capture new information about changes in 3D deformation which occur during RVH.

4.2 Biventricular Model Geometry

The complex shape of the RV does not lend itself well to geometric modeling. An accurate geometric model is necessary, however, for reconstructing the 3D motion and for shape analysis. Since the septum plays an important role in the function of both ventricles, our approach is to create a biventricular geometric model. Rather than fitting a predefined model to contour data, we generate a volumetric finite element mesh directly from contours extracted from end-diastolic images.

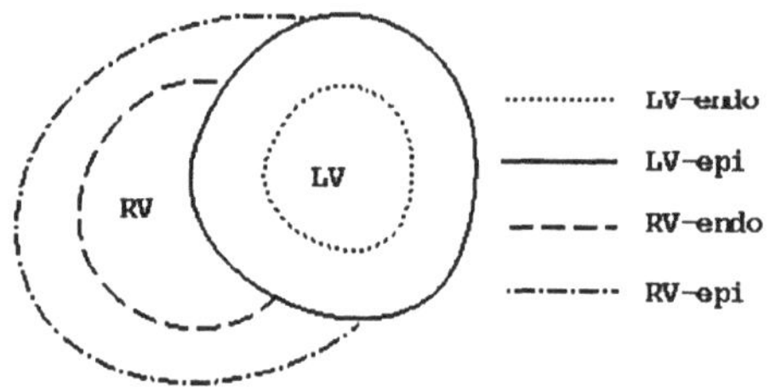

Figure 4.2: Heart walls are segmented into 4 contours labeled LV-epi, LV-endo, RV-epi, and RV-endo.

The result is a piecewise definition of the ventricular geometry with finite elements, where the number and type of element is altered according to the local geometry. The use of existing finite element mesh generation packages would not have provided this control and may have required additional pre- and post-processing. With our approach, the geometry-building phase and fitting phase are integrated into one program. The finite element mesh geometry is defined in two stages:

1) Partition the contours into the set of model points (nodes) in order to set up the topology, and

2) Generate the finite elements that connect these nodes.

4.2.1 RV Contour Segmentation

In order to build the geometric model, heart wall borders, or contours, must be segmented from the tagged images at end-diastole. The endocardial and epicardial borders of the RV and LV were segmented semi-automatically using active contours [1, 8], or snakes. As shown in Fig. 4.2 two closed, circular contours were first used to define the LV walls. Next, two open contours were used for the RV: the ends of open contours can either be free or constrained to slide along the LV epicardial contours (Fig. 4.3(a)) . This allowed us to follow the insertion of points of the RV and LV through successive images. Fig. 4.2 shows that the ends of the open RV-endo and RV-epi contours are contiguous with the LV-epi contour at the insertion of the RV into the LV.

4.2.2 Processing Contour Data

In order to make the problem of tessellating a 3D volume more tractable, the algorithm calls for tessellation of cross-sections having the same topology for generating volumetric elements to connect those sections. Since the cross-sectional

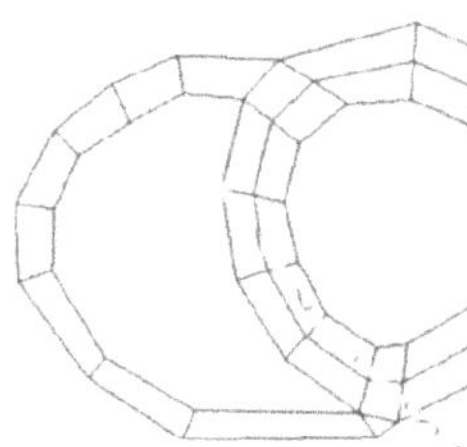

(a)

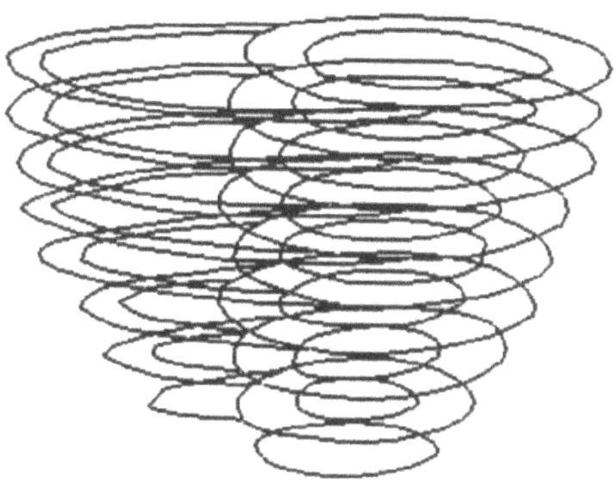

(b)

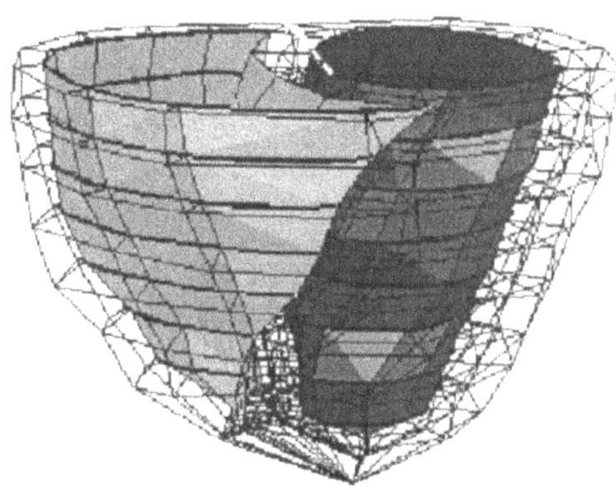

(c)

Figure 4.3: Finite element mesh geometry. **(a)** Cross-sectional layout of elements. **(b)** Short-axis contours from stacked set of MR images. **(c)** Final mesh with shaded endocardial walls. The RV is on the left in all figures.

topology in the main portion of the biventricular unit remains more or less constant in the short-axis (rather than long-axis) views, short-axis contours are used for the mesh generation. The stacked set of short axis contours is shown in Fig. 4.3b. The contours must be sampled in such a way that elements of the RV and LV elements are continuous at the insertion points. The RV and LV endocardial contours are equally sampled. The connection with the appropriate outer wall is found by intersecting the local normal with the epicardial contours. As shown in Fig. 4.3a, the elements are arranged in two concentric layers in the LV free wall and septum, and are one layer thick in the RV.

4.2.3 Finite element mesh generation

The geometry of a finite element is defined by the location of its vertices, or nodes, and its shape functions, which determine the position (and the value of other parameters) of points within the element. The shape functions and elements used in the mesh are shown in the Appendix. Given the complexity of the RV shape, a large number of smaller elements with linear shape functions are used, rather than larger elements with higher-order shape functions. The nodes of the finite elements are points from the sampled contours described in the previous section. Eight-noded elements connect nodes across the wall and between tessellated levels while six-noded wedge-shaped elements are used to prevent the elements from getting too skewed and to taper the mesh to a point at the apex. In order to be able to visualize the endocardial or epicardial surface of either ventricle, the faces of the finite elements that lie on these surfaces are labeled during this mesh-building step and later triangulated for shaded surface display and curvature calculation. The finite elements will later play a role in both the fitting method and the calculation of strains. The total number of elements varies with heart size and number of intervals used in partitioning the contours. The number of intervals can be adjusted to provide a desired number of elements and number of model degrees of freedom. The final finite element mesh shown in Fig. 4.3c has 222 elements and 336 nodes.

4.3 3D RV and LV motion reconstruction

We use a deformable model to reconstruct the 3D motion of the RV from multiple tag plane orientation data. The deformable modeling technique is a commonly-used approach in which a model deforms to fit the data using energy minimization or a classical physics-based equation of motion [10]. The specifics of how to deform the model and apply the deformation constraints vary with the particular application. The motion reconstruction algorithm we describe can be applied to any organ for which CINE-MRI tagged images have been acquired. Having a model of the heart ventricles allows us to incorporate *a priori* geometric information. The RV-LV mesh building method we describe provides model of each subject's heart.

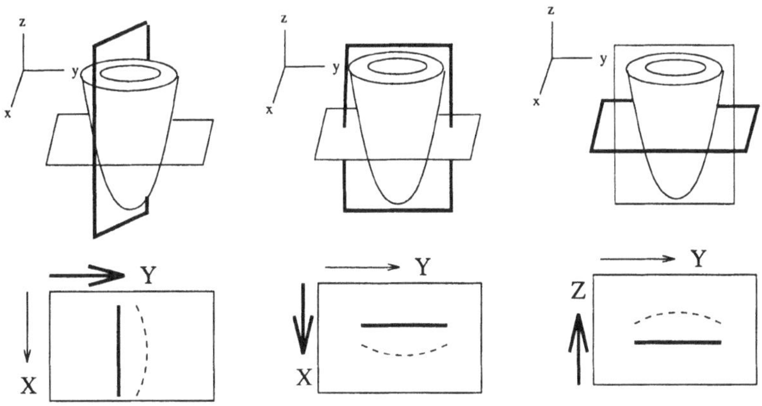

Figure 4.4: 1st row: Schematic LV with image (light) and tag (dark) planes. 2nd row: 2D images with examples of tag motion from initial (dark lines) to final (dashed lines) times. Highlighted arrows indicate for which direction in the coordinate system shown motion information is provided.

4.3.1 MRI Input Data

Tagged MR images were acquired to provide 3D motion information. Since the tag planes only provide information about motion in the direction perpendicular to the initial tag planes, three mutually perpendicular tag plane orientations must be combined to capture 3D motion. The fact that each tag plane must be perpendicular to the image planes requires the use of multiple image views. The current method makes use of two sets of stacked short-axis (transverse) image planes with tag planes that appear as vertical or horizontal stripes, and a set of long-axis (longitudinal) images with tag planes appearing as horizontal stripes in the images. The schematic in Fig. 4.4 shows these combinations along with the motion information that each combination provides.

Tags were semi-automatically tracked in successive images using an interlocking grid of active contours. The tag stripes were sampled at points lying approximately 2mm apart.

4.3.2 Model Dynamics

The deformable model was fit to both tag and contour data from successive images. The current application of the deformable model fitting technique is suited to the RV since local (rather than global) smoothing and a relatively large number of degrees of freedom are used.

The RV-LV model deforms towards the data according to the *Lagrangian* equation equation of motion:

$$\mathbf{M}\ddot{\mathbf{q}} + \mathbf{D}\dot{\mathbf{q}} + \mathbf{K}\mathbf{q} = \mathbf{f}_q \,. \tag{4.1}$$

The degrees of freedom are stored in the displacement vector $\mathbf{q}$, while the velocity and acceleration are stored in $\dot{\mathbf{q}}$ and $\ddot{\mathbf{q}}$, respectively. The matrices $\mathbf{M}$, $\mathbf{D}$, and $\mathbf{K}$ are the mass, damping, and stiffness matrices, and the vector $\mathbf{f}_q$ contains the image-derived forces.

In this case, since the model is to come to rest once reaching the data, the inertia term $\mathbf{M}\ddot{\mathbf{q}}$ is neglected. With the damping matrix $\mathbf{D}$ set to the identity, Eq. 4.1 is simplified to:

$$\dot{\mathbf{q}} + \mathbf{K}\mathbf{q} = \mathbf{f}_q \,. \tag{4.2}$$

In previous work, the degrees of freedom were converted to parameter functions which were chosen using previous knowledge about typical patterns of LV deformation [14]. However, a frame of reference is necessary for describing parameters such as radial shortening and contraction. Since the RV shape is too complex to readily define such a global frame of reference and there are currently no simple parameters that describe RV contraction, the current model has localized, more general degrees of freedom: the 3D displacement $\mathbf{q}$ of each node in the finite element mesh. Due to the relative sparsity of the data available from tagged images, localized spatial smoothing is also added through the finite element stiffness matrix $\mathbf{K}$. Stiffness can also be viewed as an internal resistance which results in a force equal to $\mathbf{K}\mathbf{q}$. Using these considerations, *Lagrange's* equation of motion is written for each node i as

$$\dot{\mathbf{q}}_i = \mathbf{f}_{i,internal} + \mathbf{f}_{i,external}, \tag{4.3}$$

where $\mathbf{q}_i$ is the 3D nodal displacement, $\mathbf{f}_{i,internal} = [\mathbf{K}\mathbf{q}]_i$ is an internal stiffness force, and $\mathbf{f}_{i,external}$ is an external, image-derived force. It is important to note that these forces are only used to deform our model and are not meant to replicate the actual forces or material properties of cardiac tissue.

Similarly, spring-like external forces (which do not occur in cardiac tissue) are used to deform the model to the image-derived data. In previous work [6, 15], separate spring constants were used for the contour and tag data. The Euler integration used a constant step size so that damping effects caused the model to come to rest before it reached the data positions and manual control of these forces was required. With the current work, the fitting is automated as follows:

1. All forces are directly proportional to the distance between the model and image-derived data: $\mathbf{f}_{data} = \mathbf{d}_{data}$, where $\mathbf{d}_{data}$ is the distance from a point on the model to the location of the appropriate data.

2. Equation 4.3 is integrated using the adaptive Euler method [17]. The discretized equation is:

$$\mathbf{q}_{i,t+1} = q_{i,t} + h \sum f_i \,, \tag{4.4}$$

where h is the step size and the subscript t denotes iteration step. Note that the step size is multiplied by the sum of the forces, and can be seen as the effective "strength" of the forces.

3. With the adaptive Euler method, the step size h is inversely related to the integration error. Since the model is initially far from the data, the integration error will be large, and the step size will be small (it is initially 0.01). As the model moves closer to the data, the integration error is reduced and the step size increases. Thus, the forces and step size are inversely related.

With this framework, the adaptive step sizing effectively modulates the strength of the forces.

The model is fit sequentially to data from each image time phase, with five or more phases imaged through systole. Fitting errors, ϵ_{data}, are equal to the magnitude of the image-derived forces $\mathbf{f}_{data}$, and their convergence determines whether the fitting to image data from a particular time phase should be terminated. This process is repeated for each image time phase.

In the following, we describe the calculation of the internal forces and two types of external image-derived forces: contour ($\mathbf{f}_{contour}$) and SPAMM ($\mathbf{f}_{SPAMM}$) forces. Since contours are defined at heart wall boundaries, contour forces are only calculated and applied to boundary nodes b belonging to the endocardial or epicardial surfaces of the model. Conversely, the mid-wall nodes m will only have SPAMM forces acting on them: $\mathbf{f}_{m,external} = \mathbf{f}_{m,SPAMM}$. Therefore, to keep the forces between the mid-wall and the boundaries balanced, contour forces at the boundary nodes are combined with the SPAMM forces according to: $\mathbf{f}_{b,external} = w\mathbf{f}_{b,contour} + (1 - w)\mathbf{f}_{b,SPAMM}$. Since contour data tends to be less accurate than tag data, w is set to 0.25.

4.3.3 External Forces from SPAMM data

The SPAMM markers provide information about motion within the myocardium. We refer to these markers in general as "tag surfaces", and to the initially planar tags as "tag planes". The SPAMM force calculation is based on the fact that the tag data provide information about the time evolution of the deformation of markers in the actual heart muscle. Since the initial position of both the model and the tags are known, simulated tag planes that coincide with the initial tag plane positions can be "hooked on" to the model. Since these planes are registered to the deformable model, we call them material surfaces. The material surfaces are modeled as a

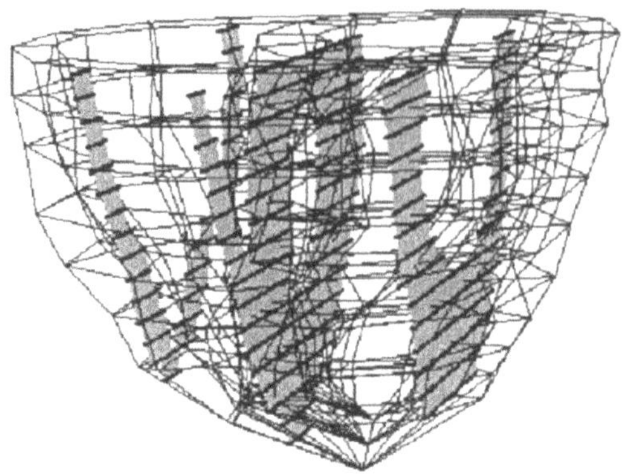

Figure 4.5: Finite element mesh with initial material planes drawn shaded and material points drawn black. Each of these points is registered to the element in which it lies.

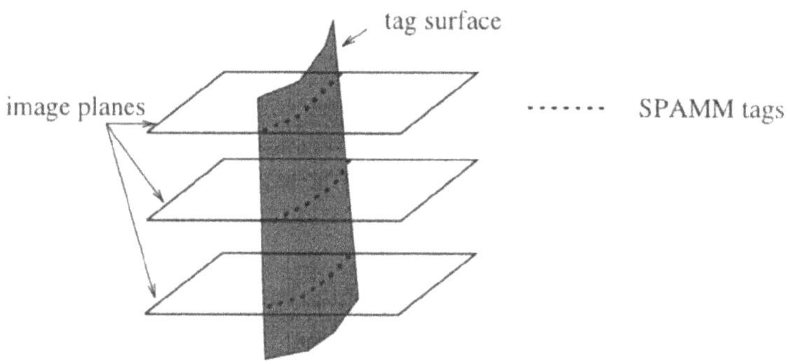

Figure 4.6: The intersection of each tag surface with the image planes produces dark bands in the images.

triangulated set of points (Fig. 4.5), and the SPAMM forces are then calculated between these points and tag data from the images. The forces are then distributed to the nodes of the finite elements, so that the model is pulled towards this data. By simultaneously fitting the deformable model to tag data provided in three mutually perpendicular directions, the 3D motion can be reconstructed.

Although we have a 3D motion model, the original tag data exists only at the locations of the original image planes. The material point locations, on the other hand, are not limited to these planes. In order to calculate the forces on all material points, the position of the tags between the image planes must be approximated. As seen in Fig. 4.6, the stripes seen in MRI images are the intersections of the tag surfaces with the image planes . If the image plane separation is small enough (about 8mm in our case), there will be only a small variation in the shape of the tag surface between each image plane. Therefore, the position of the entire tag surface can be reconstructed from the tag stripe positions at each image time phase. The

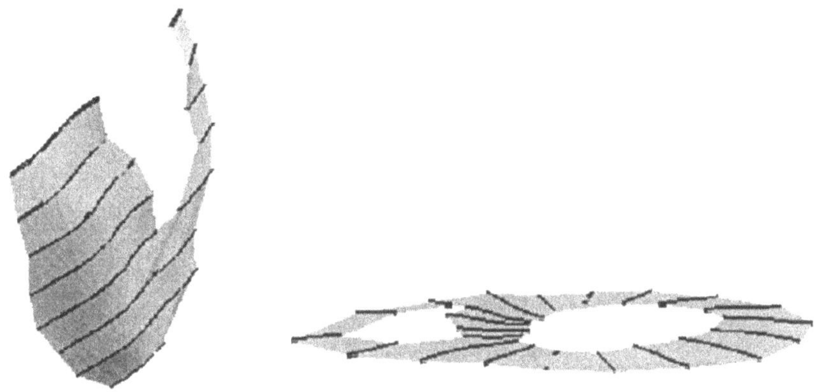

(a) (b)

Figure 4.7: Reconstructed tag surfaces (shown shaded) along with original tag stripes (black lines). **(a)** Stripes originating from stacked, short-axis image planes. **(b)** Stripes originating from a set of rotating long-axis image planes. It may be helpful to compare this figure to Fig. 4.6.

reconstruction results in the availability of tag data irrespective of the image plane locations. Tag surfaces along with their original stripes are shown in Fig. 4.7.

The SPAMM forces are designed to pull the model material surfaces towards the reconstructed tag surfaces as shown in Fig. 4.8. Thus, a force is calculated between each material point, $\mathbf{mp}$, and the appropriate reconstructed tag surface. The force direction is determined by keeping in mind that, as the tagging planes deform into surfaces, they only provide motion information normal to their original orientation. We also keep track of the SPAMM error, ϵ_{SPAMM}, which is the RMS average of the distance forces, $\mathbf{f}_S$, from all material points defining sets of material surfaces in all three orientations.

4.3.4 External forces From Contour Data

If the current image resolution allows for a 6mm minimum tag separation, few or no tags may fall on portions of the 3-5mm thick RV free wall. This issue is less problematic in the long-axis views, since the 1D tags are parallel to the normals to the heart walls and can therefore traverse the thickness of those walls (Fig. 4.9a). In short-axis views, the curvature of the RV wall is more variant and some regions may receive one or fewer tags (Fig. 4.9b). In order to adequately constrain the motion of the model, contour forces are calculated from short-axis contour data. These forces are then combined with the components of the SPAMM forces, which constrain motion within the short-axis image planes.

Since each portion of a contour provides motion information in the direction of the local normal, the contour forces are calculated in the direction normal to the

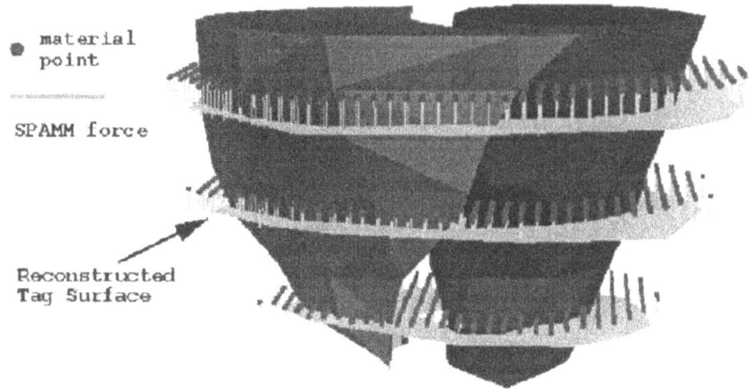

Figure 4.8: Each collection of material points defining a material surface (not drawn) is attracted to the corresponding tag surface via the SPAMM forces. Several tag surfaces reconstructed from the long-axis view are shown along with model endocardial walls.

model boundary and within planes parallel to short-axis images. The boundary normals are calculated from the triangulated surfaces generated during the geometry generation phase. Although the boundary normal may not initially be equal to the contour normal, the model normals are recalculated as the model is being pulled closer to the contours, causing the two normals to gradually coincide. Since the normal heart exhibits twisting, boundary forces are not activated until $\epsilon_{SPAMM} < 1.0$mm in order to ensure that these normals will have more or less the same orientation.

If the node lies between two image planes, the forces from each plane are combined. This force is then projected onto the original node normal, $\mathbf{n}$, in order calculate the contour force, $\mathbf{f}_{contour}$. The contour error $\epsilon_{contour}$ is the RMS of the contour forces calculated on all boundary nodes.

4.3.5 Internal Forces Due To Stiffness

The degrees of freedom of our model are the 3D displacements of the finite element nodes. Forces calculated from segmented contours and tags, may have inaccuracies in the data due to human error during segmentation or image noise. In order to account for the discrete sampling of motion data due to the tags and factors which cause inaccuracies in the input data, a stiffness component adds smoothing to the deformable model. In our formulation, stiffness is considered to be an internal force, $\mathbf{f}_{i,internal}$. In order to impose a continuity and smoothing constraint between image time phases, each element is considered to consist of a material that is isotropic, linear, and compressible.

The element force vector $\mathbf{f}_e$ contains the forces on the element nodes. It is cal-

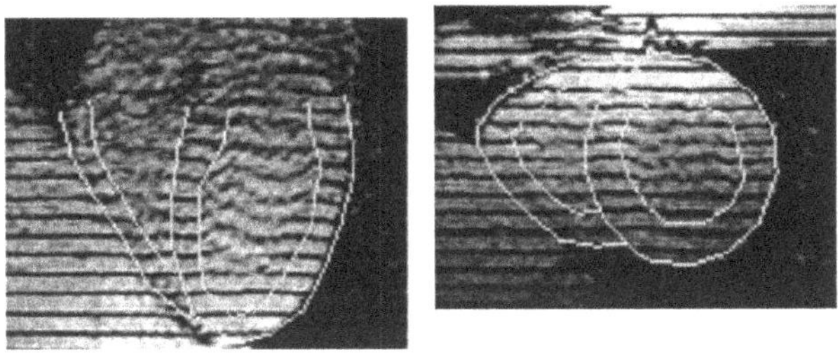

(a) (b)

Figure 4.9: Representative segmented tagged images. **(a)** In the long-axis view, most horizontal tags fall across the heart walls. **(b)** The curvature of the RV varies in the short-axis view. In this case, only one stripe falls on the anterior and posterior portions of the RV.

culated for each element as:

$$\mathbf{f}_e = \mathbf{K}\mathbf{d}_e\,, \tag{4.5}$$

where $\mathbf{d}_e$ contains the nodal displacements. The stiffness matrix, $\mathbf{K}$, incorporates the geometry and material properties of the element and is computed from

$$\mathbf{K} = \iiint \mathbf{B}^T\mathbf{D}\mathbf{B}\,dV\,. \tag{4.6}$$

The matrix $\mathbf{D}$ contains the material property information and relates nodal stresses σ to nodal strains ε as follows

$$\sigma = \mathbf{D}\varepsilon. \tag{4.7}$$

The matrix $\mathbf{B}$ relates nodal strains to displacements according to

$$\varepsilon = \mathbf{B}\mathbf{d}_e\,. \tag{4.8}$$

Once the element forces are calculated, each element contributes to the total internal force of its nodes, $\mathbf{f}_{i,internal}$. A detailed derivation of the finite element formulation for calculating the stiffness matrix $\mathbf{K}$ can be found in [24]. A Poisson's ratio of 0.4 and a Young's modulus of 0.02 are used for the material model. Since heart muscle is nearly incompressible, a Poisson's ratio of 0.4 provides a constraint on the maximum amount that each element in the model can decrease its volume. The Young's modulus was chosen empirically to provide computational stability under the assumption that there were no significant human errors (such as misdirecting the snakes mesh) introduced during the tag and contour extraction process. The Young's modulus can be altered to increase the smoothing needed to resolve the latter issue and/or an increase in noise due to poor image quality. In order to prevent element distortions of the linear elements, the stiffness matrix is recalculated after fitting to each time phase, thereby making the smoothing piecewise linear.

4.4 Motion and Deformation Analysis

The 3D motion reconstruction provides the estimated nodal displacements of the ventricular model. Using the finite element shape functions, an effective dense set of displacement data within the finite elements representing the ventricles can be interpolated between the nodes. However, since simply viewing the motion of a finite element mesh is of little use to researchers and clinicians, an important area of research is to be able to quantify the motion and visualize the results in an efficient manner. The motion quantities are then visualized with plots on the endocardial or epicardial wall surfaces. Statistical analysis is performed to compare similar regions in each heart.

4.4.1 Motion Parameters

In a previous study [15], LV motion was described in terms of variables that clinicians are already familiar with for the ventricle – – – for example, twisting and radial contraction. Due to the complex shape of the RV, however, it is difficult to find a single axis about which to calculate twisting and radial contraction. Therefore, we calculate twisting of the RV about the long-axis of the LV. An area of future research will be to apply the 3D motion reconstruction technique described in this chapter to a significant number of normal RVs and work closely with clinicians to determine variables that succinctly describe RV motion in health.

Due to the lack of an obvious frame of reference for the RV, we prefer to use motion variables that are independent of the coordinate system being used. Both the 3D regional displacement and deformation of the biventricular model during systole are calculated. Displacement results are presented by showing the paths of model points along with a plot on the appropriate wall. A still better indicator of the degree of muscle contraction is a quantity that describes differential motion, such as the strain tensor [19].

We use *Lagrangian* strain $\mathbf{E}$ to describe systolic deformation in a region surrounding a point in the heart relative to its position at end-diastole. It is defined by

$$\mathbf{E} = \frac{1}{2}(\mathbf{F}^T\mathbf{F} - \mathbf{I}), \tag{4.9}$$

where $\mathbf{I}$ is the identity matrix and $\mathbf{F}$ is the deformation gradient tensor, whose elements are given by

$$F_{pq} = \frac{\partial x_p}{\partial X_q}. \tag{4.10}$$

(see Chapter 1 for a detailed derivation).

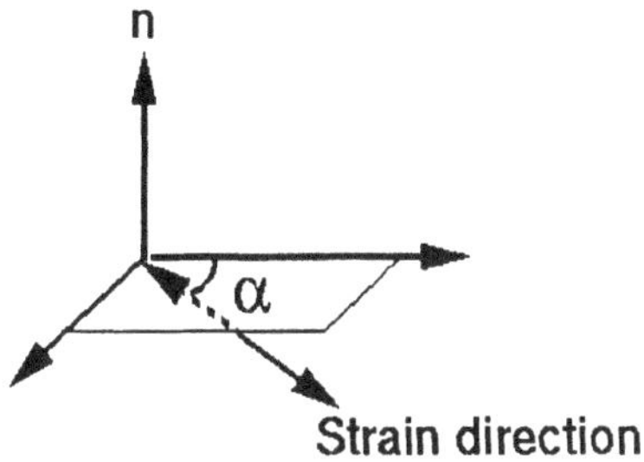

Figure 4.10: Definition of α: the angle that the strain direction, makes with the short-axis image planes. The normal, $\mathbf{n}$, to the short axis image planes is shown along with two vectors in the plane.

Since the 3D motion reconstruction only provides discrete motion information, and no explicit functions relating $\mathbf{X}$ and $\mathbf{x}$ exist, finite elements are used to compute strains numerically. In order to do so, the derivatives in Eq.(4.10) are expanded by using the chain rule:

$$F_{pq} = \frac{\partial x_p}{\partial X_q} = \frac{\partial x_p}{\partial \xi_i}\frac{\partial \xi_i}{\partial X_q}, \tag{4.11}$$

where ξ_i is a component of the local finite element coordinate system (see the Appendix for details).

Since the *Lagrangian* strain is a tensor, which includes orientation information, it is defined relative to a reference coordinate frame. Since the issue of defining a coordinate frame for the RV remains an open research question, we report coordinate-system-independent principal strains and directions. These quantities are derived by finding the eigenvalues and eigenvectors of the *Lagrangian* strain tensor, respectively. The eigenvalues of $\mathbf{E}$ are the principal strains, where a positive value indicates extension while a negative value indicates compression [19]. The eigenvector corresponding to the eigenvalues is that principal strains direction. Since the minimum principal strain, E_3, is negative in the normal heart, we use it as a measure of the magnitude and direction of contraction.

The parameter α is used to describe an orientation of a principal strain with respect to short axis image planes (Fig. 4.10). This parameter ranges from 0 to 90 degrees, with a value of zero indicating that the strain direction is completely circumferential (aligned with the short-axis images), and a value of 90 indicating that the strain direction is longitudinal.

4.4.2 Data Analysis

The regional variation of several motion quantities was studied in normals and patients with RVH. Motion quantities were calculated at elements and averaged

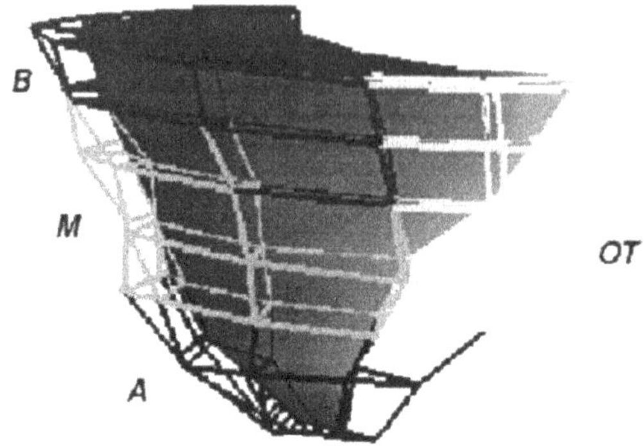

Figure 4.11: Subdivision of free wall into 4 regions. Anatomical landmarks from original images were used to locate the outflow tract (OT). The rest of free wall (and the septum) were divided based on normalized height, h, along a septal axis. Apex (A): $0 \leq h < 0.35$, mid-ventricle (M): $.35 \leq h < 0.6$, and base (B): $0.6 \leq h \leq 1.0$.

for each region of the free wall and septum. Anatomical landmarks defined in the original images were used to demarcate these regions. First, the outflow tract was separated from the rest of the free wall by defining the parietal and septal bands. A septal long-axis was defined between a point on the basal septum and the insertion of the RV into the LV at the epicardial apex. The initial normalized height h of points with respect to this long-axis were used to separate the rest of the free wall, as well as the septum into 3 regions (Fig. 4.11). Deformation and motion quantities for each region were calculated as the weighted average (according to element volume) of the strains in the elements belonging to those regions.

We analyzed 5 normals and 4 patients who were diagnosed with RVH with echocardiography. Regional variations in the RV free wall and septum within each group of normals and RVH patients were analyzed using repeated measures ANOVA with Scheffé subtesting. A p-value less than 0.05 was considered significant. Comparisons between corresponding regions in the free wall and septum were performed with multiple paired t-tests with the significance adjusted for multiple comparisons. Furthermore, corresponding regions in the walls of normal and RVH groups were compared with unpaired t-tests, with significance adjusted for multiple comparisons (e.g., the number of regions in the free wall or septum).

4.5 Results

In this section, we present results related to the 3D motion reconstruction technique. First, we demonstrate model convergence and fitting behavior. Next, we present the results of the validation studies. Finally, we detail the application of the motion reconstruction technique to clinical data.

4.5.1 Model fitting behavior

The 3D motion reconstruction technique was applied to synthetic data and data from 9 human subjects, with the same smoothing parameters used for all cases. During the fitting, the RMS errors between the material surfaces and reconstructed tag data, ϵ_{SPAMM}, and between surface nodes and contour data, $\epsilon_{contour}$, were measured. Fig. 4.12a shows the convergence of ϵ_{SPAMM} for all image time phases for representative normal data. Fig. 4.12b shows the relationship between ϵ_{SPAMM}, $\epsilon_{contour}$, and the adaptive step size as the model is fit to data from one image time phase. As described in Sec. 4.3.4, the contour forces were only applied when $\epsilon_{SPAMM} < 1.0$, and the figure shows that these errors also converged once the fitting was applied.

In Sec. 4.3.2, we pointed out that the goal of the adaptive step sizing was to modulate the effective strength of the distance-equivalent forces. It can be seen that an inverse relationship exists: as the fitting errors decrease (i.e., the model gets closer to the data), the step size increases automatically. The inverse relationship ensures that the model does not come too rest too early. Considering the convergence behavior of the system, the fitting for data from a certain image time phases was terminated when the changes in ϵ_{SPAMM} and $\epsilon_{contour}$ were both smaller than 2%. The total fitting time for the clinical experiments was about 40 minutes (8 minutes for the synthetic data) on an SGI 0^2 RS10000 workstation (Mountain View, CA). Since several algorithms have not yet been optimized, we estimate that the fitting time can be reduced to 15 minutes. The time for the automatic mesh generation was relatively small, about 15 seconds.

4.5.2 Validation studies

Synthetic tag and contour data from a motion simulator were used as input to the 3D motion reconstruction. The goodness of the fit was evaluated by comparing the analytically calculated displacements with the reconstructed displacements. The displacement errors and tag fitting errors (ϵ_{SPAMM}) were about 0.6mm RMS, or an average of 2%. Since the pixel size in the MR images is only about 1mm, the accuracy of the model fitting in this case is less than the accuracy that can be obtained in locating the tags. In addition, the largest errors occurred in the 'base' of the model which was above the top simulated image plane, and therefore less constrained. The maximum simulated displacement of 25mm was at the base of the model.

Next, we compared the results of the 3D motion reconstruction to the original images from which the data was derived. The in-vivo validation results are presented for a representative normal study which had 5 time phases through systole and a tag plane separation of 6mm in Figs. 4.13 and 4.14. For each image plane, we show the end-diastolic and end-systolic images with an overlay of the model material plane/ image plane intersections. Fig. 4.13 shows the short-axis images of a mid-ventricular slice. A slight mismatch appears in the end-systolic horizontal

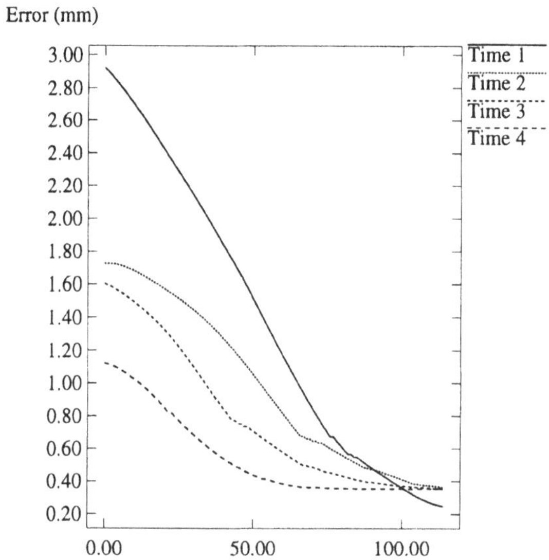

(a)

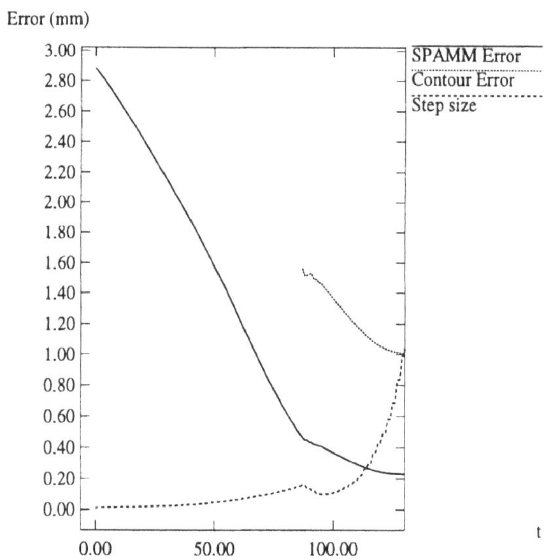

(b)

Figure 4.12: Convergence behavior of fitting technique for a representative study. **(a)** Decrease in ϵ_{SPAMM} versus iteration, t, for all 4 image time phases. **(b)** ϵ_{SPAMM}, $\epsilon_{contour}$, and step size versus t while fitting to data from an initial time phase.

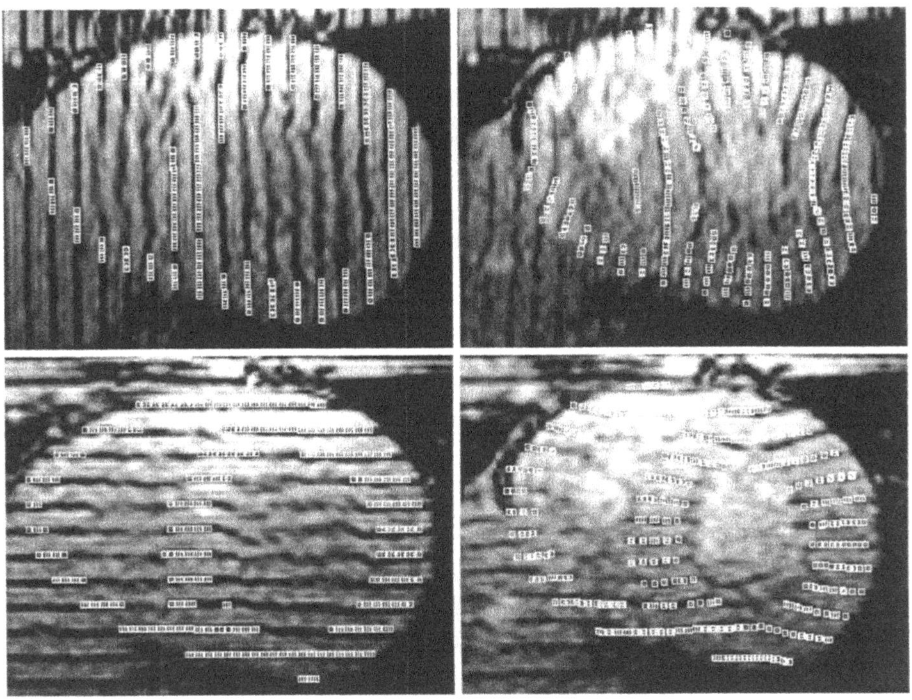

(a) (b)

End-diastole End-systole

Figure 4.13: Short-axis end-diastolic and end-systolic images with **(a)** horizontal and **(b)** vertical tags. The intersections of model material surfaces are shown along with the original images.

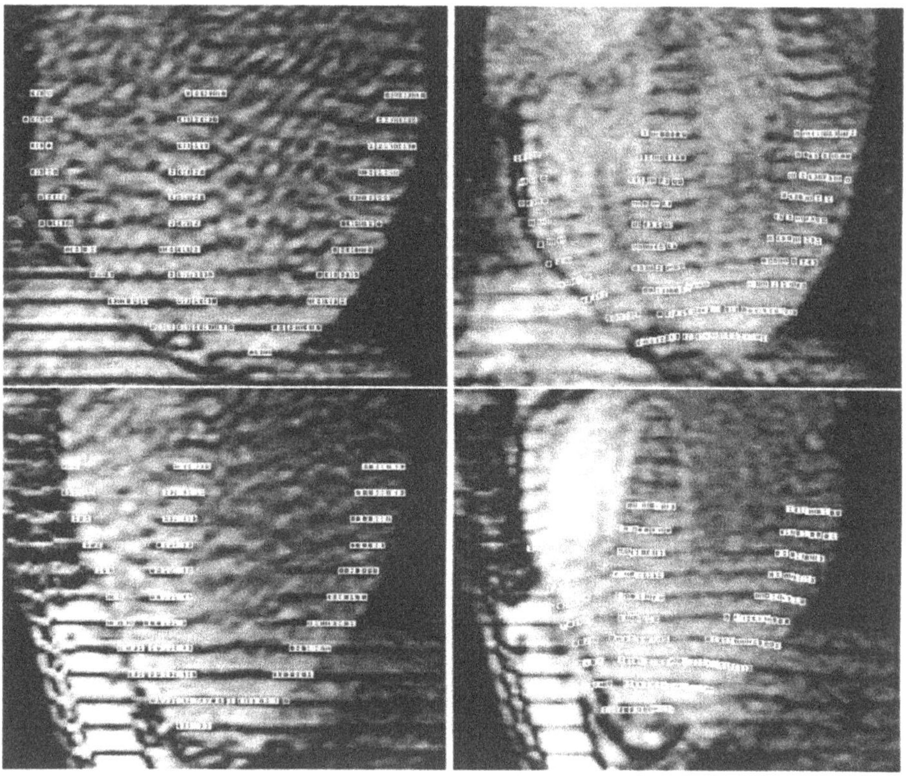

End-diastole End-systole

Figure 4.14: Long-axis end-diastolic and end-systolic images with each row showing two different locations. The intersections of model material surfaces are shown along with the original images.

tagged images (Fig. 4.13a) at the anterior septum and in the anterior portion of the RV. It appears that the model was too stiff at those points to fit the entire curvature of those tags. In addition, portions of the model RV free wall appear not to have moved sufficiently towards the LV. This is again apparent in the deformed vertical tag images (Fig. 4.13b), where we see a mismatch in the anterior-lateral free wall. Two long-axis image views, shown in Fig. 4.14(a,b), show a good agreement between the model and corresponding images. The location in the top row shows the same mismatch in the RV free wall which was shown for short-axis images.

4.5.3 Clinical Data

Normals

All 5 normals exhibited similar qualitative and quantitative behavior. Fig. 4.15 shows the motion of points in the RV-LV for several element "slices". The angular displacements about the LV long-axis for each wall at each level are plotted. Within each level, the angular displacement is similar for the RV free wall, LV free wall, and septum. When comparing basal, mid-ventricular, and apical levels, it can be seen that all regions initially rotate clockwise. The basal slice subsequently changes direction and rotates in a counterclockwise (CCW) direction while the apex continues to rotate clockwise (CW).

Fig. 4.16 shows the motion of the model (looking at the free wall) over all time phases for a typical normal study. The path of points in the center of the RV free wall are plotted along with a plot of point displacement on the endocardial wall. It can be seen that the paths of most points in the free wall are anterior and towards the apex. The plot of displacement in Fig. 4.16 reveals a nonuniform distribution. The greatest amount of both total and axial displacement in the biventricular unit occurs in the basal free wall of the RV. Linear regression was used to assess the presence of decreased base-apex displacement in the RV free wall (outer wall) (R = .724).

In order to quantify the magnitude of the greatest muscle contraction between end-diastole and end-systole, we calculated the minimum principal strain, E_3. Fig. 4.17 shows a plot on the endocardial surface of the RV free wall of E_3 at end-systole for all 5 normal subjects. The associated principal directions are plotted at the mid-ventricular, with lengths normalized according to the maximum contraction at those locations. We can see a decreasing trend base to apex contraction. Basal E_3 was significantly smaller than in other regions ($p < .002$). This suggests that mid and apical portions of the heart have the greatest contraction to pull the base of the heart towards the apex.

Right Ventricular Hypertrophy (RVH)

A common reaction of the right ventricle to elevated blood pressures or volumes is to increase its mass, a process called hypertrophy. Increased pressures are usually

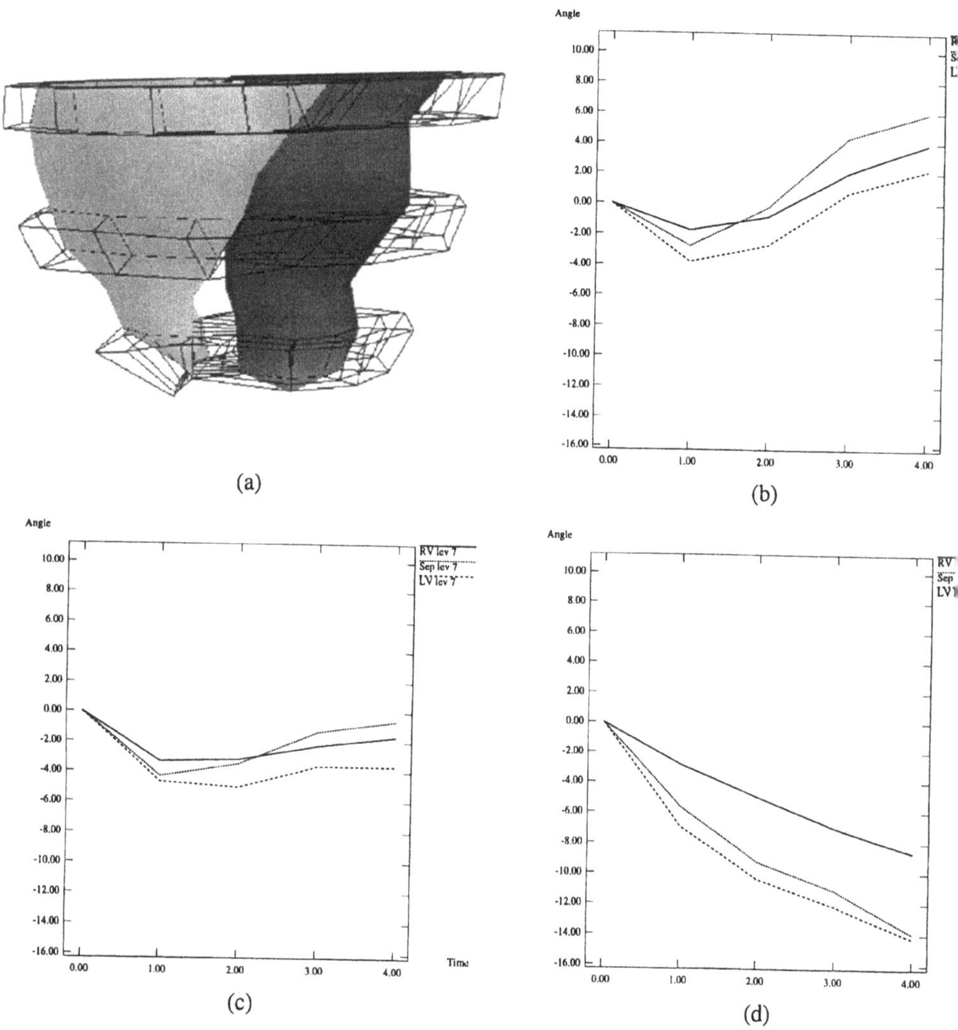

Figure 4.15: Motion about the LV long-axis at 3 levels, or slices, in the model. **(a)** Slices relative to endocardial walls (shown shaded). Slices are **(b)** basal, **(c)** mid, and **(d)** apical. Angular position as a function of image time phase is shown. CCW is positive.

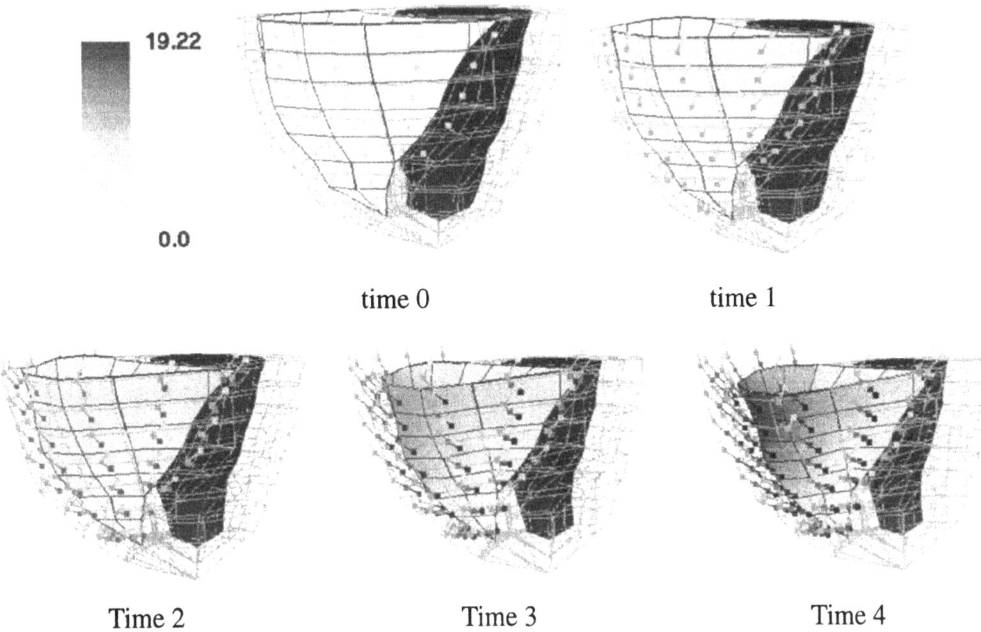

Figure 4.16: Normal heart displacement through systole: Plot of displacement on the RV endocardial free wall. The paths of points located in the centers of the elements are shown from end-diastole (light blue) to end-systole (dark blue). See color Plate 1.

a result of some sort of blockage in the lung (e.g., embolism). Volume overload is usually a result of over-circulation due to congenital heart disease [2]. Both types of hypertrophy can alter cellular contractile function [20], produce prolonged action potentials [4], and result in a lowered ejection fraction [2]. Furthermore, increased pressures in the RV cavity can cause the septum to bulge into the LV cavity, thereby decreasing left ventricular ejection fraction [13]. The changes in the actual pumping mechanisms in the heart are not well-characterized.

The paths of points in the RV free wall is displayed along with a plot of the displacement for a representative RVH study in Fig. 4.18a. It can be seen that the paths of the point are different from the normals, with no anterior motion of points in the free wall. When compared to normals, we found that average displacement was decreased in most regions of the free wall and septum for RVH patients ($p < .01$). The strains also decreased, as can be seen in Fig. 4.18b. Note that the scales are the same as that for the normals. Regional differences are better seen in the bar plot in Fig. 4.19. The average value of $|E_3|$ decreased for all regions in both the free wall and septum during RVH and was significantly different in most regions. It can also be seen that the angles of the minimum principal strain directions are more '"horizontal' for the RVH case compared to the normals. Although statistically significant changes could not be found for the current number of subjects, this is an indication that the direction of maximal contraction has actually altered. Al-

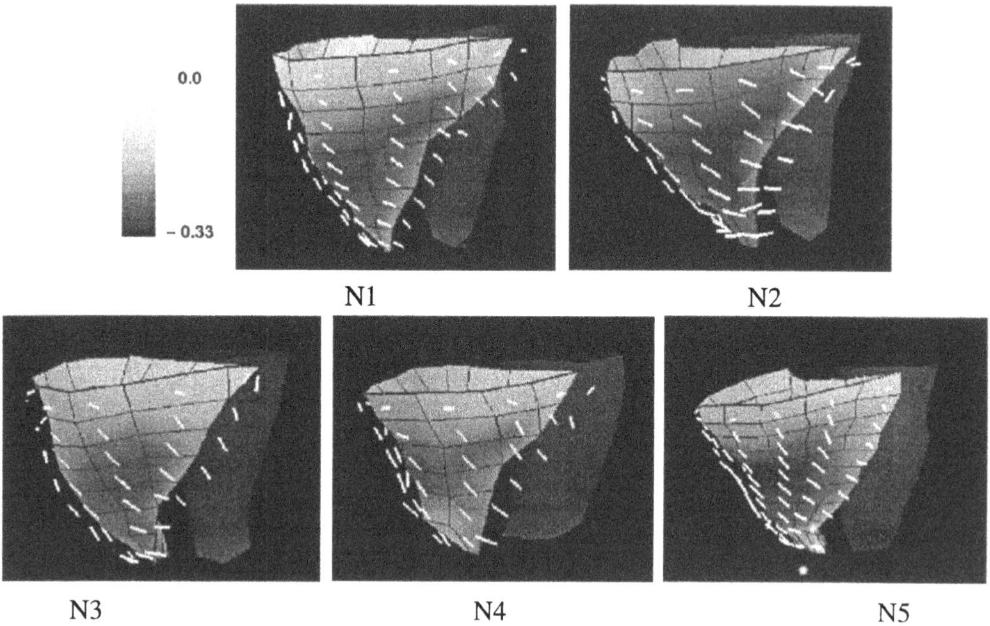

Figure 4.17: Normal E_3: Recovered end-systolic position of all normal studies. A plot of minimum principal strain is on the RV endocardial free wall. The minimum principal strain directions are drawn as lines at the centers of the elements, with lengths normalized by the strain magnitude.

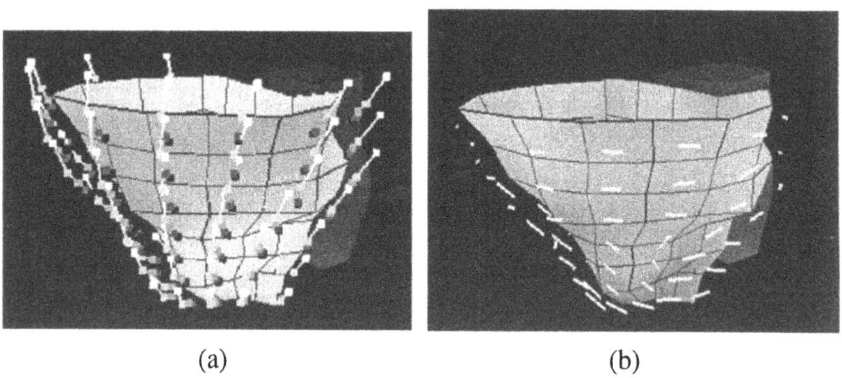

Figure 4.18: Motion reconstruction of RVH. RV shown at end-systole with plots on the endocardial walls. Scales are the same as in normals. **(a)** Displacement plot along with the paths of points located in the centers of the elements are shown from end-diastole (white) to end-systole (blue). **(b)** Strain map of minimum principal strain. Bright lines are the minimum principal strain directions.

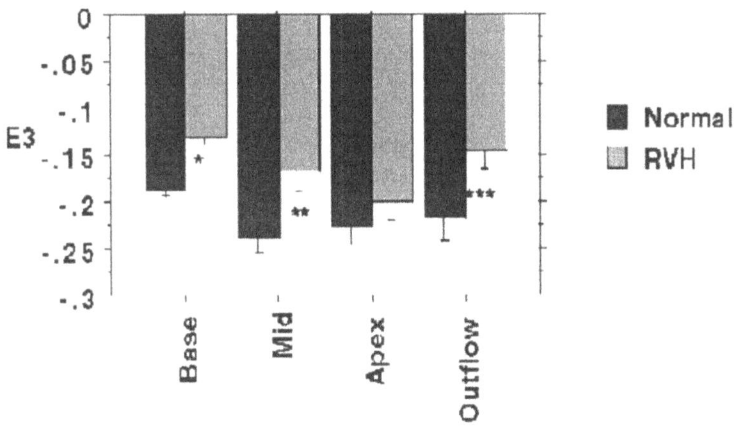

(a)

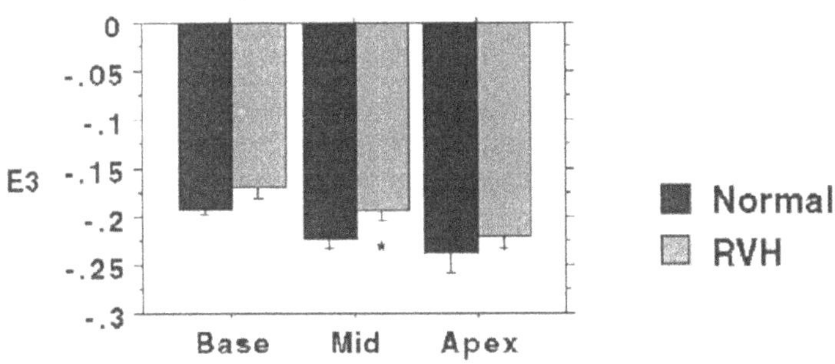

(b)

Figure 4.19: Strain in normals vs. RVH: comparison between regions. **(a)** In the free wall, all regions had an average decrease in $|E_3|$, with significant differences in the base ($^*p < .0001$), mid-ventricle ($^{**}p < .002$), and outflow tract ($^{***}p < .002$). **(b)** In the septum, all regions had an average decrease in $|E_3|$, with significant differences in the mid-ventricle ($^*p < .008$). Significance levels were adjusted from .05 by the number of regions within each wall. Values are mean$\pm$SD

though changes in muscle cell orientation during hypertrophy has been observed, the consequences of these changes have not been measured until now.

4.6 Discussion

Some of the concepts in this chapter were used in previous 3D motion reconstruction techniques. As we mentioned earlier, we use the deformable model fitting framework of Park, et al. [15] for the fitting process. In a recent paper dealing with LV 3D motion reconstruction using least squares, Young [21], used the idea of registering the entire surface of the tags to the model [22] (as opposed to the tag stripes [6], or tag intersections [15,22]). In that paper, the constraints were limited to image plane locations: material surfaces were intersected with image planes and the distance to the tags in that image plane was calculated. Our experience during preliminary work [6] was that limiting the degrees of freedom to the image planes resulted in too few constraints being applied to the model.

In order to constrain the entirety of material planes, we had to interpolate the tag data between image planes by reconstructing the tag surfaces. In the 3D reconstruction technique of Moulton, et. al. [11], the tag data was reconstructed using B-spline surfaces and material points were limited to the intersections of the B-spline surfaces. The topology of the LV sections in short and long-axis views allowed for parameterization of the B-spline such that no portion of the spline had to pass through the cavity (where there is not data). Since the biventricular topology is more complex, rather than dealing with possible numerical instabilities of fitting higher-order surface through the cavities (large regions with no data) with B-splines or with thin-plate splines [9], we triangulate the surfaces between the tags. Although this does not allow for smoothing of the tag data, a smoothing constraint is already incorporated in the form of stiffness forces in our through the finite elements. In the new methodology, material surface registration and tag surface reconstruction are incorporated into the deformable modeling framework. In addition, the current technique allows for:

1) The use of short-axis contour data to compensate for lack of stripes in the RV free wall.

2) The application of local, piecewise linear smoothing.

3) The automation of the fitting.

4) The generation of a detailed geometric model.

The accuracy of the technique described in this chapter was limited by the image quality and tag spacing. Better image quality would have decreased the noise of the input data and more closely spaced tag data would have provided more constraints for the model. Our method included local smoothing to account for image noise and discrete sampling of motion. With probable future improvements in image resolution, more closely-spaced tags will provide a greater number of constraints. The finite element mesh generation procedure described in this chapter can be extended to increase the degrees of freedom of the deformable model by generating a larger number of elements or using higher-order element shape functions. In addition, we did not model a portion of the RV outflow tract, which is oriented obliquely in both short and long-axis data, due to the limitation of building the geometric mesh from short-axis contours only. However, once the RV outflow tract is accurately modeled, the reconstruction method described in this chapter can be directly applied to a model that encompasses the outflow tract.

4.7 Conclusions and Future Work

In this chapter, we present an approach to 3D motion reconstruction which captures both right and left ventricular deformation from tagged MRI. The differential motion of the tags allow for calculation of both displacement and deformation strain. With motion reconstruction, we can get a full picture of the motion of the RV, not just what is seen in the image planes. The results of the 3D motion reconstruction were then used to demonstrate the pattern of strain in the RV free wall and septum, as well as changes found during RVH.

Acknowledgments

The authors are thankful to Victor Ferrari, Zahi Fayad, Doug Decarlo, Alistair Young, and Jonathan Kaye for their help in various aspects of this work. This research has been funded by grants from the NSF (Career Award 96-24604), the Whitaker Foundation, the NIH (HL 43014) and the NIH/NLM (LM06638-01).

Appendix: Finite Element Shape Functions

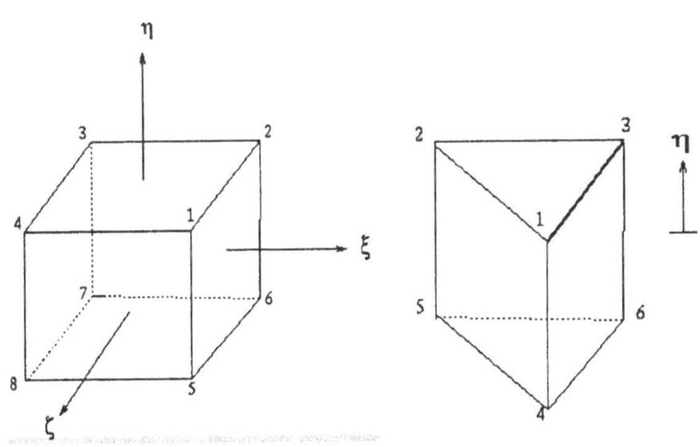

(a) (b)

Figure 4.20: Elements used to build deformable model are shown along with the local coordinate system and node numbering. **(a)** 8-noded parallelepiped. **(b)** 6-noded wedge.

The shape functions are used to interpolate a motion variable (displacement, position) from the nodes to a point within the element. Fig. 4.20 shows the eight-noded and six-noded elements used in the finite element mesh [24]. The shape functions for an eight-noded parallelepiped are:

$$N_1 = (1+\xi)(1+\eta)(1+\zeta)\,, \tag{4.12}$$
$$N_2 = (1+\xi)(1+\eta)(1-\zeta)\,, \tag{4.13}$$
$$N_3 = (1-\xi)(1+\eta)(1-\zeta)\,, \tag{4.14}$$
$$N_4 = (1-\xi)(1+\eta)(1+\zeta)\,, \tag{4.15}$$
$$N_5 = (1+\xi)(1-\eta)(1+\zeta)\,, \tag{4.16}$$
$$N_6 = (1+\xi)(1-\eta)(1-\zeta)\,, \tag{4.17}$$
$$N_7 = (1-\xi)(1-\eta)(1-\zeta)\,, \tag{4.18}$$
$$N_8 = (1-\xi)(1-\eta)(1+\zeta)\,. \tag{4.19}$$

The shape functions for a six-noded wedge-shaped element are:

$$N_1 = 0.5L_1(1-\eta)\,, \tag{4.20}$$
$$N_2 = 0.5L_2(1-\eta)\,, \tag{4.21}$$
$$N_3 = 0.5L_3(1-\eta)\,, \tag{4.22}$$
$$N_4 = 0.5L_1(1+\eta)\,, \tag{4.23}$$
$$N_5 = 0.5L_2(1+\eta)\,, \tag{4.24}$$
$$N_6 = 0.5L_3(1+\eta)\,, \tag{4.25}$$

where L_1, L_2, and L_3 are the area coordinates of triangle 1-2-3 and 4-5-6 in Fig. 4.20b [24].

Appendix: Strain Calculation Using Finite Elements

Due to significant deformation in the heart wall during systole, we must use finite deformation theory for our strain calculations. A more detailed description of this theory can be found in [19]. The deformation of a point in a continuum is defined as

$$\mathbf{x} = \mathbf{x}(\mathbf{X}, t)\,, \tag{4.26}$$

where $\mathbf{X}$ and $\mathbf{x}$ are the initial and final positions, respectively, of a point in the continuum. This vector equation can be written for each coordinate direction. For example, a uniform extension is written as:

$$x = \lambda_x X,\ y = \lambda_y Y,\ z = \lambda_z Z\,, \tag{4.27}$$

Since we are concerned with relative deformation, we calculate the 3×3 deformation gradient tensor, $\mathbf{F}$. The components of $\mathbf{F}$ are

$$F_{pq} = \frac{\partial x_p}{\partial X_q}, \tag{4.28}$$

where x_p is one of the three components of $\mathbf{x}$. In our model, we calculate the *Lagrangian* strain, $\mathbf{E}$, which is a measure of the deformation of a point in the model with respect to its initial position.

$$\mathbf{E} = \frac{1}{2}(\mathbf{F}^T\mathbf{F} - \mathbf{I}), \tag{4.29}$$

where $\mathbf{I}$ is the identity matrix.

Since the derivatives in Eq. 4.28 cannot be calculated directly, the chain rule is used:

$$F_{pq} = \frac{\partial x_p}{\partial X_q} = \frac{\partial x_p}{\partial \xi_i}\frac{\partial \xi_i}{\partial X_q}, \tag{4.30}$$

This equation is written in matrix form as the product of 2 matrices, $\mathbf{S}$ and $\mathbf{T}$:

$$\begin{bmatrix} \frac{\partial x}{\partial X} & \frac{\partial x}{\partial Y} & \frac{\partial x}{\partial Z} \\ \frac{\partial y}{\partial X} & \frac{\partial y}{\partial Y} & \frac{\partial y}{\partial Z} \\ \frac{\partial z}{\partial X} & \frac{\partial z}{\partial Y} & \frac{\partial z}{\partial Z} \end{bmatrix} = \underbrace{\begin{bmatrix} \frac{\partial x}{\partial \xi} & \frac{\partial x}{\partial \eta} & \frac{\partial x}{\partial \zeta} \\ \frac{\partial y}{\partial \xi} & \frac{\partial y}{\partial \eta} & \frac{\partial y}{\partial \zeta} \\ \frac{\partial z}{\partial \xi} & \frac{\partial z}{\partial \eta} & \frac{\partial z}{\partial \zeta} \end{bmatrix}}_{\mathbf{S}:3\times 3} \underbrace{\begin{bmatrix} \frac{\partial \xi}{\partial X} & \frac{\partial \xi}{\partial Y} & \frac{\partial \xi}{\partial Z} \\ \frac{\partial \eta}{\partial X} & \frac{\partial \eta}{\partial Y} & \frac{\partial \eta}{\partial Z} \\ \frac{\partial \zeta}{\partial X} & \frac{\partial \zeta}{\partial Y} & \frac{\partial \zeta}{\partial Z} \end{bmatrix}}_{\mathbf{T}:3\times 3}. \tag{4.31}$$

This matrix is the derivative of the position of a point in the element with respect to the local coordinates of that element. We recall that positions can be expressed as functions of the local coordinates through the shape function equations. These equations are used to interpolate the position of a point in the element from the positions of the nodes. For example, the x-coordinate of a position within the element is:

$$x = \sum_{i=1}^{n} N_i x_i = N_1 x_1 + N_2 x_2 + \cdots + N_n x_n. \tag{4.32}$$

Where (x_i, y_i, z_i) is the deformed position of the ith node.

The derivative with respect to a local coordinate, ξ for example, is

$$\frac{\partial x}{\partial \xi} = x_{,\xi} = \sum_{i=1}^{n} N_{i,\xi}\, x_i = N_{1,\xi}\, x_1 + N_{2,\xi}\, x_2 + \cdots + N_{n,\xi}\, x_n. \tag{4.33}$$

In matrix form, the relations for all 3 displacement derivatives taken with respect to the 3 local coordinates is:

$$\mathbf{S} = \begin{bmatrix} x_{,\xi} & x_{,\eta} & x_{,\zeta} \\ y_{,\xi} & y_{,\eta} & y_{,\zeta} \\ z_{,\xi} & z_{,\eta} & z_{,\zeta} \end{bmatrix}$$

$$= \begin{bmatrix} x_1 & x_2 & x_3 & x_4 & \dots & x_n \\ y_1 & y_2 & y_3 & y_4 & \dots & y_n \\ z_1 & z_2 & z_3 & z_4 & \dots & z_n \end{bmatrix} \begin{bmatrix} N_{1,\xi} & N_{1,\eta} & N_{1,\zeta} \\ N_{2,\xi} & N_{2,\eta} & N_{2,\zeta} \\ N_{3,\xi} & N_{3,\eta} & N_{3,\zeta} \\ N_{4,\xi} & N_{4,\eta} & N_{4,\zeta} \\ \vdots & \vdots & \vdots \\ N_{n,\xi} & N_{n,\eta} & N_{n,\zeta} \end{bmatrix}. \quad (4.34)$$

It is easier to calculate the inverse of $\mathbf{T}$, which we call $\mathbf{U}$:

$$\mathbf{U} = \mathbf{T}^{-1} = \begin{bmatrix} X_{,\xi} & X_{,\eta} & X_{,\zeta} \\ Y_{,\xi} & Y_{,\eta} & Y_{,\zeta} \\ Z_{,\xi} & Z_{,\eta} & Z_{,\zeta} \end{bmatrix}. \quad (4.35)$$

The initial coordinates, (X, Y, Z), can also be interpolated with the shape functions. For the X coordinate,

$$X = \sum_{i=1}^{n} N_i X_i = N_1 X_1 + N_2 X_2 + \cdots + N_n X_n. \quad (4.36)$$

Where (X_i, Y_i, Z_i) are the initial positions of the ith node. The derivative with respect to a local coordinate, ξ for example, becomes

$$\frac{\partial X}{\partial \xi} = X_{,\xi} = \sum_{i=1}^{n} N_{i,\xi}\, X_i = N_{1,\xi}\, X_1 + N_{2,\xi}\, X_2 + \cdots + N_{n,\xi}\, X_n. \quad (4.37)$$

The nine equations (similar to the one above) for the derivatives of the 3 initial coordinates with respect to the natural coordinates can be summarized in matrix form:

$$\mathbf{U} = \begin{bmatrix} X_{,\xi} & X_{,\eta} & X_{,\zeta} \\ Y_{,\xi} & Y_{,\eta} & Y_{,\zeta} \\ Z_{,\xi} & Z_{,\eta} & Z_{,\zeta} \end{bmatrix},$$

$$= \begin{bmatrix} X_1 & X_2 & X_3 & X_4 & \dots & X_n \\ Y_1 & Y_2 & Y_3 & Y_4 & \dots & Y_n \\ Z_1 & Z_2 & Z_3 & Z_4 & \dots & Z_n \end{bmatrix} \begin{bmatrix} N_{1,\xi} & N_{1,\eta} & N_{1,\zeta} \\ N_{2,\xi} & N_{2,\eta} & N_{2,\zeta} \\ N_{3,\xi} & N_{3,\eta} & N_{3,\zeta} \\ N_{4,\xi} & N_{4,\eta} & N_{4,\zeta} \\ \vdots & \vdots & \vdots \\ N_{n,\xi} & N_{n,\eta} & N_{n,\zeta} \end{bmatrix} \quad (4.38)$$

For the case of linear elements, we calculate the strain at the center of the each element. In order to calculate the strain at the nodes, we average the strains from all the elements that contain that particular node.

References

[1] Axel, L. and Dougherty, L. (1989). Heart wall motion: Improved method of spatial modulation of magnetization for MR imaging. Radiology, 172(2):349–50.

[2] Barnard, D. and Alpert, J. (1987). Right ventricular function in health and disease. Curr Probl Cardiol, 12(7):422–29.

[3] Boxt, L. (1999). Radiology of the right ventricle. Radiologic Clinics of North America, 37(2):379–400.

[4] Chouabe, C., Espinosa, L., Megas, P., Chakir, A., Rougier, O., Freminet, A., and Bonvallet, R. (1997). Reduction of I(Ca,L) and I(to1) density in hypertrophied right ventricular cells by simulated high altitude in adult rats. J Molec and Cell Cardiology, 29(1):193–206.

[5] Czegledy, F. and J.Katz (1993). A new geometric description of the right ventricle. J Biomed Eng, 15:387–91.

[6] Haber, E., Metaxas, D., and Axel, L. (1998). Motion analysis of the right ventricle from MRI images. In Medical Image Computing and Computer-Assisted Intervention - MICCAI, pages 177–188, Cambridge, MA.

[7] Hurst, J. (1988). Atlas of the Heart. Gower Medical, New York.

[8] Kass, M., Witkins, A., and Terzopoulos, D. (1987). Snakes: active contour models. Int J Comput Vision, 1(4):321–31.

[9] Kerwin, W. and Prince, J. (1998). Cardiac material markers from tagged MR images. Medical Image Analysis, 2(4):339–53.

[10] McInerney, T. and Terzopoulos, D. (1996). Deformable models in medical image analysis: A survey. Medical Image Analysis, 1(2):91–108.

[11] Moulton, M., Cresswell, L., Downing, S., Actis, R., Szabo, B., Vannier, M., and Pasque, M. (1996). Spline surface interpolation for calculating 3-D ventricular strains from MRI tissue tagging. Am J Physiol, 39:H281–H297.

[12] Nielsen, P., Grice, I. L., Smaill, B., and Hunter, P. (1991). Mathematical model of geometry and fibrous structure of the heart. J Appl Physiol, 260:H1365–H1378.

[13] Noordegraaf, A., Marcus, J., Roseboom, B., Postmus, P., Faes, T., and de Vries, P. (1997). The effect of right ventricular hypertrophy on left ventricular ejection fraction in pulmonary emphysema. Chest, 112(3):640–45.

[14] Park, J. (1996). Model–based shape and motion analysis: Left ventricle of a heart. PhD thesis, University of Pennsylvania, Philadelphia.

[15] Park, J., Metaxas, D., and Axel, L. (1996). Analysis of left ventricular wall motion based on volumetric deformable models and MRI-SPAMM. Med Image Analysis, 1(1):53–71.

[16] Pirolo, J., Bresina, S., Creswell, L., Myers, K., Szabo, B., Vannier, M., and Pasque, M. (1993). Mathematical three-dimensional solid modeling of biventricular geometry. Annals of Biomed Eng, 21:199–219.

[17] Press, W., Teukolsky, S., Vetterling, W., and Flannery, B. (1992). *Numerical Recipes in C: The Art of Scientific Computing*. Cambridge University Press, Cambridge.

[18] Sacks, M., Chuong, C., Templeton, G., and Peshock, R. (1993). *In vivo* 3-D reconstruction and geometric characterization of the right ventricular free wall. Annals of Biomed Eng, 21:263–275.

[19] Spencer, A. (1980). Continuum Mechanics. Longman, London.

[20] Tsutsui, H., Tagawa, H., Kent, R., McCollam, P., Ishihara, K., Nagatsu, M., and 4th, G. C. (1994). Role of microtubules in contractile dysfunction of hypertrophied cardiocytes. Circulation, 90(1):533–55.

[21] Young, A. (1998). Model tags: Direct 3D tracking of heart wall motion from tagged MR images. In Medical Image Computing and Computer-Assisted Intervention - MICCAI, pages 92–101, Cambridge, MA.

[22] Young, A. and Axel, L. (1992). Three-dimensional motion and deformation of the heart wall: estimation with spatial modulation of magnetization - a model-based approach. Radiology, 185:241–47.

[23] Young, A., Fayad, Z., and Axel, L. (1996). Right ventricular mid-wall surface motion and deformation using magnetic resonance tagging. J Appl Physiol, 271(6):H2677–88.

[24] Zienkiewicz, O. and Taylor, R. (1989). The Finite Element Method. McGraw-Hill, New York, fourth edition.

Chapter 5

Motion Analysis of the Whole Heart

Cengizhan Ozturk
Bogazici University,
Institute of Biomedical Engineering,
80815 Bebek, Istanbul, Turkey
cozturk@boun.edu.tr

Elliot R. McVeigh
Laboratory of Cardiac Energetics, NHLBI,
Building 10, Room B1D416,
Bethesda, MD 20892-1061
mcveighe@zeus.nhlbi.nih.gov

5.1 Motivation and Background

In this chapter, we present a brief overview of our research on cardiac motion analysis. MRI of the whole heart, at an adequate temporal resolution, produces significant number of images. Over the past years, the main goals of cardiac MR research have been to develop not only faster and better pulse sequences, but also mathematical techniques and end-user software to analyze the ever-increasing number of images. In fact, one important reason that some of the cardiac MR techniques have not become a part of a routine cardiac examination is certainly the deficiency of appropriate analysis tools that can be used by clinicians.

One focus of our research is to analyze the motion of the heart as a whole, which encompasses the motion of all chambers. It might require the use of different imaging and analysis techniques, but the final aim is to attain a comprehensive analysis of the motion of the whole heart. This final goal remains to be achieved, but significant progress has been made on several fronts. In this chapter, we will present our research in two areas:

1) Development of a general motion field to depict simultaneously the motion of both ventricles.

A.A. Amini and J.L. Prince (eds.),
Measurement of Cardiac Deformations from MRI: Physical and Mathematical Models, 91–117.

2) Surface based analysis tools to describe the atrial motion.

The heart is routinely divided into four chambers, two atria and two ventricles, but there is a strong functional interdependence between all of them. This is the result of close anatomic and functional association: some are connected to others with valves that open during certain cardiac phases, others are encircled by common muscle fibers or enclosed fully or partly with a common pericardium. Independent increases in the volume of each of the four chamber shifts the pressure-volume relationship of the other three chambers upward and to the left in an isolated heart [1]. This close relationship is especially true between right and left ventricle, where it is believed that 20-40% of the right ventricular (RV) systolic pressure may result from left ventricular (LV) contraction and about 4-10% of the LV systolic pressure may result from RV contraction [2]. Although a significant portion of the common cardiac symptoms is ventricular in origin, coexistence of atrial pathologies might also play a role in the outcome in a significant portion of primarily ventricular diseases [3]. These chamber-to-chamber interactions are shown in various *in vitro* studies and known to be more significant *in vivo* when pericardium is intact and further increased in certain pathologies [4].

This chapter is organized as follows: In Section 5.2, some brief background on physiology and cardiac motion analysis is given, only to emphasize the clinical relevance and our motivation. In the last part of Section 5.2, we have included a short overview of our motion tracking technique for tagged MRI analysis. Section 5.3 contains information about our imaging and analysis methods. Although our ventricular and atrial motion fields are both 4D and B-spline based, there are significant methodological differences between them. A slightly detailed description of atrial motion tracking technique is given at the end of Section 5.3. Section 5.4 contains examples of biventricular motion tracking from three normal volunteers and results of an atrial motion tracking from one of them. This is followed by a discussion (Section 5.5) and a final summary (Section 5.6).

5.2 Introduction and Background

Magnetic resonance imaging (MRI) is a powerful noninvasive technique for mechanical analysis of the heart. We have mainly used cardiac-gated, fast gradient echo (FGRE) images of the heart, both for ventricular and atrial analysis. A specific MRI technique, *tagging* [5, 6], is used in the ventricular analysis while atrial analysis relies on surface based object registration. In the past, several methods have been used in the motion analysis of the left ventricle (LV) for tagged MRI (see [7, 8, 25] and Chapter 2) Our ventricular method allows us to examine right ventricle (RV) in addition to LV and our atrial technique presents the preliminary results of the first surface tracking method for the atria. In this section, we focus on the RV and atria, and do not provide a description of our LV analysis. Please refer to Chapters 3-4 and 6-8 for detailed descriptions on LV analysis.

This section is further subdivided for convenience: First, we briefly describe the relevant anatomy and physiology. Rather than to provide a comprehensive overview, our aim is to stress the unique features that make biventricular and atrial motion analysis difficult. The next section provides a brief overview of the imaging and mechanical analysis of the ventricles and atria. The third section reviews the studies that employed MRI for RV and atrial analysis. The last section gives a basic overview of our motion field fitting method with references to other similar 3D and 4D-motion field fitting techniques.

5.2.1 Anatomy and Physiology

Although several methods exist for the analysis of tagged MRI images of the left ventricle (LV), analysis of the right ventricle (RV) remains challenging due to its complex anatomy and significant through plane motion. The RV receives its deoxygenated blood from the right atrium and pumps it through the pulmonary artery into the lungs. The RV has relatively thin (3-5 mm) walls in comparison to the LV and partly wraps around the LV, forming a crescent shape in cross sections of the heart (see Figures 5.1 and 5.6). As a result, the RV has a large surface-area-to-volume ratio; small changes in the septum-to-free-wall displacement will cause a large volume displacement.

Not only is the geometry of the RV complex, but so is its contraction pattern. The ejection of blood from the RV is achieved by combined action of the RV free wall, septum, and conus. It is believed that the free wall contracts in a peristaltic fashion starting at the base and progressing to the apex. The conus, which is the outflow tract of the RV, contracts 30-50 ms after the rest of the RV [10, 11]. It is therefore considered to be a functionally different part, as also supported by its different embryological origin.

RV function can be altered by several conditions without or (more commonly) with varying degrees of LV pathology [12]. The RV appears to be relatively resistant to infarction and has a remarkable ability to recover even after a prolonged occlusion [13]. On the other hand, acute ischemia, pulmonary hypertension, and spill-over effects from chronic left heart diseases provide a complex variety of RV dynamics.

The atrial chambers serve as reservoirs and conduits for blood returning from the systemic and pulmonary circulation to the heart. In a normal sinus rhythm, the reservoir and conduit phases represent the majority of the atrio-ventricular flow volume. A "booster" pump activity arises from the atrial systole, which sends additional blood into the ventricular cavity at the end of diastole [14]. Most obvious reason for the pathologies of atrial shape and dynamics is valve dysfunction, these can be valvular stenosis or regurgitation or both. In addition, myocardial disorders are usually accompanied by diastolic dysfunction, which subsequently leads to increased atrial pressure and size. Increased size and depressed motion of the left atrium have been linked to increased risk of cardiogenic embolism and stroke [15]. Although ventricular diseases mostly cause the shape changes and alterations in the

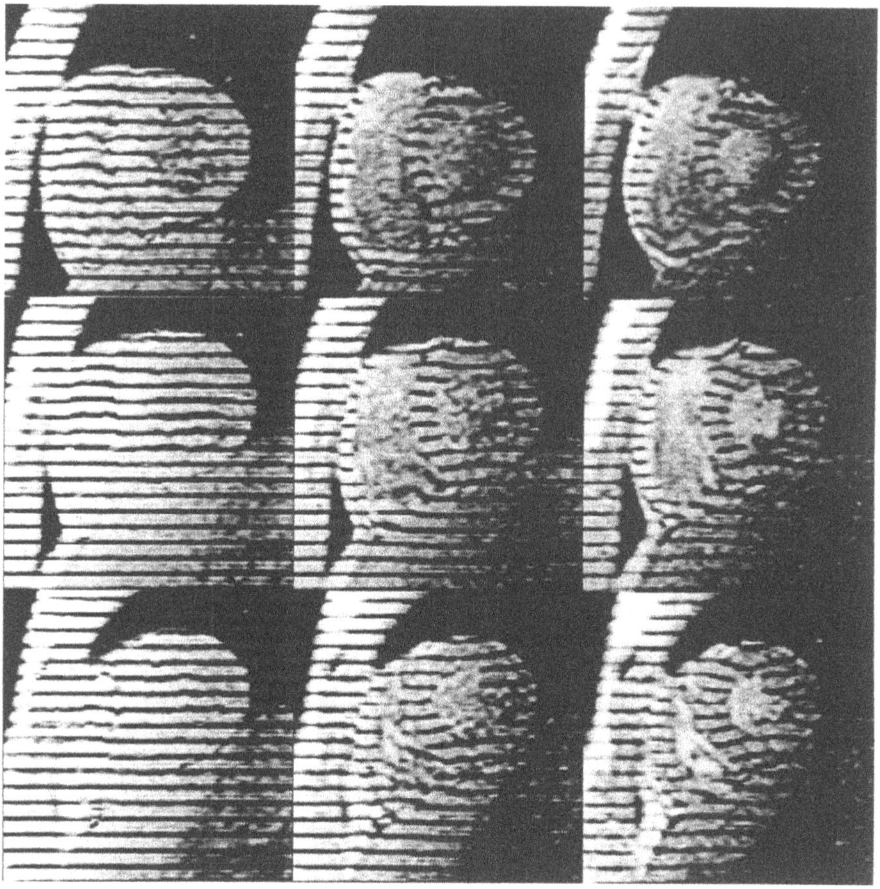

Figure 5.1: Sample tagged MRI images. Each row is taken from the same short axis image plane at end diastole (left column), mid systole (mid column) and end systole (right column). From top to bottom the 3 SA image planes are arranged from base to the apex of the heart.

dynamics of atrial function, there are also reported cases of idiopathic dilation of both atria. The usual presenting symptom of these patients is atrial fibrillation [16]. Atrial morphology is very dynamic; increased atrial size, one of the major risk factors for atrial fibrillation, has been shown to diminish with restoration of the sinus rhythm [17].

5.2.2 Studying Right Ventricular and Atrial Dynamics

Earlier studies of the RV have been restricted to the discrete measurements of the global dimensions or local segment lengths [11, 18]. On the other hand, different studies have urged caution in using a single or a few chord dimensions as a measure of global RV dynamics [19]. These discrete measures are also insensitive to local variations in ventricular function in normal and pathological cases. The 2D strain measurements were achieved on selected regions of the RV by using multiple markers [20,21]. These markers are usually designed for cine fluoroscopic [20] or ultrasonic imaging [21]. An extension of this approach had also been achieved using a 2D array of markers for the analysis of a relatively larger section of the RV free wall [22]. Although these studies are important in a laboratory setting, their invasive nature precludes them from routine clinical use.

Left atrial dynamics were first studied indirectly by observing the aortic root motion using echocardiography [23]. In those studies, the aortic root motion correlated well with the expected changes in left atrial volume during the cardiac cycle both in the normal subjects and in patients with heart disease. Examination of right atrial wall motion using sub-costal M-mode echocardiography has been shown to be an effective method of discriminating various types of arrhythmias when the P-waves are hidden or flat on standard electrocardiograms [24]. This is especially helpful in the follow-up and evaluation of certain pacemakers. In a more detailed study, which also included patients with tachyarrhythmias and atrial flutter, it has been concluded that recording of atrial wall motion provides information which is otherwise available only by esophageal ECG or by invasive means [25].

In another study, the left atrial shape and wall changes have been found to be significantly different in the permanent ventricular pacing group in comparison to the atrial and sequential paced group [26]. It is proposed that enlargement of left atrium and a decrease in its contraction might account for the increased predisposition to embolic events for the ventricular only paced cases. Left atrial wall motion abnormalities have also been shown for systemic hypertension [27] and left ventricular diastolic dysfunction [28]. In heart transplant patients it has been discovered that atrial abnormalities represent a major contributing factor to altered mitral and pulmonary venous flow patterns [29].

5.2.3 MR Imaging of Right Ventricular and Atrial Function

Advantages of MRI are high spatial resolution, excellent soft tissue contrast, intrinsic 3D acquisition and absence of ionizing radiation. It has been previously shown that the RV volume can be measured reliably using MRI in spite of its complex geometry [30]. Although some attempts are made to quantify the RV function using cine imaging and local surface properties like curvature [31], most of the current research revolves around a special MR imaging technique, known as MR tagging. MR imaging is based on selectively disturbing tissue magnetization in a high magnetic field and observing the subsequent inductive effects. Tags are voids in the regular MRI images created by spatially selective presaturation pulses. These move with the tissue and provide temporary internal fiducial markers (see Figure 5.1).

MR tagging has been applied to the RV to track a midwall surface motion based on a finite element model using both the tag and contour information [32]. In a different approach, only the intersection points of a tagging grid have been tracked in 2D and subsequent changes of the distance between them have been evaluated [33]. In a similar study, the feature points have been defined as the tag points at mid RV wall and percent change in segmental length has been calculated over the heart cycle [34]. Although several methods exist for the LV [7, 8], no motion field fitting method has been previously implemented for RV.

As it was noted in the previous section, there is a wide spectrum of clinical cases where detailed analysis of the atrial dynamics can be beneficial. In the past, these studies have been restricted to 1D or 2D due to intrinsic limitations of the conventional ultrasound. On the other hand, although increasingly utilized in ventricular mechanical analysis, MRI has not been used fully in studying the atrial dynamics. Use of MRI has been widely accepted for congenital diseases [35], which could contain some of the most severe pathologies of the atria. Excluding these, there are few studies that investigated the normal atrial function and even fewer studies that included patients. There have been several studies that investigated atrial dynamics in the presence of different valve diseases [36–38]. Examining valve pathologies is well established using echocardiography, so for most of the cases, an additional MRI exam is not justified for the diagnosis of valve pathology, but it might come "free" during a cardiac MRI exam done for another purpose. Our focus here is to measure the normal dynamics of the atrium rather than those occurring in valve disease.

It was shown some time ago that all chamber volumes of the heart can be studied reliably using *cine* MRI [39]. Studies done by Jarvinen et al. [14, 40–42] provided the first comprehensive series that systematically dealt with the atrial dynamics. In the first study [40], which used cadaveric atrial casts and normal volunteers, it was shown that right atrial volumes can be measured reliably using MRI. A similar conclusion was reached about the left atrium in a subsequent study [14]. The same group later correlated selected 2D area measurements with 3D volume calculations for the left atrium [41] and found that the specificity of area based analysis was 92% and the sensitivity was 65% in identifying atrial shape and contractile disturbances in individual patients. They still preferred the 3D method for atrial conduit and stroke volume calculations.

In terms of atrial motion analysis in the cardiac patient population, right and left atrial phasic volumetric changes have been assessed in mildly symptomatic dilated and hypertrophic cardiomyopathy. Filling and emptying rates of either atrium were found to be decreased in both pathologies [42]. In another study, atrial function has been assessed in patients with transplanted hearts [43]; the atrial filling and emptying rates were found to be lower, reservoir and conduit volumes were larger and minimal volumes were much larger in the transplant patients in comparison to the normal group. In patients with myocardial infarction (14 patients, no valve disease, in sinus rhythm), left atrial end-diastolic and systolic volumes were higher, emptying fraction was lower, right atrial end-diastolic volume were higher, and emptying fraction was lower than those in the control group [43].

In all of these studies, the atrial dynamics were studied using global indices calculated from volumes that were derived from image plane contours. We believe that local mechanical analysis would provide further insight into the pathophysiology of some of the atrial diseases. Calculation of local mechanical properties requires both fast imaging pulse sequences with adequate spatial resolution, as well as computational methods for registering material points in subsequent time frames using surface matching techniques. Fortunately, over the past few years significant advances have been made on both fronts, enabling us to calculate a parametric motion field that can be used to track surface points on the atria over time.

5.2.4 B-Spline based Motion Tracking

B-splines are piecewise polynomial functions that can describe both scalar and vector fields of higher dimensions as tensor products (e.g., 2D for the image plane, 3D for a volume-of-interest, or 4D for the space-time continuum). They are widely used in computer graphics for curve and surface representations [44], and they have several very useful properties including parametric continuity, compact representation of the information, local support, and differentiability [44, 45].

B-spline based methods have been previously used in the analysis of cardiac MR images to describe the *tag* lines and planes. Moulton et al. [46] utilized them to describe the deformed tag planes as surfaces; and in the first approach of Amini et al. [3, 47], tags were segmented using a two-dimensional coupled B-snake grid. They later provided a general framework for the extension of their approach to a 4D B-spline based analysis for left ventricular motion [1, 50].

The observed tag deformation at a tag point contains information only about one component of its past motion, from tagging to imaging time [51]. In order to achieve a full 3D tracking of any point through time, the information coming from different tagging sets must be combined and interpolated in space and time.

As a brief summary, in our approach we go through the following steps in order to obtain a final motion field:

a) From the detected tag points, 1D deformation samples are collected for each image.

b) Two 1D, B-spline displacement fields are computed at every short axis (SA) image for the two tagging directions.

c) Through-plane motion information is derived and incorporated from long axis (LA) images as follows. First, a displacement field is fit at each of the LA slices. Then, these fields are evaluated at the LA-SA intersection lines. Finally, a through-plane displacement field is fit for each SA image plane.

d) The matching reference position of each tag point at tagging time is computed using the two SA displacement fields (from step b) and the through-plane displacement field (from step c).

e) A forward motion field is computed that maps these reference points from tagging time to their deformed locations.

f) After repeating steps (a)–(e) for each time frame, a time smoothing is done to the motion parameters to achieve a final 4D B-spline based motion description.

We then represent the final cardiac motion field for a volume of interest that encompasses RV and LV as:

$$\phi(\mathbf{P}, t) = \sum_{u,v,w,t} B_u(x)B_v(y)B_w(z)B_t(t) \cdot \mathbf{C}_{u,v,w,t}. \tag{5.1}$$

In this equation, the displacements for a given material point $\mathbf{P}(x, y, z)$ are obtained by summing over the 4D tensor product of the basis functions B and control points $\mathbf{C}$. Basis functions for a given location can be computed once a control point density is chosen using a standard iterative formula [44]. The result of this motion field is a vector pointing to the new location from the material point $\mathbf{P}$. Further details of this algorithm were previously presented [51]; it has been validated *in vivo* [52] and compared with other methods for the LV [53].

The motion of the atria is described using two additional four-dimensional B-spline deformation fields separately computed for each atrium. Earlier, we provided a brief overview of the computation of a four-dimensional motion field for tagged MRI. Unfortunately, this cannot be used for the atria due to its thin walls making MR tagging impossible. Therefore, the correspondence problem has been solved by a surface matching technique that uses both physical closeness of candidate points and similarity of local surface properties (see Section 5.3.4).

5.3 Methods

5.3.1 MR Imaging

Tagged MR images were acquired from three normal human volunteers using a cardiac gated and breath-hold gradient echo sequence, with partial k-space acquisition and no echo-sharing or interpolation, in a 1.5 T GE cardiac scanner. Subjects' ages were 24, 26 and 32 (two male and one female) and their heart rates were 65, 53, and 70 beats per minute, respectively. After determining the long axis of the heart, 8–10 parallel cine short axis (SA) images of the heart were acquired with two sets of orthogonal planar tags. Next, 9 long axis (LA) images were acquired, perpendicular to the SA images, every 20 degrees around the LV center. For all LA images, the tags were arranged in such a way that their displacements provided motion information orthogonal to SA images. Other MR imaging parameters employed in this study were as follows: TR = 3.3 ms, TE = 1.2 ms, flip angle = 12°,

160 frequency encoding steps, 120 phase encoding steps, field of view = 32 cm, slice thickness 8 mm, 8 phase encoding steps per cardiac phase (NVP), tag spacing = 7.5 mm (6 pixels). The first 11–15 time frames within systole comprising 8–10 SA slices and 9 LA slices were chosen for subsequent motion analysis. The average time resolution was 30 ms, and the first time frame was approximately 40 ms after the tagging.

For the atrial analysis, separate sets of cardiac gated, fast spin echo (FSE) and fast gradient echo (FGRE) MRI images were acquired from one of the subjects. FSE images provided a high contrast black blood images at a mid-diastolic phase. For the same image planes, cardiac gated *cine* images were acquired, giving different atrial phases for the same imaging planes. For the right atrium, a stack of FSE images are shown in Figure 5.2. FGRE images for a selection of slices are shown in Figure 5.3.

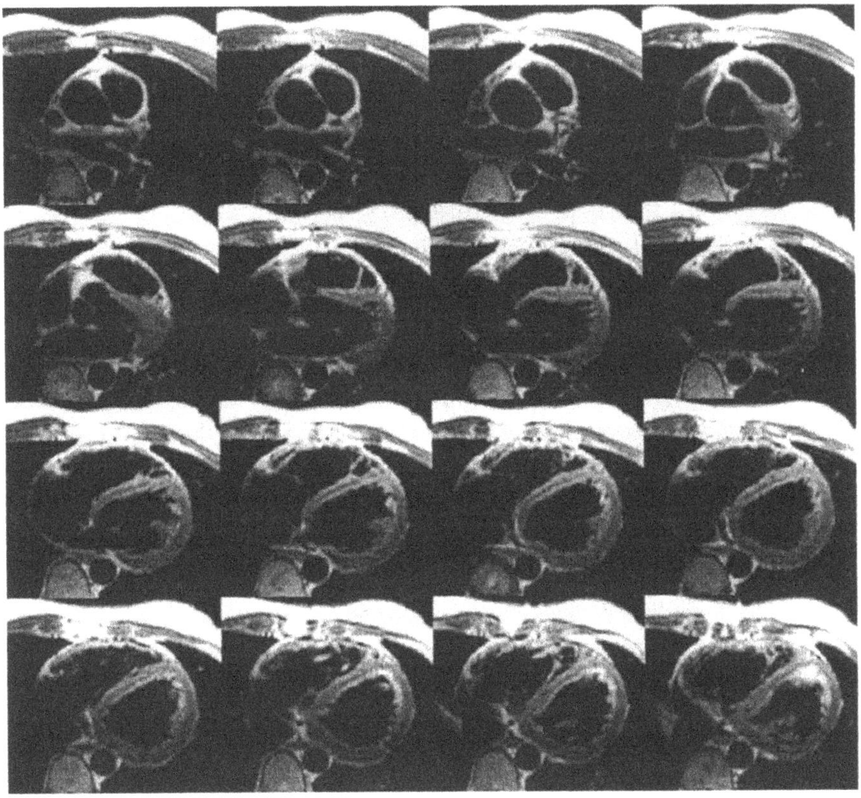

Figure 5.2: A set of contiguous FSE images to be used for right atrium template generation. Top left is the most superior slice, moving inferior left-to-right and down.

The imaging planes for the right atrium (RA) were prescribed graphically using the centers of inferior and superior vena cava. This is essentially very close to a

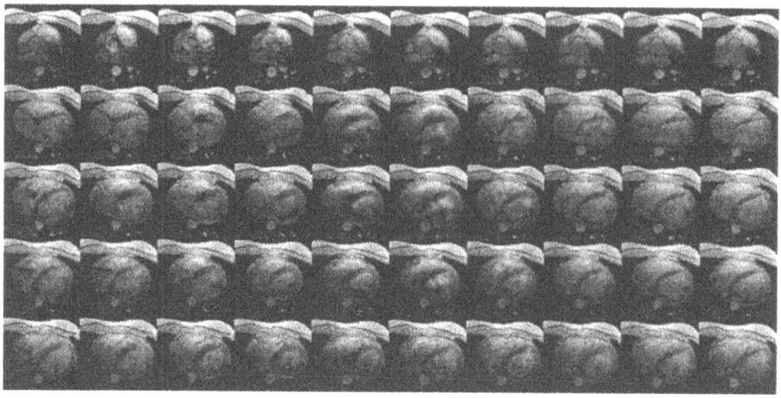

Figure 5.3: Five sample slices of *cine* FGRE images for the right atrium. Each row displays the same slice over the heart cycle at selected phases. At the top, the slices start at the superior vena cava, and moves towards inferior vena cava. Ten phases are chosen at equal intervals over the heart cycle.

true axial acquisition. This gave a better depiction of anatomy and greater white blood contrast than the simple extension of basal short axis imaging planes for ventricular tagging to cover the atria. On the other hand, standard sagittal imaging planes were adequate for the left atrium. Sample FSE and FGRE images for left atrium are given in Figures 5.4 and 5.5, respectively.

The imaging parameters for the FSE acquisitions were: cardiac gated, separate breath-hold for each slice, flow comp on, blood suppression on, Auto TI, TE = 68ms, TR = 2RR, flip angle = 13 degrees, BW = 62.5kHz, ETL = 16, a 256 $\times$ 128 matrix, 5mm slice thickness, and a field-of-view = 32 cm. The imaging parameters for the fast gradient echo (FGRE) images were: cardiac gated, separate breath hold for each slice, 27 phases with time resolution of 50 ms, no view sharing, multi-echo acquisition with ETL = 4 and VPS = 8, field-of-view = 30cm, 256 $\times$ 160 matrix, slice thickness = 8mm, flip angle = 10 degrees, and BW = 125kHz.

5.3.2 Ventricular Motion Analysis

Following myocardial and tag segmentation, a 4D B-spline based parametric motion field was computed for a volume of interest encompassing both ventricles, as overviewed in section 5.2.4. In this study, control point densities of 8x8 and 7x7x7 were employed for the inverse and forward fields respectively. The cardiac region of interest was roughly 100 x 100 x 80 mm for each case. A final time smoothing was done using a number of control points equal to roughly 50% of the number of cardiac phases.

Separate B-spline surface representations were computed for LV and RV surfaces. Although these were not used for the displacement field calculations, they

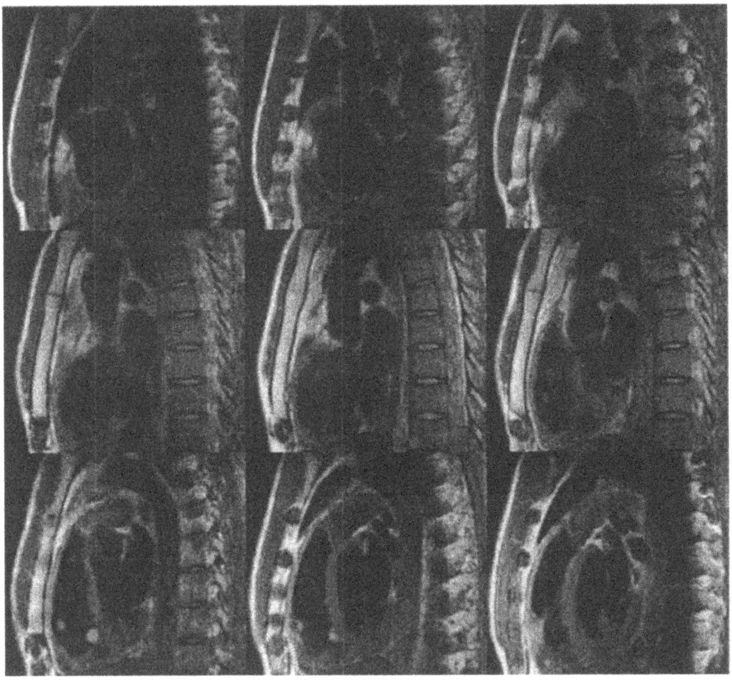

Figure 5.4: Sample sagittal FSE images for the left atrium arranged row by row from top to bottom, starting from left and moving towards right side.

provided an excellent way of presenting the results. Using the motion field, 3D displacements and strains were calculated at the RV and LV mid-wall surfaces (see Figure 5.6). The circumferential strain (E_{cc}) is commonly used for the analysis of LV function. Both for RV and LV, we chose the E_{cc} direction to be tangential to the midwall surface and parallel to the short axis image plane.

5.3.3 Atrial Surface Fitting

The first step in atrial motion analysis is to create templates for each atrium. The surface fitting described below is essentially the same as that used in the ventricles, except that the coordinate system is local for both atria. This can be converted easily to the scanner coordinate system for a combined motion display.

Atrial templates are generated by contouring the individual slices of the FSE images, and subsequently fitting a 2D surface B-spline (see Figure 5.7). The 2D-tensor product of a B-spline surface representing the inner wall of the atrium can be written as:

$$A = \sum_u \sum_v B_u(\ell) B_v(z) \cdot \mathbf{C}_{u,v} \, . \tag{5.2}$$

In the above equation, B represents the B-spline basis function and C is a 3D

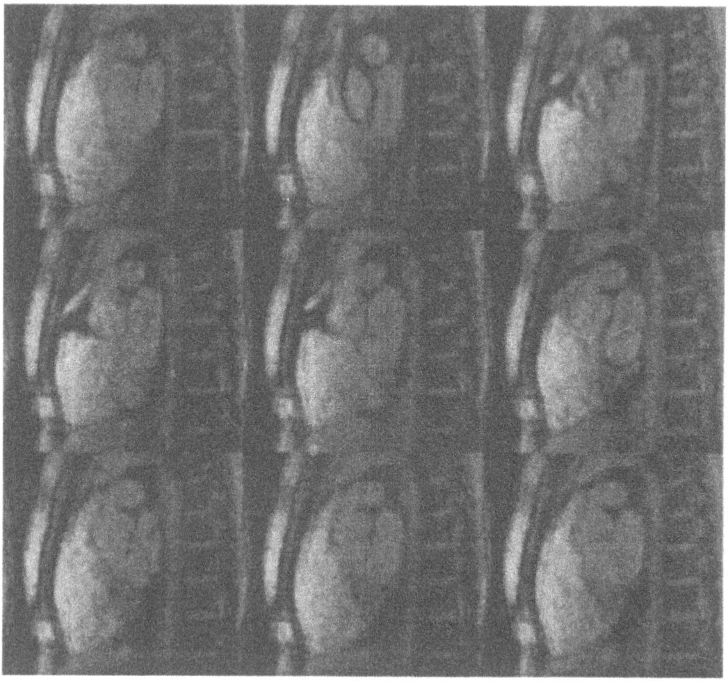

Figure 5.5: Time evolution of a single slice for the left atrium.

surface control point. The summation is carried out over the 2D-tensor product of basis functions. The surface is designated with two parameters: z and ℓ. z is the parameterization perpendicular to the imaging planes, so every contour point in an image plane has the same z value. The second parameter ℓ is a chord length parameterization along the contours:

$$\ell(k) = \frac{\sum_{i=2}^{k} \|P_i - P_{i-1}\|}{\sum_{i=2}^{n+1} \|P_i - P_{i-1}\|} \qquad \text{for } 1 < k \leq n\,, \tag{5.3}$$

where k is an index of points along the contours and n is the total number of points in a given contour line. This makes the denominator of (5.3) equal to the total length of the curve for each slice. For the initial point, $\ell(1) = 0$. We have to also make sure to incorporate circularity in the angular direction; i.e., the point $n+1$ is the same as the first point.

Periodicity must also be considered when calculating the basis function at a particular location. To prevent twisting of the closed surfaces, the chord length parameterization of subsequent slices must be adjusted to compensate for the in-plane shift of the starting point. All the contours must be contoured either clockwise

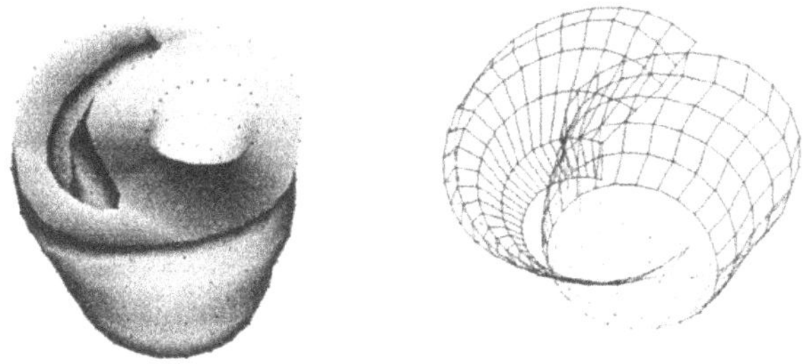

Figure 5.6: An example of RV-LV surface model generated from MRI images. **(Right)** Corresponding RV-LV midwall surface mesh, which is used in the calculation of the E_{CC} strain values (oriented slightly differently for better visualization). **(Left)** Shading comes from regular light sources and has no other significance.

or counter-clockwise. At the end, for a given choice of control point density, the control points are found by least square minimization. We employed a similar approach in the past for ventricular surface fitting [51].

Once the parametric atrial surface is found, it is sampled homogeneously giving a relatively dense mesh. This mesh is then transferred to the *cine* image set and adjusted for each time frame to correctly segment underlying anatomy. A second surface fitting and smoothing is done following the interactive refinement of the template. This decreases the variability of the adjusted surfaces among different operators.

The parametric surfaces can be used to directly calculate some of the local surface properties, like surface normal, at every location. On the other hand, they cannot be used to follow the trajectory for the points on the atrial wall, because due to the nature of their parameterization, all points will stay at the same z level. In other words there is no through-plane motion. However, these surfaces are adequate in calculating global shape changes and volumes. Now, we are ready to address the material point-tracking problem of the atria by a combined motion field fitting and point matching technique.

5.3.4 Calculation of the Atrial Motion Field

We employed a four-dimensional, tensor-product of B-splines motion field to transform the volume of interest (which encompasses the atrial surface) from the first time frame to the later time frames. This motion field is described mathematically as follows:

$$T : \mathbb{R}^3 \times \mathbb{R} \rightarrow \mathbb{R}^3,$$

$$T(\mathbf{P}, k) = \sum_{u,v,w,t} B_u(x) B_v(y) B_w(z) B_k(k) \cdot \mathbf{C}_{u,v,w,k} \,. \tag{5.4}$$

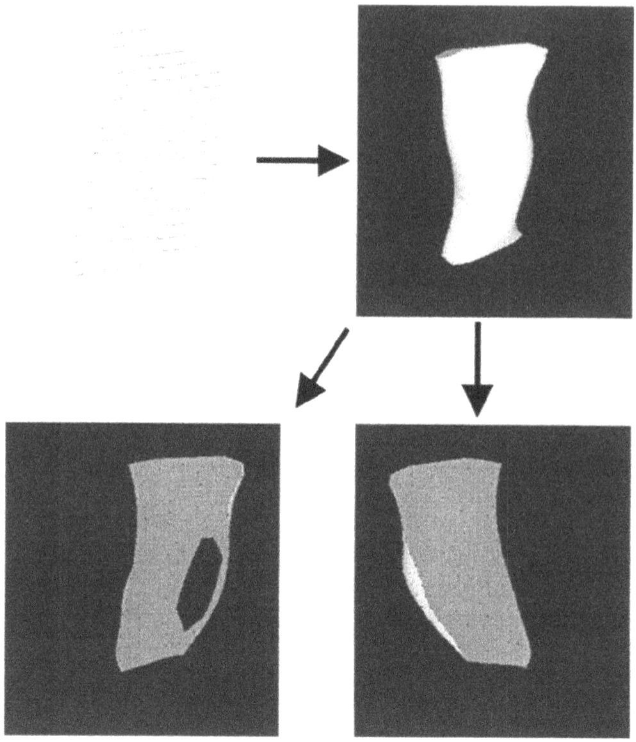

Figure 5.7: **(Top Left)** A sample of contours drawn on FSE images. **(Top Right):** B-spline surface corresponding to these contours (oriented slightly differently). **(Bottom Left):** Posterior half of RA. (Bottom Right) Anterior half of RA. For orientation see text [section 5.4.2]

In this equation, the sum for a given material is done over the 4D-tensor product of basis functions and control points. The 1D basis function for a given location is calculated using the standard iterative formula, given the knot sequence and the degree of the B-spline [45]. We employed quadratic B splines and chosen a knot sequence of 6 by 6 by 6 by 12. Please note that the result of this motion field for a given point P is the coordinates of the new location P^k at time k. (We prefer to use k for time to avoid confusion with the transformation T.) This motion field representation is slightly different from our previous implementations for tagged MRI analysis, where a similar field was used to describe the displacement field. In that implementation the result of the motion field was a 3D vector pointing from the original point to the new location [52].

In order to select the best parameters we use a least-squares criterion, which tries to minimize an error function between the transformed points of the first set and the corresponding points of the later time frames. The corresponding points at later time frames are selected iteratively based on their closeness in a 6 dimensional space which includes — in addition to the regular 3 space components — 3 more dimensions coming from the surface normal at each point. The distance between two points in this space can be thought of as a weighted sum with two components: the first part is the residual Euclidean distance between matching points and the second component is the length of the difference vector of the two surface normals at those locations:

$$E = \sum_{k=1}^{k_{max}} \sum_{i=1}^{n_K} \left(\alpha \cdot \|Q_{i,k}\left(T(\mathbf{P}_i, k)\right) - T(\mathbf{P}_i, k)\| + (1-\alpha) \cdot \left\|\mathbf{n}_{\mathbf{P}_i} - \mathbf{n}_{Q_{i,k}}\right\|\right) . \tag{5.5}$$

In this equation, $\|v\|$ is the L^2 norm (=length) of a vector v, n_k is the total number of points that are reliably matched for the time frame k, and $Q_{i,k}$ is the "closest" point among the points of time k to the transformed point P_i (see the pseudo-algorithm of iterative closest point matching below). The coordinates are normalized so that the coordinates of the points and of the vectors are between -1 and 1. The weighting factor α has been determined empirically. The initial match between transformed first time frame points and points at a later time frame are assigned by their physical closeness. A fast k-D tree search was implemented for quick point matching. In the past, a similar distance metric was successfully implemented for matching endocardial and epicardial points of the left ventricle in a gated-SPECT image sequence using a planispheric coordinate system [54].

The optimization is done using the iterative closest point approach; for each time frame k a simple flow diagram is as follows:

1) Start with an initial transformation T (unitary transform or previous time frame's final T).

2) Find the closest points Q_k to the transformed points $T(P^1)$.

3) Calculate the best T (best set of B-spline control points) which describes a motion from the first time point locations (P^1) to the matched point locations (Q_k).

4) Calculate the error function and check the finishing criterion.

5) Go to step 2.

The finishing criterion is either:

1) No decreases in the error function.

2) No significant change in the calculated control point parameters.

Equations (5.3) and (5.4) are defined for the whole space, but the information we have is limited to the points on the atrial surfaces. Therefore, an additional smoothing term for the control point parameters is necessary when calculating the control points in Step 3).

5.4 Results

5.4.1 Motion Analysis of Right and Left Ventricles

The circumferential strain (E_{cc}) is commonly used in the analysis of the LV [53,55]. For both the RV and LV, we chose the E_{cc} direction to be tangential to the surface and parallel to the short axis image plane. In this paper, the time course of E_{cc} was examined for mid-myocardial surfaces of both the RV and LV for three normal human volunteers. In Figure 5.8, these are shown for the LV in an 8 by 12 arrangement of time-strain plots. Each row represents a short axial cut through the LV. Moving along the rows is equivalent to clockwise rotation on the LV when viewed from apex to base. The right column of the graph is essentially connected to the left column.

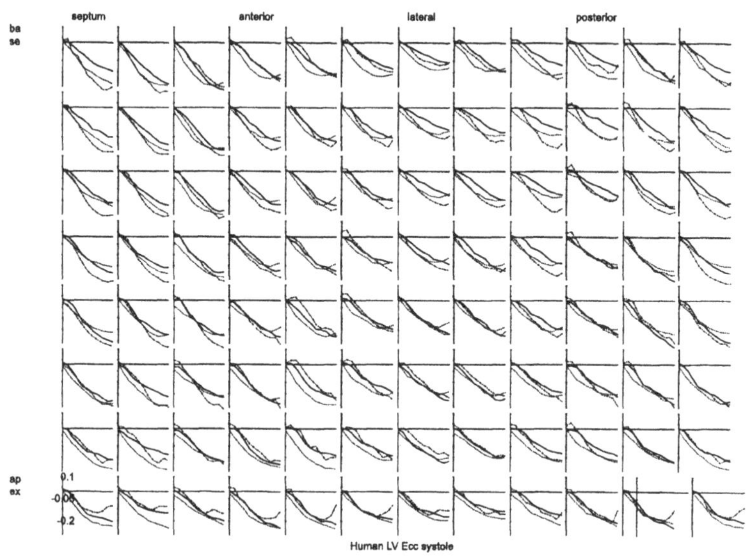

Figure 5.8: Circumferential strain values (E_{CC}) of three normal human volunteers for the left ventricle. Each row represents a short axis slice of the LV; it starts at septum and travels clockwise when it is viewed from apex of the heart toward its base. Time (x-axis) is normalized for different systolic intervals of each subject.

For the LV of three subjects, the mean end-diastolic and end-systolic circumferential strain difference (ΔE_{cc}) values were -0.22 ± 0.04, -0.22 ±0.03 and –0.28 ± 0.03. Everywhere on the LV, the time evolution of the strain showed a linear progression. For each subject, the spatial heterogeneity of E_{cc} over the LV was evaluated using its coefficient of variation (CV):

$$\text{C.V. } (\%) = \frac{(\text{standard deviation of } \Delta E_{cc})}{(\text{mean } \Delta E_{cc})},$$

where the standard deviation is evaluated over the whole LV surface for each subject (or over the RV surface below). The C.V. values of the ΔE_{cc} for the LV were 19%, 14%, and 13% for the three subjects.

The spatial distribution and time evolution of the RV circumferential strain is shown in Figure 5.9. Here, as in Figure 5.8, the columns are arranged in clockwise direction (from posterior through free wall ending in anterior RV). Unlike Figure 5.8, the first and last columns are not connected, but instead form the two attachment sides of the RV to the LV. For the RV free wall, we found ΔE_{cc} values of -0.17 ± 0.03, -0.17 ± 0.06, and -0.21 ± 0.05, with coefficient of variability (C.V.) values of 19%, 34%, and 24%, respectively. When we eliminate two slices, one from the base and one from the apex, the C.V. improves slightly to 18%, 21%, and 21%, respectively.

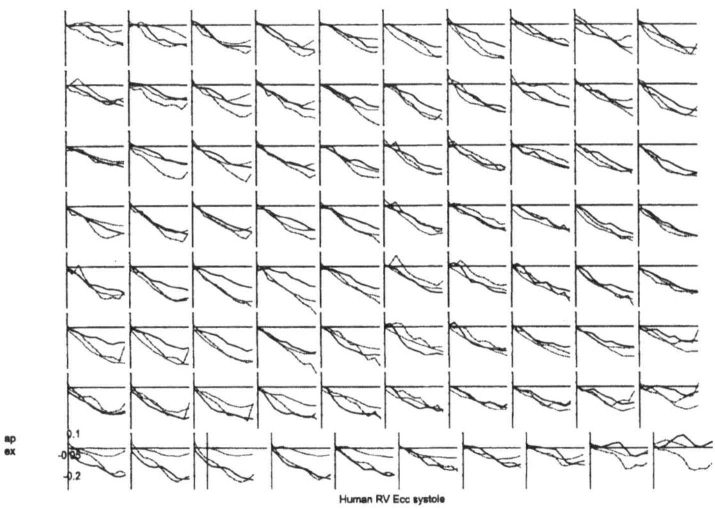

Figure 5.9: Circumferential strain values (E_{cc}) of three normal human volunteers for the right ventricle. Each row represents a short axis slice of the RV; it starts at posterior attachment and travels clockwise toward the anterior attachment when it is viewed from apex of the heart toward its base. X-axis is the time, normalized for different heart rates.

5.4.2 Motion Analysis of Atria

The right atrium displayed different patterns of motion depending on location. The time evolution of total displacement values at selected locations is shown in Figure 5.10. At several locations the dual motion pattern of the atrium is quite visible. The first prominent component is due to the passive movement arising from the ventricular contraction followed by the active atrial systole.

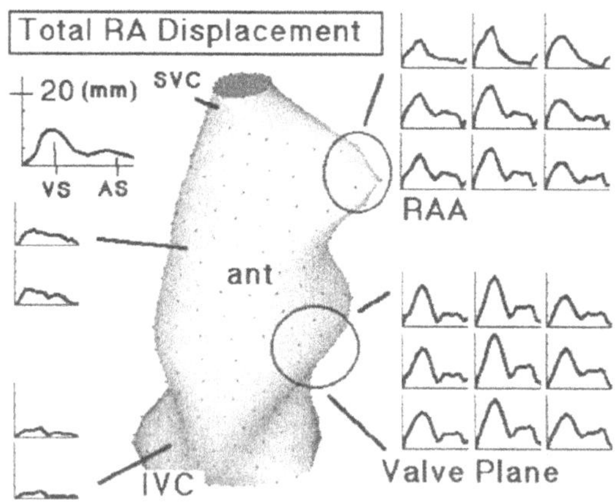

Figure 5.10: A spectrum of right atrial motion patterns. Total displacement values are shown for selected locations over the full heart cycle. **RAA**: right atrial appendage, **IVC**: inferior vena cava, **SVC**: superior vena cava, **ant**: anterior wall of RA, **VS**: ventricular systole, **AS**: atrial systole.

For a more detailed visualization, the right atrium is cut in half approximately in a coronal plane (see Figure 5.7). In Figures 5.11 and 5.12, the 3D trajectories of atrial surface points are shown separately for the anterior and posterior halves of the surface, respectively. The anterior half is observed from a posterior vantage looking at the inside of RA anterior surface. In this perspective, the left part of the surface is the lateral wall of RA and the hole corresponds to the tricuspid valve. The posterior half of right atrium is displayed so that the trajectories will be observed from an anterior vantage looking towards the inside of the RA posterior surface. In this case, the lateral wall of the RA is on the right side, and the inter-atrial septum is on the left side.

We analyzed the central part of the left atrium between the pulmonary vein origins. The shape and motion of the left atrium were found to be much less complex than the RA, but there was still a significant inter-regional difference in motion (see Figure 5.13). It displayed the greatest motion in the anterior and inferior walls. We did not observe any significant through-plane (right-to-left) motion.

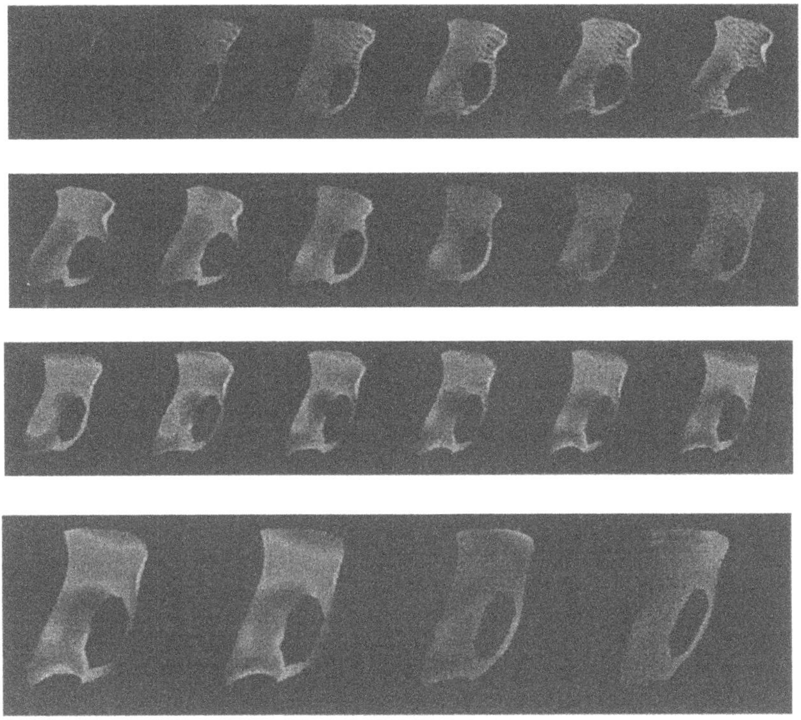

Figure 5.11: **(Top Row)** Right atrial anterior section's motion during ventricular systole. **(Second Row)** Early diastole. **(Third Row)** Mid diastole. **(Bottom Row)** Atrial systole. In Figures 5.11 and 5.12, for all images, the surface color-coding represents the total Euclidean displacement from the initial time frame. The lines are trajectories of the points from the start of each row. The last image of the previous row is the same as the first image of the subsequent row. See color Plate 2.

5.5 Discussion

The results for the LV show expected homogeneity and pattern within the range that was shown before for normal volunteers [55]. For the RV, the individual values and time courses of E_{cc} did not vary significantly over the ventricle. There is a slight trend of increased E_{cc} at the free wall in comparison to the RV attachment sites. Also, the lower variability after eliminating the top and bottom slices suggest that RV free wall behaves more homogeneously than the rest of the RV. There may be several factors involved, some of which are:

1) Rapid changes of the fiber structure and surface at the apical parts of the RV,

2) Increased trabeculation especially at the apical locations,

3) Interactions from the LV at the attachment sites.

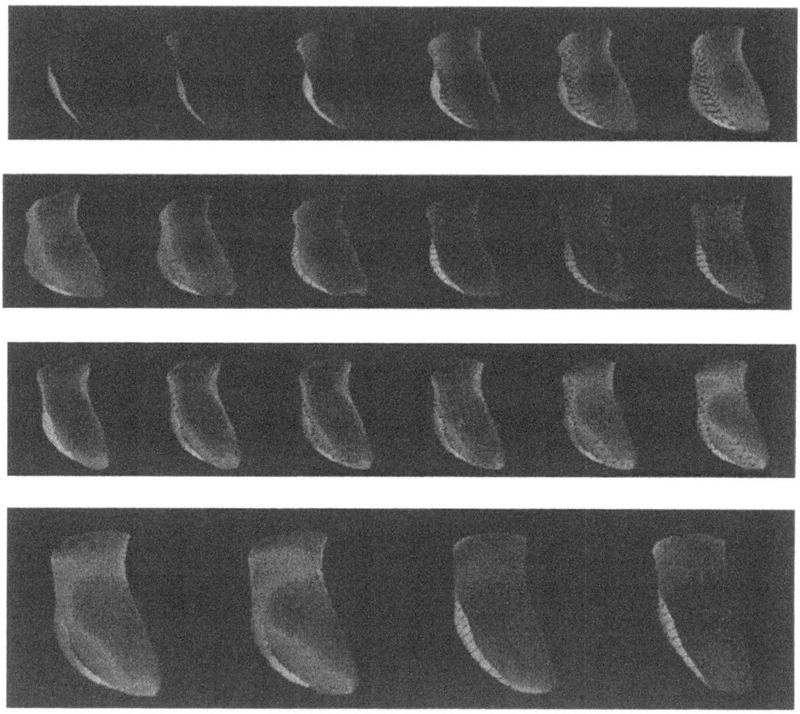

Figure 5.12: **(Top Row)** Right Atrium Posterior Section's motion during ventricular systole. **(Second Row)** Early diastole. **(Third Row)** Mid diastole. **(Bottom Row)** Atrial systole. For further infofmation see the caption of Figure 5.11. See color Plate 3.

The coefficient of variation (C.V.) values for ΔE_{cc} provided a good measure of synchrony.

For ventricular analysis, we have used the difference of E_{cc} (strain range) between two time frames in our analysis. If abnormal initial stretch had been present, this parameter would have been more sensitive for picking ventricular asynchrony — e.g., in pathologies of cardiac electrical conduction or during pacing. Also, note that this parameter is very closely associated with strain rate.

Circumferential strain values are calculated using the 4D-motion field, but the calculated E_{cc} values are evaluated in 2D image planes. These values are in good agreement with previously calculated values from the literature [34, 56]. The small differences from these studies can be due to several factors:

1) We calculate the strains in true material points as we track them over time,

2) We do not use RV contour/area centroids for the determination of the circumferential direction; we only use local surface properties.

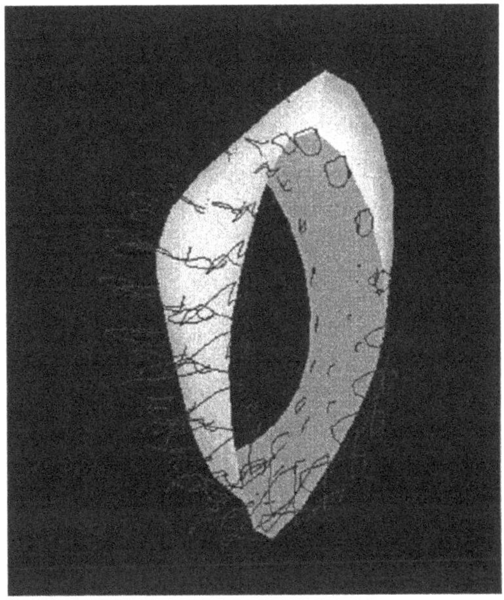

Figure 5.13: Left atrium, looking left to right. The anterior wall is on the left side. The mitral valve has not been carved out. The red lines are trajectories of selected atrial material points over the full heart cycle.

Our field fitting approach provides a practical solution for tracking the RV in addition to the LV. An important implementation area of the noninvasive RV dynamics research is congenital malformations [57, 58]. Only a "model free" approach, such as the one used in this paper, can be of any use in assessing the disease progress for highly variable RV geometry and dynamics found in congenital heart pathologies.

Segmentation is currently the most time consuming part of our analysis, taking approximately 120 minutes for a midsize atrial dataset (27 phases, 15 slices). The ventricular analysis requires segmentation of endocardial and epicardial contours of both ventricles and subsequent tag detection, which could take the same amount of time. The motion field fitting for tagged analysis and atrial surface tracking takes 15 minutes each on a desktop PC.

We have used FSE image sets to generate our first surface templates of both atria. These were later transferred to the *cine* FGRE image sets and fine-tuned. The remaining images of both atria are segmented using interactive, template-based segmentation starting at the corresponding time frame and proceeding towards both time directions [59]. In this approach, time interpolation techniques can be employed where the motion of the atria is diminished or regular. Only minor manual adjustment of the surface was necessary for this dataset when five key frames were segmented carefully and the rest is constructed via interpolation. Once a template is generated, it can be used on subsequent imaging of the same or even different subject; making the FSE set unnecessary and saving a significant amount of imaging time.

For both atria, the displacement values showed high spatial variability. During ventricular systole, the right atrial appendage (RAA), the anterior wall and the valve plane of right atrium showed the most displacement. Significant through plane motion was present in axial slices for RA. The time resolution used here ($\sim$50 ms) was found to be adequate to capture the full atrial dynamics including atrial systole.

We have previously validated our motion tracking algorithm *in vivo* for the left ventricle of a normal healthy volunteer [50]. In that study, the mean tracking error of selected points stayed less than the image resolution at all times. We expect our technique to perform equally well for the RV; this is supported by the consistent circumferential strain values. Strain values in other directions showed less consistency for the RV, and even less than LV (results not shown here). We have also applied our technique to a variety of human and canine hearts as part of a study comparing different cardiac motion analysis techniques [53]. Our technique displayed a nice balance of noise robustness and spatial resolution.

We have not yet provided a validation for our atrial surface tracking algorithm. There is no other noninvasive method available to track atrial points with the same coverage and SNR provided by MRI. Invasive studies and markers will change the normal dynamics of atria dramatically. Unlike ventricular tracking where material points are tagged magnetically, our surface tracking method infers material properties from physical closeness and surface properties. Therefore, atrial surface tracking relies heavily on its model of correspondence assignment, which is represented by various parameters in its error function (Eq. 5.5). We believe that the intrinsic smoothness of B-spline functions and the careful balance of surface and distance properties provide us a solution that is very close to the real one.

A noninvasive method of atrial wall motion analysis, such as the one presented here, could provide additional information to predict when a particular atrial shape change is prone to atrial fibrillation or a particular atrial arrhythmia is inclined to thrombo-embolic events [60]. Previous studies with ultrasound failed to show any consistent findings, but this can be attributed to the limitation of the analysis to 2D [15]. On the other hand, clinical use of our atrial analysis during atrial fibrillation is limited due to multiple beat averaging difficulties.

5.6 Conclusion

Tagged MRI with our new motion field analysis gave consistent RV circumferential strain results. The spatial coefficient of variation for E_{cc} provided a good parameter for the right and left ventricular synchrony. Tagged MRI based RV mechanical analysis can be used along with LV results for a more complete evaluation of cardiac pathologies and a better understanding of the inter-ventricular dynamics.

The fast MR imaging techniques, in conjunction with special surface fitting and registration methods can describe the complex 3D motion of both atria. This might provide a helpful tool where a detailed mechanical analysis is needed for the diagnosis and evaluation of treatment protocols in a wide variety of clinical conditions.

We are now ready to put all the pieces of the puzzle together for a comprehensive motion field of the heart. A combined motion field that incorporates tag analysis and surface based registration is the current direction of our research.

Acknowledgments

Dr. Ozturk was supported by Falk Fellowship and Medtronic Corporation. The authors would like to thank Jerome Declerck Ph.D. for his enormous and continuing support during this project, which involved the modification of his earlier surface tracking techniques for atrial motion analysis.

References

[1] Maruyama, Y., K. Ashikawa, and S. Isoyama,. Mechanical interactions between four heart chambers with and without the pericardium in canine hearts. Circulation Research, 1982. 50: p. 86-100

[2] Yamaguchi, S., et al. Comparative significance in systolic ventricular interaction. Cardiovasc Res, 1991. 25(9): p. 774-83.

[3] Gordon, S., et al. Atrial infarction complicating an acute inferior myocardial infarction. Arch Intern Med, 1984. 144(1): p. 193.

[4] Santamore, W.P. and L.J. Dell'Italia. Ventricular interdependence: significant left ventricular contributions to right ventricular systolic function. Prog Cardiovasc Dis, 1998. 40(4): p. 289-308.

[5] Zerhouni, E.A., et al. Human heart: tagging with MR imaging–a method for noninvasive assessment of myocardial motion. Radiology, 1988. 169(1): p. 59-63.

[6] McVeigh, E.R. and E.A. Zerhouni. Noninvasive measurement of transmural gradients in myocardial strain with MR imaging. Radiology, 1991. 180(3): p. 677-83.

[7] O'Dell, W.G., et al. Three-dimensional myocardial deformations: calculation with displacement field fitting to tagged MR images. Radiology, 1995. 195(3): p. 829-35.

[8] Declerck, J., N. Ayache, and E.R. McVeigh, Use of a 4D planispheric transformation for the tracking and the analysis of LV motion with tagged MR images. Proc. SPIE Medical Imaging, 1999. 3660 p. 69-80.

[9] Young, A., et al. Tracking and Finite Element Analysis of Stripe Deformation in Magnetic Resonance Tagging. IEEE Trans on Medical Imaging, 1995. 14(3): p. 413-421.

[10] Dell'Italia, L.J. and W.P. Santamore. Can indices of left ventricular function be applied to the right ventricle? Prog Cardiovasc Dis, 1998. 40(4): p. 309-24.

[11] Raines, R.A., M.M. LeWinter, and J.W. Covell. Regional shortening patterns in canine right ventricle. Am J Physiol, 1976. 231(5 Pt. 1): p. 1395-1400.

[12] Barnard, D. and J.S. Alpert. Right ventricular function in health and disease. Curr Probl Cardiol, 1987. 12(7): p. 417-49.

[13] Goldstein, J.A. Right heart ischemia: pathophysiology, natural history, and clinical management. Prog Cardiovasc Dis, 1998. 40(4): p. 325-41.

[14] Jarvinen, V., et al. Assessment of left atrial volumes and phasic function using cine magnetic resonance imaging in normal subjects. Am J Cardiol, 1994. 73(15): p. 1135-8.

[15] Gustafsson, C., et al. Echocardiographic findings and the increased risk of stroke in nonvalvular atrial fibrillation. Cardiology, 1992. 81(4-5): p. 189-95.

[16] Arima, M., et al. Clinical manifestation and survival of patients with idiopathic bilateral atrial dilatation. Intern Med, 1999. 38(2): p. 112-8.

[17] Manning, W.J. and D.I. Silverman. Atrial anatomy and function postcardioversion: insights from transthoracic and transesophageal echocardiography. Prog Cardiovasc Dis, 1996. 39(1): p. 33-46.

[18] Armour, J.A., J.B. Pace, and W.C. Randall, Interrelationship of architecture and function of the right ventricle. Am. J. Physiology, 1970. 218: p. 174-179.

[19] Chin, K.W., et al. Asynergy of right ventricular motion in man. L Throc Cardivasc Surg, 1989. 97: p. 104-9.

[20] Meier, G.D., et al. Contractile function in canine right ventricle. Am J Physiol, 1980. 239(6): p. H794-804.

[21] Chuong, C.J., et al. Regional deformation and contractile function in canine right ventricular free wall. Am J Physiol, 1991. 260(4 Pt 2): p. H1224-35.

[22] Waldman, L.K., et al. Distributed mechanics of the canine right ventricle: effects of varying preload. J Biomech, 1996. 29(3): p. 373-81.

[23] Akgun, G. and C. Layton. Aortic root and left atrial wall motion. An echocardiographic study. Br Heart J, 1977. 39(10): p. 1082-7.

[24] Drinkovic, N., B. Ferek, and M. Jursic. Subcostal M-mode echocardiography of the right atrial wall in evaluation of cardiac arrhythmias and pacing. Pacing Clin Electrophysiol, 1985. 8(1): p. 110-22.

[25] Egeblad, H. and V. Rasmussen. Analysis of arrhythmias based on atrial wall motion. Usefulness and feasibility of recording left and right atrial systole by echocardiography. Acta Med Scand, 1986. 219(3): p. 283-9.

[26] Kubica, J., et al. Left atrial size and wall motion in patients with permanent ventricular and atrial pacing. Pacing Clin Electrophysiol, 1990. 13(12 Pt 2): p. 1737-41.

[27] Rubler, S., et al. Effects of systemic hypertension and left ventricular hypertrophy on posterior left atrial wall motion. Am J Cardiol, 1986. 58(11): p. 1115-7.

[28] Yoshikawa, J., et al. Study of posterior left atrial wall motion by echocardiography and its clinical application. Jpn Heart J, 1975. 16(6): p. 683-93.

[29] Spes, C.H., et al. Doppler analysis of pulmonary venous flow profiles in orthotopic heart transplant recipients: a comparison with mitral flow profiles and atrial function. Z Kardiol, 1996. 85(10): p. 753-60.

[30] Jauhiainen, T., et al. MR gradient echo volumetric analysis of human cardiac casts: focus on the right ventricle. J Comput Assist Tomogr, 1998. 22(6): p. 899-903.

[31] Sacks, M.S., et al. In vivo 3-D reconstruction and geometric characterization of the right ventricular free wall. Ann Biomed Eng, 1993. 21(3): p. 263-75.

[32] Young, A.A., Z.A. Fayad, and L. Axel. Right ventricular midwall surface motion and deformation using magnetic resonance tagging. Am J Physiol, 1996. 271(6 Pt 2): p. H2677-88.

[33] Klein, S.S., T.P. Graham, Jr., and C.H. Lorenz. Noninvasive delineation of normal right ventricular contractile motion with magnetic resonance imaging myocardial tagging. Ann Biomed Eng, 1998. 26(5): p. 756-63.

[34] Fayad, Z.A., et al. Right ventricular regional function in normal subjects using magnetic resonance tissue tagging. Book of abstracts, Society of MR, 1994: p. 1504.

[35] Higgins, C.B., et al. Magnetic resonance imaging in patients with congenital heart disease. Circulation, 1984. 70(5): p. 851-60.

[36] Aurigemma, G., et al. Evaluation of mitral regurgitation by cine magnetic resonance imaging. Am J Cardiol, 1990. 66(5): p. 621-5.

[37] Higgins, C.B., et al. Evaluation of valvular heart disease with cine gradient echo magnetic resonance imaging. Circulation, 1991. 84(3 Suppl): p. I198-207.

[38] Pflugfelder, P.W., et al. Noninvasive evaluation of mitral regurgitation by analysis of left atrial signal loss in cine magnetic resonance. Am Heart J, 1989. 117(5): p. 1113-9.

[39] Matsuoka, H., et al. Measurement of cardiac chamber volumes by cine magnetic resonance imaging. Angiology, 1993. 44(4): p. 321-7.

[40] Jarvinen, V.M., et al. Right atrial MR imaging studies of cadaveric atrial casts and comparison with right and left atrial volumes and function in healthy subjects. Radiology, 1994. 191(1): p. 137-42.

[41] Jarvinen, V.M., et al. A simplified method for the determination of left atrial size and function using cine magnetic resonance imaging. Magn Reson Imaging, 1996. 14(3): p. 215-26.

[42] Jarvinen, V.M., et al. Right and left atrial phasic volumetric function in mildly symptomatic dilated and hypertrophic cardiomyopathy: cine MR imaging assessment. Radiology, 1996. 198(2): p. 487-95.

[43] Lauerma, K., et al. Assessment of right and left atrial function in patients with transplanted hearts with the use of magnetic resonance imaging. J Heart Lung Transplant, 1996. 15(4): p. 360-7.

[44] Farin, G. Curves and Surfaces for Computer Aided Geometric Design: A Practical Guide. 1990:Academic Press.

[45] deBoor, C. A prectical guide to splines. 1978: Springer-Verlag.

[46] Moulton, M.J., et al. Spline surface interpolation for calculating 3-D ventricular strains from MRI tissue tagging. Am J Physiol, 1996. 270(1 Pt 2): p. H281-97.

[47] Amini, A.A., et al. MR Physics-Based Snake Tracking and Dense Deformations from Tagged Cardiac Images. AAAI Symposium on Applications of Computer Vision in Medical Image Processing, Stanford University, March 1994. : pp. 126-129.

[48] Amini, A.A., et al. Coupled B-snake grids and constrained thin-plate splines for analysis of 2-D tissue deformations from tagged MRI. IEEE Trans Med Imaging, 1998. 17(3): p. 344-56.

[49] Radeva, P., A.A. Amini, and J. Huang. Deformable B-Solids and Implicit Snakes for 3D Localization and Tracking of SPAMM MRI Data. Computer Vision and Image Understanding, May 1997. 66(2): pp. 163-178.

[50] Huang, J., et al. Spatio-temporal tracking of myocardial deformations with a 4-D B-spline model from tagged MRI. IEEE Trans Med Imaging, 1999. 18(10): p. 957-72.

[51] Ozturk, C. and E.R. McVeigh. Four Dimensional B-spline Based Motion Analysis of Tagged Cardiac MR Images. in Medical Imaging 1999. San Diego: SPIE.

[52] Ozturk, C. and E.R. McVeigh. Four Dimensional B-Spline Based Motion Analysis of Tagged MR Images: Introduction and In Vivo Validation. Physics in Medicine and Biology, 2000. 45(6): p. 1683-1702.

[53] Declerck, J., et al. Left ventricular motion reconstruction from planar tagged MR images: a comparison. Phys Med Biol, 2000. 45(6): p. 1611-32.

[54] Declerck, J., J. Feldmar, and N. Ayache. Definition of a 4D continuous planispheric transformation for the tracking and the analysis of LV motion. Medical Image Analysis, 1998. 2(3): p. 197-213.

[55] Moore, C.C., et al. Three-dimensional systolic strain patterns in the normal human left ventricle: characterization with tagged MR imaging. Radiology, 2000. 214(2): p. 453-66.

[56] Stuber, M., et al. Assessment of right ventricular function. Proceedings of the society of magnetic resonance in medicine, 1994. 3: p. 1502.

[57] Geva, T. Introduction: magnetic resonance imaging. Pediatr Cardiol, 2000. 21(1): p. 3-4.

[58] Powell, A.J. and T. Geva. Blood flow measurement by magnetic resonance imaging in congenital heart disease. Pediatr Cardiol, 2000. 21(1): p. 47-58.

[59] Shechter, G., C. Ozturk, and E.R. McVeigh. Interactive Four-Dimensional Segmentation of Multiple Image Sets. Proc. SPIE Medical Imaging 2000: Image Display and Visualization, 2000. 3976: p. 165-173.

[60] Jalife, J., et al. Mechanisms of atrial fibrillation: mother rotors or multiple daughter wavelets, or both? J Cardiovasc Electrophysiol, 1998. 9(8 Suppl): p. S2-12.

Chapter 6

Harmonic Phase MRI

Nael F. Osman
Department of Radiology,
Johns Hopkins University,
3400 N. Charles St.,
Baltimore, Maryland 21218
nael@jhu.edu

Jerry L. Prince
Electrical and Computer Engineering,
Johns Hopkins University,
3400 N. Charles St.,
Baltimore, Maryland 21218
prince@jhu.edu

6.1 Introduction

MR tagging has not become a standard clinical tool in large part because it has required excessive imaging and processing time. Harmonic phase (HARP) MRI addresses this issue by exploiting the unique Fourier spectrum of tagged MR images in fast, automatic computations of cardiac motion requiring very little Fourier data. To date these methods have been used in two-dimensional (2-D) cardiac motion analyses [1–3], have been validated in human and animal studies [4, 5], and have been extended to three dimensions [6]. HARP-MRI requires very little Fourier data, so that real-time, 2-D imaging should be possible in the near future and breath-hold, 3-D imaging may be possible as well.

HARP-MRI exploits the fact that tagged images have regularly distributed patches of energy in their Fourier spectra. Each patch corresponds to a complex harmonic image, which undergoes specific changes due the motion of the heart. The magnitude of a harmonic image provides the morphology of the heart without the presence of tags, while the phase is tightly related to the underlying motion at pixel resolutions. Two *harmonic phase* images acquired from horizontal and vertical

A.A. Amini and J.L. Prince (eds.),
Measurement of Cardiac Deformations from MRI: Physical and Mathematical Models, 119–150.

tagged images can be used to calculate two-dimensional motion, which is mathematically related to the true three-dimensional cardiac motion.

Computation of harmonic phase (HARP) images is accomplished through the use of bandpass filters applied to the observed tagged images followed by a phase angle computation. HARP images are used in two distinctly different ways. The first approach, which we refer to as *CINE-HARP*, requires a time sequence of HARP image pairs. In this approach, the HARP angles are tracked using an optical flow-like (cf., [7]) technique producing pathlines of selected points. This approach is used to generate Lagrangian strain and to display material properties throughout a time series. A fast, but approximate, optical flow calculation can produce a sequence of velocity fields between image frames, a result similar to that produced by 2-D phase contrast methods (see Chapters 9 and 10). The CINE-HARP framework is also used to synthesize tag lines, which provides a high-resolution grid for motion visualization.

The second approach, which we refer to as *Single-shot HARP* requires only one pair of HARP images acquired at a single phase in the cardiac cycle, generally end-systole. Single-shot HARP uses the slope of HARP images to compute dense strain maps, in the Eulerian sense, which represents the total strain from the moment the tags were placed in the tissue. These computations are fast and require no human interaction.

This chapter is organized as follows. In Section 6.2 we develop a harmonic model of tagged MR images, and in Section 6.3 we describe the principles of motion estimation using HARP images. Section 6.4 describes the CINE-HARP methods while Section 6.5 describes the Single-shot HARP methods. We provide a brief summary in Section 6.7, which concludes the chapter. Instead of providing a single section for demonstrating how the algorithms work — e.g., Results or Experiments — we instead demonstrate each method as it is described.

6.2 A Harmonic Model of Tagged MR Images

In this section we review the basics of HARP. Further details can be found in conference papers [8, 9] and journals [1–3]. Clinical validations can be found in [4, 5].

Figures 6.1(a) and (b) show horizontal and vertical MR tagged short-axis images of the left ventricle of a canine heart at end systole. The left ventricle appears as an annulus at the center of the images, and the tag lines, which are straight at end-diastole, are bent due to the motion of the heart. The magnitudes of the Fourier transforms of these images are shown in Figures 6.1(c) and (d). The spectral peaks in these images arise because of tagging, which modulates the underlying image with a truncated cosine series. The value of a tagged image at image coordinate $\mathbf{y}$

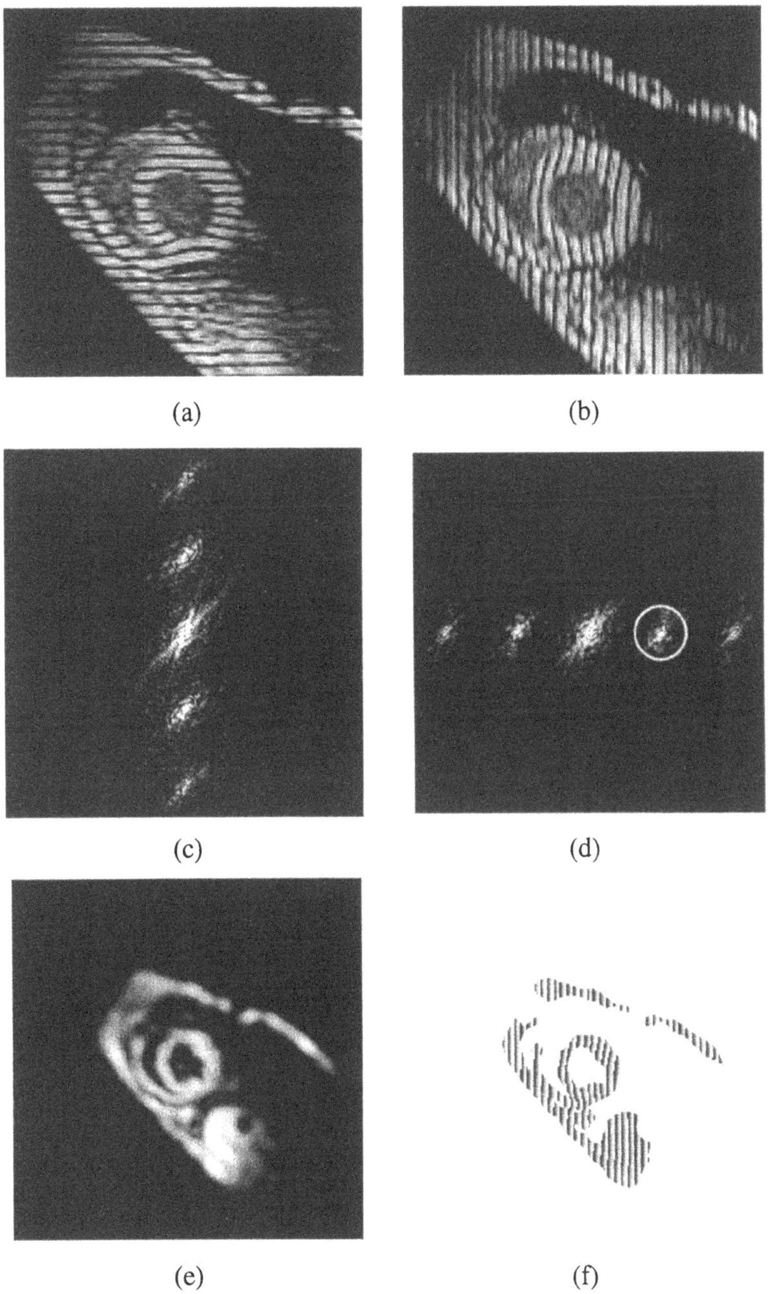

Figure 6.1: MR images with horizontal **(a)** and vertical **(b)** tag lines. The corresponding Fourier spectra are shown in **(c)** and **(d)**, respectively. The **(e)** magnitude and **(f)** phase of the harmonic image whose peak is circled in (d).

and time t can be written as a summation

$$I(\mathbf{y},t) = \sum_{l=-L}^{+L} I_l(\mathbf{y},t), \tag{6.1}$$

where $L = 2$ in this case. Each *complex* image $I_l(\mathbf{y},t)$ corresponds to a separate spectral peak [9], with the *DC peak* at the origin and the *harmonic peaks* at the other positions.

Harmonic images are the inverse Fourier transforms of isolated harmonic peaks. Because they do not have conjugate symmetric Fourier transforms, harmonic images are complex-valued. The magnitude and phase of the harmonic image corresponding to the spectral peak circled in Figure 6.1(d) are shown in Figures 6.1(e) and (f). We refer to these images as the *harmonic magnitude* and *harmonic phase* images respectively. Since the spectrum corresponding to a harmonic image is localized, it is possible to extract a harmonic image using a bandpass filter that captures the peak. In fact, the harmonic image represented by the magnitude and phase in Figures 6.1(e) and (f) was extracted using a filter whose bandpass region is bound by the circle in Figure 6.1(d). The best shape and location of the bandpass filter is determined by the tagging frequency, the size of the harmonic peak, and its relation to the other peaks [10].

Two spectral peaks, a first-order harmonic from each of the horizontal and vertical tagged images, are required to describe (and measure) 2D motion. Despite the abuse of notation, we will refer to these two harmonic images as $I_l(\mathbf{y},t)$, $l = 1, 2$, which are represented mathematically as

$$I_l(\mathbf{y},t) = D_l(\mathbf{y},t)e^{j\phi_l(\mathbf{y},t)} . \tag{6.2}$$

A harmonic magnitude image $D_l(\mathbf{y},t)$ is a real-valued image that resembles the morphology of the untagged MR image. Because tagging is a temporary feature, $D_l(\mathbf{y},t)$ fades over time and is eventually overwhelmed by noise. We can see in Figure 6.1(e) that its intensity is higher within tissue than in the background; therefore, $D_l(\mathbf{y},t)$ can be used to segment tissues from background using a simple threshold. This is useful for visualization purposes. For example, the harmonic phase image shown in panel (f) of Figure 6.1 is masked by a thresholded version of the magnitude image in (e) in order to give a representation of the underlying anatomy for reference.

A harmonic phase image is the inverse tangent of the ratio of the imaginary part of $I_l(\mathbf{y},t)$ to its real part. Because the inverse tangent operator[1] determines the phase angle modulo 2π, the computed harmonic phase image $a_l(\mathbf{y},t)$ is related to the true harmonic phase $\phi_l(\mathbf{y},t)$ by

$$a_l(\mathbf{y},t) = \mathcal{W}(\phi_l(\mathbf{y},t)), \tag{6.3}$$

1 - Refer to the atan2 routine in most math programming libraries.

where the wrapping operator $\mathcal{W}$ is given by

$$\mathcal{W}(\phi) \stackrel{\triangle}{=} \text{mod}(\phi + \pi, 2\pi) - \pi \,. \tag{6.4}$$

The resulting values of $a_l(\mathbf{y}, t)$, which we refer to as a HARP image, are in the range of $[-\pi, +\pi)$. Inspection of the harmonic phase image Figure 6.1(e) reveals crisp, sawtooth-like features, which result from phase wrapping, that deform like the tag lines in the original image Figure 6.1(b). This demonstrates that significant tissue motion information is encoded in HARP images, despite the relatively small bandwidth of the image source.

In this chapter, we use a special set of images to demonstrate HARP methods. The set is two sequences of 20 tagged MR short-axis images of a paced canine heart, one with horizontal tags and the other with vertical tags. The images were acquired at 14 ms intervals during systole during breath-hold periods with a segmented k-space acquisition. In this paper we use those acquired in a basal plane, near the location of the pacing lead. The entire image sequence for both tag orientations, cropped to the LV region, are shown in Figure 6.2(a) and (b). Details about the image acquisition scenario can be found in [11]. Strong early contraction can be seen near the pacing lead on the inferior lateral wall at about 5 o'clock. The septal wall is seen to bow outward in frames 4–8, an abnormal motion called *pre-stretching* caused by a delay in the electrical activation signal to the septal region. After this, the entire LV myocardium experiences continued contraction throughout systole in nearly normal fashion.

All images in Fig. 6.2(a) and (b) were bandpass filtered by selecting the lowest frequency harmonic image in each orientation. The HARP images computed from these harmonic images are shown in Fig. 6.2(c) and (d). Although we do not use the rough, phase-wrapping artifact to compute motion, it does provide a useful reference for visualizing the HARP images. We see in particular, that the HARP image features track the original tag lines very well through all images in both orientations; there is virtually no loss of motion information despite the drastic reduction in bandwidth. We use these HARP images in all subsequent motion calculations in this chapter.

6.3 HARP Motion Measurement Principles

The basic idea behind HARP methods is illustrated using the one-dimensional example shown in Figure 6.3. Because the bandpass filter extracts a single harmonic peak, the underlying tag pattern of each harmonic image is (a complex) sinusoidal. Figure 6.3(a) depicts a sinusoidal tag pattern and its corresponding (wrapped) phase. At a later time, this pattern might be deformed by tissue stretching and compression, for example; the effect on the tag pattern and its phase is illustrated in Figure 6.3(b). Two key points about HARP methods can be made. First, a particular piece of tissue has the same harmonic phase in the deformed state as it has in the reference state. This means that harmonic phase (wrapped

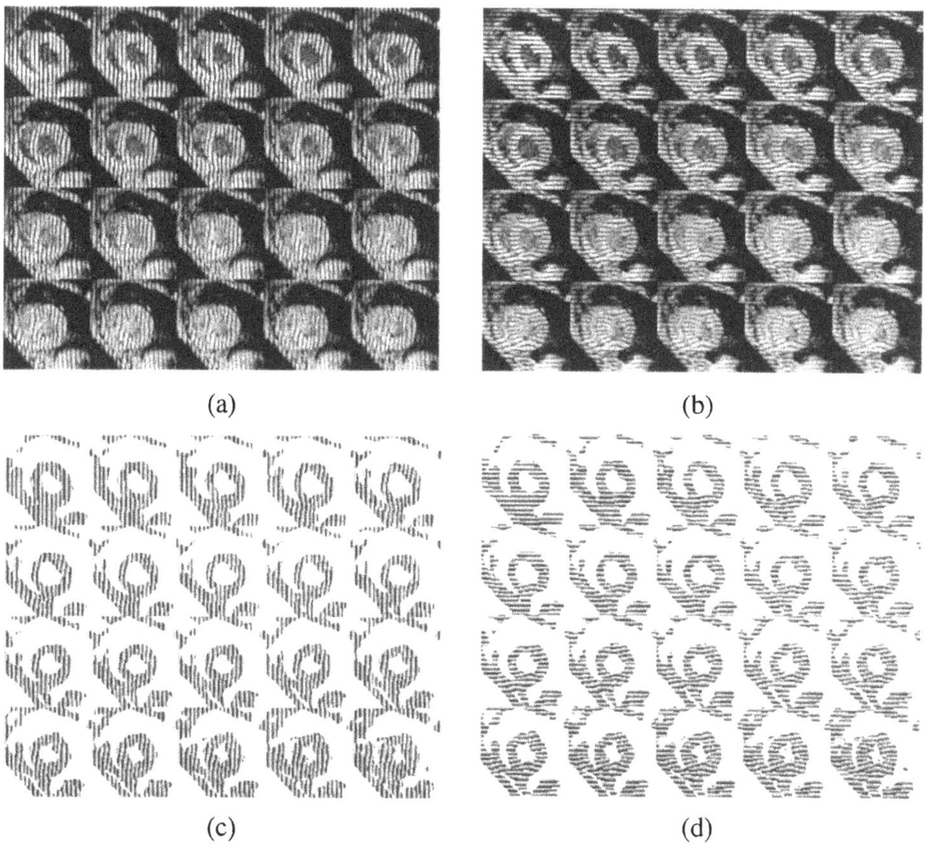

Figure 6.2: Two short-axis image sequences of a paced canine heart showing **(a)** vertical tags **(b)** horizontal tags. The sequence is ordered from end-diastole at the top-left proceeding left to right then top to bottom to end-systole at bottom-right. The corresponding HARP images are shown in panels **(c)** and **(d)**.

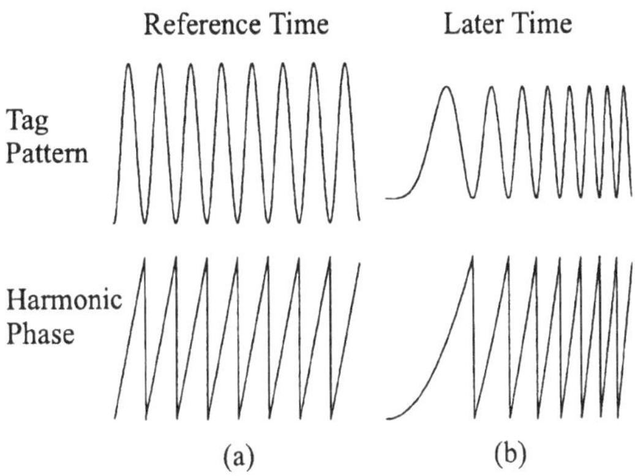

Figure 6.3: **(a)** A sinusoidal tag pattern and its harmonic phase at the reference time. **(b)** The decayed tag pattern, warped by stretching and compression, and its corresponding harmonic phase.

or non-wrapped) is a material property that can be tracked. This is the principle of CINE-HARP. Second, the slope of the harmonic phase is increased because of compression and decreased due to stretching. Therefore, the slope of harmonic phase is related to tissue strain; this is the principle of Single-shot HARP.

We note that tracking harmonic phase could be a problem due to the phase ambiguity caused by wrapping. Therefore, small motions or short time intervals are necessary in CINE-HARP. We also note that the wrapping artifact can cause a problem in calculation of the gradient. Therefore, a special gradient operator is necessary in Single-shot HARP. (It turns out that CINE-HARP also uses the gradient operator for numerical purposes.) To make all this work correctly a careful mathematical framework is required. We now lay the common foundation for all of the HARP methods.

6.3.1 Apparent Motion

Short-axis tagged images and their harmonic phase images, such as those shown in Figure 6.2, reveal tissue motion in two-dimensions. It is standard practice to track the intersection of two tag lines through an image sequence, for example. This 2-D motion is what we mean by *apparent motion*; it is characterized by an apparent reference map $\mathbf{q}(\mathbf{y}, t)$, which gives the apparent position at a reference time t_r of a material point located at $\mathbf{y}$ at time t. In standard planar tagging, the apparent reference position is precisely the projection of the actual, 3-D reference position onto the image plane.

Motion changes the phase of the underlying sinusoidal tag pattern. In fact, it produces a phase modulation given by

$$\phi_l(\mathbf{y}, t) = \boldsymbol{\omega}_l^{\mathrm{T}} \mathbf{q}(\mathbf{y}, t) , \quad l = 1, 2 , \tag{6.5}$$

where ω_l represents the position of the l-th harmonic peak (vertical or horizontal). It is convenient to write the two harmonic phase images arising from vertical and horizontal tagging using the vector

$$\phi(\mathbf{y},t) \triangleq \begin{bmatrix} \phi_1(\mathbf{y},t) \\ \phi_2(\mathbf{y},t) \end{bmatrix} . \tag{6.6}$$

This leads to the compact matrix expression

$$\phi(\mathbf{y},t) = \Omega^{\mathrm{T}} \mathbf{q}(\mathbf{y},t) , \tag{6.7}$$

where

$$\Omega \triangleq [\omega_1 \quad \omega_2] . \tag{6.8}$$

The relationship between the apparent reference map and harmonic phase, Equation (6.7), is the mathematical basis of HARP. Essentially, HARP methods are phase demodulation methods, and if we were able to measure $\phi(\mathbf{y},t)$ *itself*, these methods would be quite straightforward. Unfortunately, we can only measure the HARP images $a_l(\mathbf{y},t)$, $l = 1,2$, which are wrapped versions of the true phase. Still, much can be accomplished with only HARP images since their spatial and temporal derivatives are identical to those of the true phase under the right conditions. We now describe the numerical computations of these derivatives, which are used in most of the HARP methods described in the following section.

6.3.2 Spatial and Temporal Derivatives

Taking the gradient of both sides of (6.3) yields

$$\nabla a_l = \mathcal{W}'(\phi_l) \nabla \phi_l ,$$

where ∇ is the gradient operator with respect to $\mathbf{y}$ and $\mathcal{W}'$ is the derivative of the wrapping function. From (6.4) we see that $\mathcal{W}' = 1$ except at the points of discontinuity, $\phi_l = \pi + 2n\pi$, for $n = \ldots, -2, -1, 0, +1, +2, \ldots$, where the derivative does not exist. Theoretically, we could ignore these points since they comprise a set of measure zero; however, the wrapping discontinuity will cause difficulties in numerical implementation.

The gradient of a_l is approximated using finite differences. If the pixels used to calculate each difference do not cross a phase discontinuity then the computed gradient of a_l is a suitable approximation to the gradient of ϕ_l. If there is a phase discontinuity, however, the difference will not be correct. In this case, however, if the true phase difference is not more than π, the correct approximation can be recovered by simply re-wrapping the difference. Further, this re-wrapping operation will not affect those differences that were not computed across a phase discontinuity. In light of this discussion, and since all practical HARP images will satisfy the phase difference requirement, the gradient of $\phi_l(\mathbf{y}, t)$ is approximated by $\nabla^* a_l(\mathbf{y}, t)$ where

$$\nabla^* a_l(\mathbf{y}, t) = \frac{1}{h}[\mathcal{W}(a_l(\mathbf{y} + h\mathbf{e}_1, t) - a_l(\mathbf{y}, t)) \quad \mathcal{W}(a_l(\mathbf{y} + h\mathbf{e}_2, t) - a_l(\mathbf{y}, t))] , \tag{6.9}$$

where $\mathbf{e}_1$ and $\mathbf{e}_2$ are unit vectors in the row and column directions and h is the pixel separation. In a matrix form, we can thus write

$$\nabla \phi = \nabla^* \mathbf{a} . \tag{6.10}$$

The temporal derivative of $a_l(\mathbf{y}, t)$ is also approximated by finite differences. Let Δt be the time difference between successive images. Then the partial derivative of phase with respect to t can be approximated using

$$\frac{\partial \phi}{\partial t}(\mathbf{y}, t) \approx \frac{1}{\Delta t} \mathcal{W}(\mathbf{a}(\mathbf{y}, t + \Delta t) - \mathbf{a}(\mathbf{y}, t)) . \tag{6.11}$$

This approximation is valid provided $|\phi_l(\mathbf{y}, t + \Delta t) - \phi_l(\mathbf{y}, t)| < \pi$ for $l = 1, 2$, which is a small motion assumption. Unlike the gradient computation, which is satisfied under all normal conditions, this condition generally requires that Δt is small, no larger than approximately 30-40 ms in a normal heart. Therefore, HARP calculations requiring a temporal derivative are valid only in CINE-HARP, where an image sequence is acquired.

6.4 CINE-HARP (CHARP) Methods

CINE-HARP methods require a sequence of HARP image pairs. The methods are based on the fact that HARP angle is a material property, staying with the tissue — labeling it — throughout its entire motion. The methods we present here apply to 2-D, apparent motion, and can be used directly where 2-D quantities are sufficient or can be used in conjunction with existing 3-D modeling methods.

For convenience in this and subsequent sections we use vector/matrix notation to present algorithms. The pair of vertical and horizontal HARP images is represented by the vector image

$$\mathbf{a}(\mathbf{y}, t) = \begin{bmatrix} a_1(\mathbf{y}, t) \\ a_2(\mathbf{y}, t) \end{bmatrix} .$$

6.4.1 Tracking Motion

For a given material point with two HARP angles, there are many points sharing the same HARP angles in a later image, but only one point is the correct match. If the apparent motion is small from one image to the next, then it is likely that the nearest of these points, to the early location, is the correct point. Thus, our strategy is to track apparent motion through a CINE sequence of tagged MR images. We now formally develop this approach.

Consider a material point located at $\mathbf{y}_m$ at time t_m. If $\mathbf{y}_{m+1}$ is the apparent position of this point at time t_{m+1} then we must have

$$\phi(\mathbf{y}_{m+1}, t_{m+1}) = \phi(\mathbf{y}_m, t_m)\,, \tag{6.12}$$

This relationship provides the basis for tracking $\mathbf{y}_m$ from time t_m to time t_{m+1}. We see that our goal is to find $\mathbf{y}$ that satisfies

$$\phi(\mathbf{y}, t_{m+1}) - \phi(\mathbf{y}_m, t_m) = \mathbf{0}\,, \tag{6.13}$$

and then set $\mathbf{y}_{m+1} = \mathbf{y}$. Finding a solution to Eq. (6.13) is a multidimensional, nonlinear, root-finding problem, which can be solved iteratively using the Newton-Raphson technique. After simplification, the Newton-Raphson iteration is

$$\mathbf{y}^{(n+1)} = \mathbf{y}^{(n)} - [\nabla\phi(\mathbf{y}^{(n)}, t_{m+1})]^{-1}[\phi(\mathbf{y}^{(n)}, t_{m+1}) - \phi(\mathbf{y}_m, t_m)]\,. \tag{6.14}$$

Equation (6.14) cannot be implemented directly since we do not know ϕ. We can replace the gradient of ϕ by $\nabla^*\mathbf{a}$, however. And the phase difference term on the right can be computed by re-wrapping the phase difference between the corresponding HARP images. This means that the Newton-Raphson iteration can be computed and the material point can be tracked. We call this step HARP targeting, and it is implemented using the following algorithm. Note that the target HARP vector is denoted $\mathbf{a}^*$ and for tracking from t_m to t_{m+1} it is equal to $\mathbf{a}(\mathbf{y}_m, t_m)$.

Algorithm 1: HARP Targeting. Let $n = 0$ and set $\mathbf{y}^{(0)} = \mathbf{y}_{\text{init}}$.

1. If $n > N$ or $\|\mathcal{W}(\mathbf{a}(\mathbf{y}^{(n)}, t) - \mathbf{a}^*)\| < \epsilon$ then the algorithm terminates with $\hat{\mathbf{y}} = \mathbf{y}^{(n)}$.

2. Compute a step direction

$$\mathbf{v}^{(n)} = -[\nabla^*\mathbf{a}(\mathbf{y}^{(n)}, t)]^{-1}\mathcal{W}(\mathbf{a}(\mathbf{y}^{(n)}, t) - \mathbf{a}^*)\,,$$

   using appropriate interpolation procedures.

3. Compute a step size

$$\alpha^{(n)} = \min\left\{\frac{1}{\|\mathbf{v}^{(n)}\|}, 1\right\}.$$

4. Update the estimate

$$\mathbf{y}^{(n+1)} = \mathbf{y}^{(n)} + \alpha^{(n)}\mathbf{v}^{(n)}.$$

5. Increment n and go to step 1. □

HARP targeting tracks a material point from one frame to the next. To track that point through an entire sequence of images we successively apply HARP targeting to each image in the sequence. The target vector $\mathbf{a}^*$, remains the same throughout the entire sequence so that there is no accumulation of error. This strategy finds a succession of points having the same HARP angles, but (usually) avoids jumping to the wrong solution by keeping the initial point used in HARP targeting near to the desired solution. To formally state this algorithm, suppose that we want to track $\mathbf{y}_m$ at time t_m through all images at times $t_{m+1}, t_{m+2}, \ldots$. HARP tracking is given by the following algorithm:

Algorithm 2: HARP Tracking. Set $\mathbf{a}^* = \mathbf{a}(\mathbf{y}_m, t_m)$, $\hat{\mathbf{y}}_m = \mathbf{y}_m$, and $i = m$. Choose a maximum iteration threshold N (for HARP targeting).

1. Set $\mathbf{y}_{\text{init}} = \hat{\mathbf{y}}_i$.
2. Apply Algorithm 1 (HARP targeting) with $t = t_{i+1}$ to yield $\hat{\mathbf{y}}$.
3. Set $\hat{\mathbf{y}}_{i+1} = \hat{\mathbf{y}}$.
4. Increment i and go to step 1. □

We note that HARP tracking can be used to track points backward in time in exactly the same way as forward. Therefore, it is possible to specify a point in any image at any time and track it both forward and backward in time, giving a complete trajectory of an arbitrary point in space and time. In case tracking errors are evident in a given study it is possible to use spatial continuity of motion to reduce or eliminate these errors. This approach is described in detail in [1].

Figure 6.4 shows the trajectories of a variety of manually selected points in the paced canine demonstration study. The underlying image in this figure was created by multiplying the horizontal and vertical tagged images at the first time frame to show a tagging grid. Several observations can be made from this figure. First, since several points are located in the right ventricle, this experiment demonstrates the ability for HARP to measure right ventricular motion. Second, the motion of the points within the free wall are larger than those of the septum and the free wall seems to move toward the septum during systole. Finally, the points at approximately 1 o'clock and 8 o'clock on the LV wall begin their pathline by moving away from the 10 o'clock position. This is an indication of the abnormal motion caused by the pacemaker, which is located at approximately 5 o'clock. What happens is that initially the electrical activation is limited to the myocardium near the pacemaker. Muscle on the opposing wall is actually stretched until the electrical signal arrives.

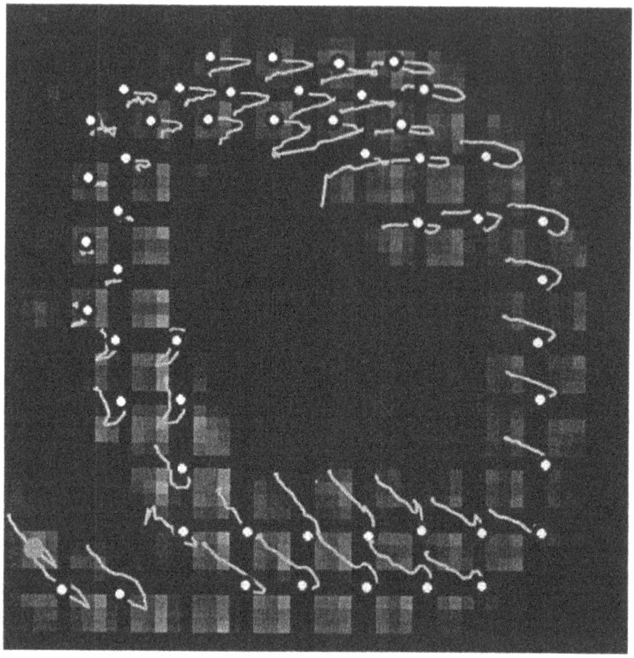

Figure 6.4: The pathlines of many manually selected points (bold circles).

6.4.2 Lagrangian Strain

Using HARP tracking, Lagrangian strain can be computed. We describe two approaches here, one based on a coarse, annular grid manually placed within the myocardium and another that is pixel-based and fully automatic.

Consider the annular grid placed within the left ventricular myocardium as shown in Figure 6.5. In this grid, there are 48 points, 16 on each circumference, characterizing the sub-endocardium, midwall, and sub-epicardium using 6 points per octant. This grid (or another with either higher or lower resolution) is placed manually on the LV myocardium at systole, when the muscle is most circular. All points on the grid are then tracked through time using CINE-HARP to identify their (apparent) trajectories throughout the heart beat.

We now consider the locations of the points at end-diastole $\mathbf{q}_i$, $i = 1, \dots, 48$ to be the reference configuration from which strain is computed. The simple strain (or elongation) at time t_m between two adjacent points $\mathbf{q}_i$ and $\mathbf{q}_j$ is given by

$$e = \frac{\|\mathbf{y}(\mathbf{q}_i, t_m) - \mathbf{y}(\mathbf{q}_j, t_m)\|}{\|\mathbf{q}_i - \mathbf{q}_j\|} - 1, \tag{6.15}$$

where $\mathbf{y}$ is the motion map resulting from HARP tracking. This quantity is zero if the distance between the points remains unchanged, negative if there is shortening,

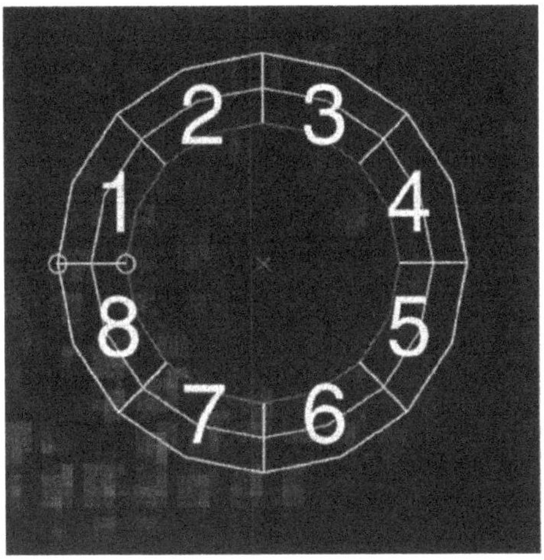

Figure 6.5: An annular grid superposed on the left ventricular wall.

and positive if there is lengthening. *Circumferential strain* is measured between points along a circumference while *radial strain* is measured between points along a radius.

All computed strains are averaged over quadrants but kept separate in annuli so that subendocardial, midwall, and subepicardial strains for each quadrant can be reported. The resulting temporal evolution of radial and circumferential strain for the paced canine data is shown in Figure 6.6.

The second approach to Lagrangian strain tracks all the pixels within the myocardium rather than just those on the annular grid. Given $\mathbf{y}(\mathbf{q}, t)$ for all points $\mathbf{q}$ within the myocardium at the reference time, we use spatial differences to compute the deformation gradient tensor $\nabla_{\mathbf{q}}\mathbf{y}(\mathbf{q}, t)$ where $\nabla_{\mathbf{q}}$ represents the gradient with respect to $\mathbf{q}$. The right Cauchy-Green strain tensor is given by $C(\mathbf{q}, t) = \nabla_{\mathbf{q}}\mathbf{y}(\mathbf{q}, t)^{\mathrm{T}}\nabla_{\mathbf{q}}\mathbf{y}(\mathbf{q}, t)$. The radial component of strain is then computed using $\mathbf{e}_R^{\mathrm{T}}C\mathbf{e}_R - 1$, and the circumferential component of strain is computed using $\mathbf{e}_C^{\mathrm{T}}C\mathbf{e}_C - 1$, where $\mathbf{e}_R$ and $\mathbf{e}_C$ the radial and circumferential unit vectors at the reference time ($t = 0$). These strains can be visualized as a movie in which the geometry remains fixed and the image grayscale depicts strain.

To demonstrate this method, we used a segmentation mask computed from the HARP magnitude image in the first frame of the paced canine series. For each point within this segmentation, a time sequence of Lagrangian circumferential strain was computed using the above method. Figure 6.7 shows images of this strain at four different times during systole. We note that the strain is presented in the reference coordinate system, which explains the rigidity of the geometry. Several observations can be made from this result. In Figure 6.7(a), the second time frame, we observe a darker region at the 5 o'clock position. This represents an early contrac-

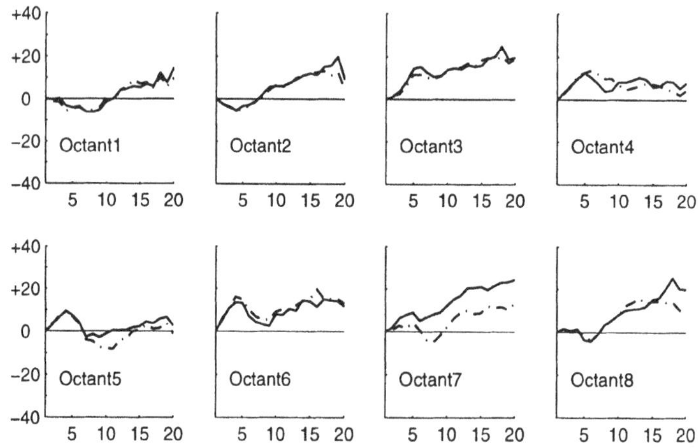

(a)

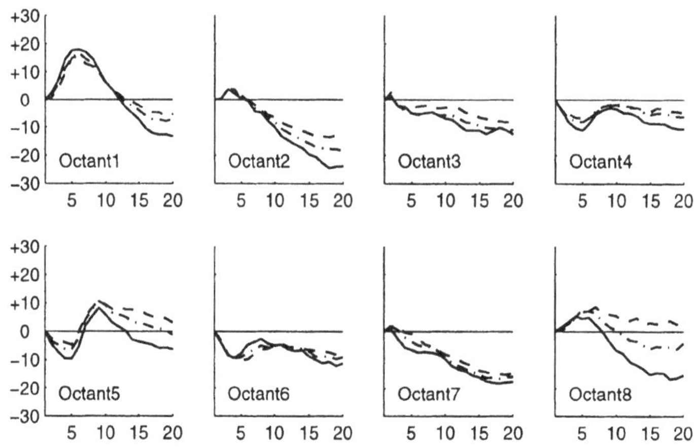

(b)

Figure 6.6: Temporal evolution of **(a)** radial and **(b)** circumferential strain in the paced canine. In **(a)**, solid lines indicate subendocardial strain while dash-dotted indicate subepicardial strain. In **(b)**, solid lines indicate subendocardial strain, dash-dotted lines indicate midwall strain, and dashed lines indicate subepicardial strain.

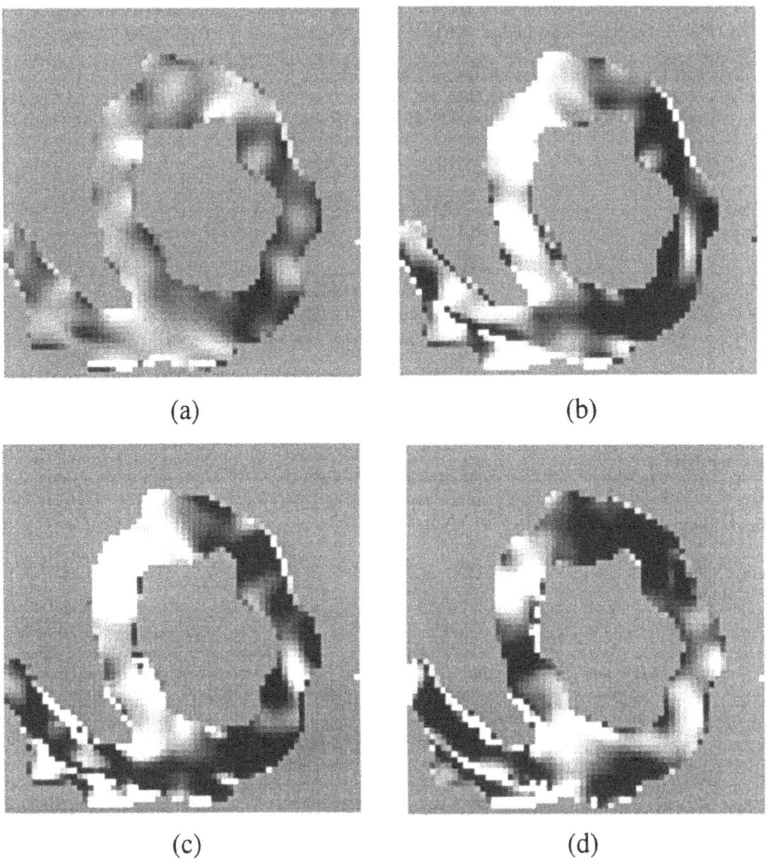

Figure 6.7: Selected frames from a movie showing Lagrangian circumferential strain. The time frames are **(a)** 2, **(b)** 4, **(c)** 6, and **(d)** 12. Dark regions indicate shortening while light regions indicate stretching.

tion at the site of the pacing lead. This contraction is larger in Figure 6.7(b) and now stretching is observed at the 10 o'clock position. In Figure 6.7(c), the sixth time frame, the early contraction is less apparent, while the prestretching is very strong. Figure 6.7(d) shows the twelfth time frame where other regions (1 and 8 o'clock) are undergoing some contraction.

6.4.3 Velocity Fields

Phase contrast MRI uses special pulse sequences to compute velocity fields which can then be used for a variety of purposes including visualization (see Chapters 9 and 10 and [12–14]). HARP tracking can be used to produce such fields by computing the apparent displacement between two successive images in a CINE tagged sequence. Applying HARP tracking to all the points in an image, however, is a computationally intensive task, and perhaps it is unnecessary if visualization is the only goal. In this section we present a fast algorithm for the computation of velocity fields in CINE tagged sequences using an optical flow method. Because the harmonic phase of a point does not change with time, optical flow can be applied to the harmonic phase images, rather than the intensity images (as in conventional optical flow). Velocity fields are then computed by adapting phase-based optical flow methods [15].

Since the harmonic phase of a material point remains constant as it moves, we have

$$\frac{d\phi}{dt} = 0\,,$$

which can be rewritten using the chain rule as

$$\nabla\phi(\mathbf{y},t)\mathbf{v}(\mathbf{y},t) + \frac{\partial\phi}{\partial t} = 0\,,$$

where ∇ is the gradient with respect to $\mathbf{y}$ and $\mathbf{v}(\mathbf{y},t)$ is the *velocity field* at time t. Solving for $\mathbf{v}$ yields

$$\mathbf{v}(\mathbf{y},t) = -[\nabla\phi(\mathbf{y},t)]^{-1}\frac{\partial\phi}{\partial t}\,. \tag{6.16}$$

We note that it can be shown that the matrix $\nabla\phi$ is always invertible. The actual harmonic phase vector ϕ is not easily calculated, however, so another approach must be taken to compute the quantities on the right-hand side of (6.16).

Using (6.10) and (6.11) yields an expression for the estimated velocity field

$$\mathbf{v}(\mathbf{y},t_n) = -\frac{1}{\Delta t}\nabla^*\mathbf{a}^{-1}(\mathbf{y},t_{n+1})\mathcal{W}[\mathbf{a}(\mathbf{y},t_{n+1}) - \mathbf{a}(\mathbf{y},t_n)]\,, \tag{6.17}$$

which can be computed rapidly using two harmonic phase images and two successive time instants in a CINE acquisition.

Figure 6.8 shows four velocity fields computed between different time frames in

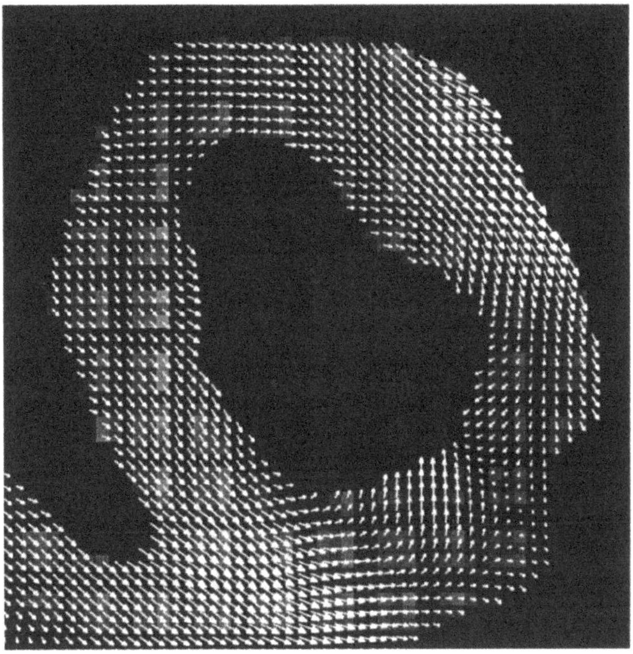

(a)

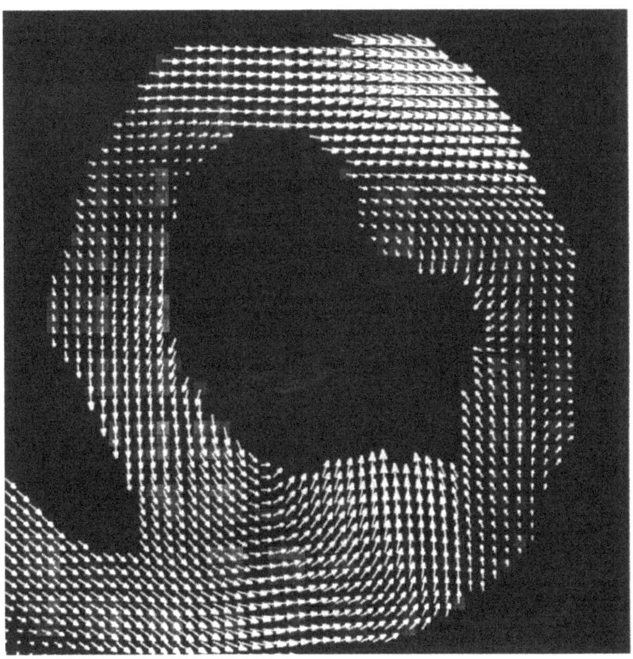

(b)

Figure 6.8: Velocity fields computed between times **(a)** 1–2, **(b)** 2–3, **(c)** 5–6, and **(d)** 6–7.

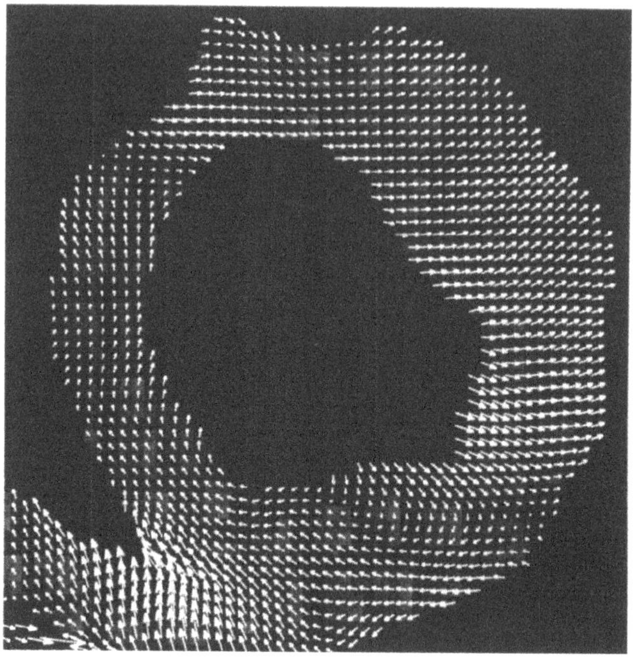

(c)

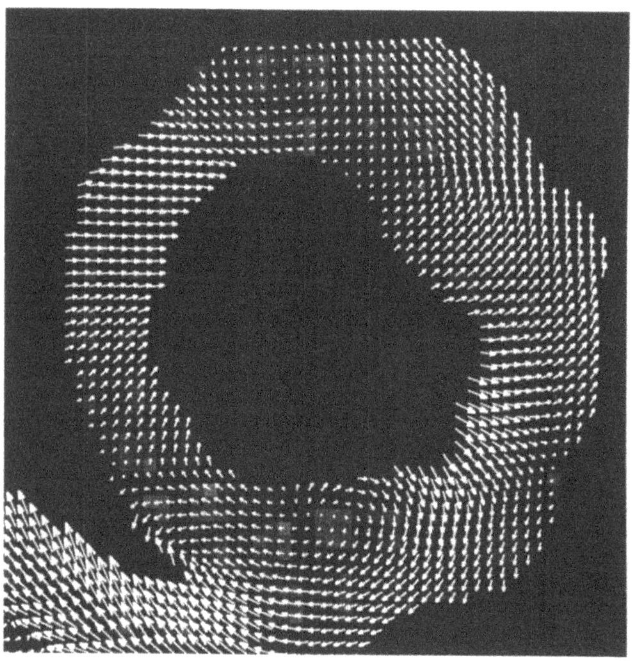

(d)

Figure 6.8 (cont.)

the cine sequence. In (a) we see a very compelling picture of an abnormal pattern of excitation. The velocity vectors at 8 and 2 o'clock are pointing circumferentially toward the pacing site, and the vectors at 10 o'clock are clearly pulling inward but separating circumferentially. Meanwhile, at the pacing site, the vectors are separating radially, indicating the thickening of the muscle, i.e., normal contraction. In (b), this general pattern continues, but evidence of radial thickening is spreading from the site of excitation. In (c) and (d), the velocity vectors show a reversal of direction as the muscle opposite the pacing site is activated. In this case, it is not so easy to discern local strain, as the overall magnitude of the vectors is quite large in most regions. An interesting rotational effect is observed in (d) at 6 and 12 o'clock. These represent the locations where the right ventricular wall joins the left, but otherwise it is not known why this effect should be present.

6.4.4 Strain-rate Maps

Strain rate, the change in strain per unit time, has also proven useful in assessing cardiac function (see Chapters 9 and 10 and [16]). It has been both directly imaged using the MR scanner [17] and calculated from phase contrast velocity fields [18]. Here, we use its fundamental relationship with velocity to calculate strain rate from HARP velocity fields.

We use the 2×2 strain rate tensor

$$S(\mathbf{y}, t) = \frac{1}{2}[\nabla \mathbf{v}(\mathbf{y}, t) + \nabla^{\mathrm{T}} \mathbf{v}(\mathbf{y}, t)], \tag{6.18}$$

as defined in [17]. To visualize this tensor, we display its radial and circumferential components. We first define the center of the LV, which can be done manually or automatically through the scanner prescription used to generate the short-axis images. The radial direction field $\mathbf{e}_R(\mathbf{y}, t)$ and the circumferential direction field $\mathbf{e}_C(\mathbf{y}, t)$ are automatically determined. These directions can be fixed to the reference position, or more appropriately, tracked to follow the annular grid orientations. The radial and circumferential strain rates are then given, respectively, by

$$S_{RR}(\mathbf{y}, t) = \mathbf{e}_R(\mathbf{y}, t)^{\mathrm{T}} S(\mathbf{y}, t) \mathbf{e}_R(\mathbf{y}, t), \tag{6.19}$$

$$S_{CC}(\mathbf{y}, t) = \mathbf{e}_C(\mathbf{y}, t)^{\mathrm{T}} S(\mathbf{y}, t) \mathbf{e}_C(\mathbf{y}, t). \tag{6.20}$$

Because of the spatial differentiation required to compute strain rate, these make very noisy images. Another way to visualize — indeed, to quantify — strain rate is to average over octants and display these averaged results. Accordingly, we averaged the strain rate over the octants depicted in Figure 6.5 in three radial bands: mid-wall, sub-endocardial, and sub-epicardial. The averaged strain rate results are shown in Figure 6.9.

In Figure 6.9(a), the early large positive radial strain rate in octant 6 coincides with the location of the pacing lead and indicates a myocardial thickening is taking place. Although difficult to discern from the velocity plots themselves, the

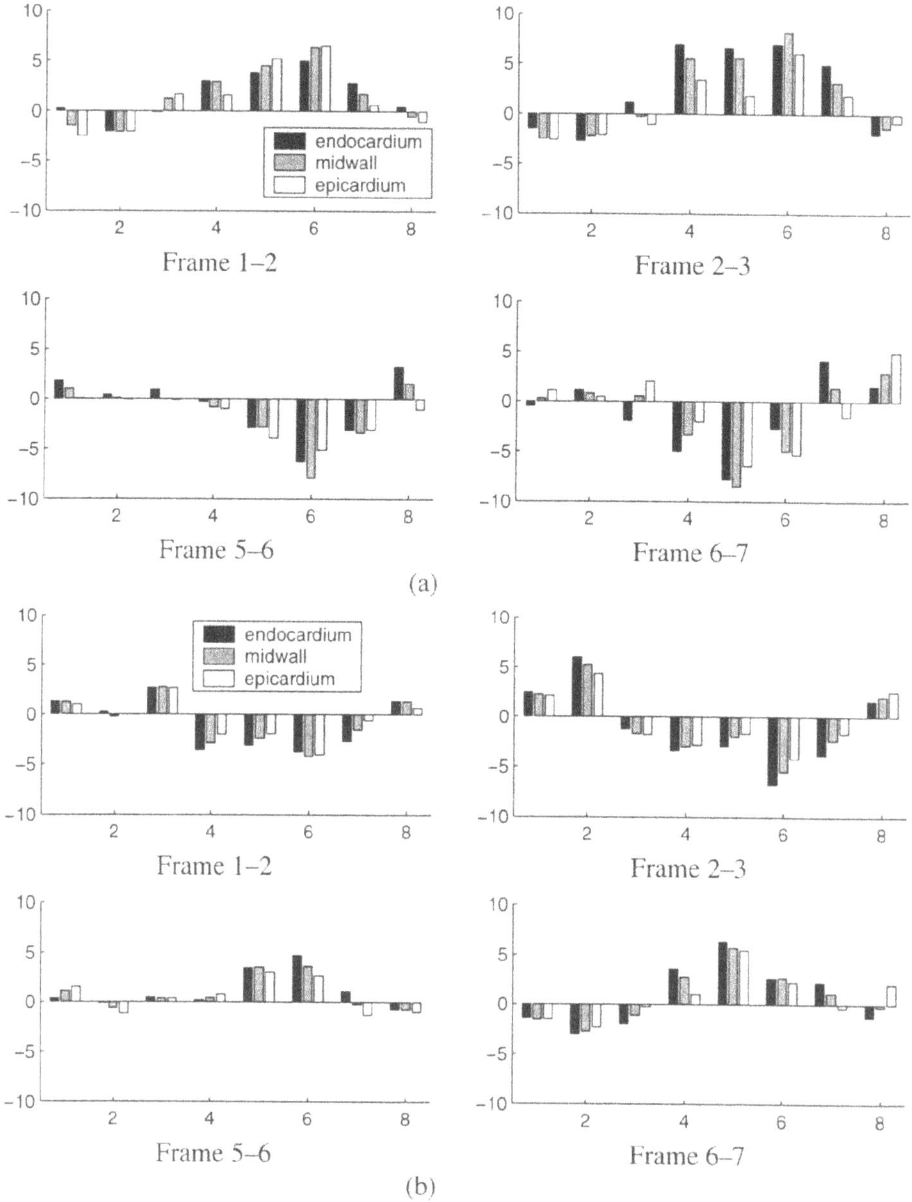

Figure 6.9: **(a)** The radial strain rate and **(b)** the circumferential strain rate for various time frames and different radial wall layers. The vertical axes indicate percentage of variation during the interval between the two time frames. Negative values indicate shortening while positive values indicate stretching.

opposite wall (octant 2) is showing a slight negative radial strain rate, indicating a myocardial thinning. At the later times, the sign of the strain rate reverses. This indicates that the opposite wall is starting to contract, while the wall nearest the pacer is starting to relax. We speculate that this is caused by a drop in tension due to muscle fatigue which is in turn caused by the prolonged stimulation around the pacing lead.

The circumferential strain rate, shown in Figure 6.9(b), agrees point-by-point with the above interpretation. The contrasting levels of strain rate, either radial or circumferential, is indicative of abnormal motion, which in this case is due to the ectopic pacing. In normal motion, a more homogeneous activity would be observed.

6.5 Single-shot HARP (SHARP) Methods

We now consider HARP motion estimation methods that require only two HARP images, typically with vertical and horizontal tag directions, acquired at the same time in the cardiac cycle. Tracking is not possible given only this data so it is not possible to associate material points between the reference time and the image time. The advantage of SHARP methods over CHARP is that the tags themselves persist much longer in the absence of imaging pulses. Therefore, acquiring high-quality HARP images well into diastole is possible using SHARP methods, but not generally possible using CHARP.

6.5.1 Tagline Synthesis

Simple visualization of tag lines has potential for use in diagnosis. It is possible to recognize abnormal patterns of motion due to infarction, abnormal electrical excitation, and ischemia. Currently, it is most common to visualize the horizontal and vertical tagged images separately or to visualize grid patterns generated by two-dimensional tagging or the superposition of vertical and horizontal tagged images (e.g., the product of Figures 6.1(a) and (b)). The resolution of this result is limited to the resolution of the tag lines, however, and this is limited by the image resolution. But HARP images have intrinsically sub-pixel resolution, so they offer the capability to "synthesize" artificial tag lines at arbitrary resolution.

Consider a single harmonic phase image $\phi_l(\mathbf{y}, t)$. Since harmonic phase is a material property (moves with the tissue), the set of points having a given target harmonic phase ϕ at a given time — an isocontour at level ϕ — is a curve. When the wrapped image $\mathbf{a}_l(\mathbf{y}, t)$ is used, the target harmonic phase $\mathbf{a}$ must be chosen in the range of the arctangent operator $[-\pi, +\pi)$ and, in principle, one curve per tag period should be selected per target phase. The presence of wrapping discontinuities, however, causes an additional curve to be selected at the phase discontinuity (see Figure 6.3), an undesirable effect.

A simple fix to this problem is to take the absolute value of the (wrapped) har-

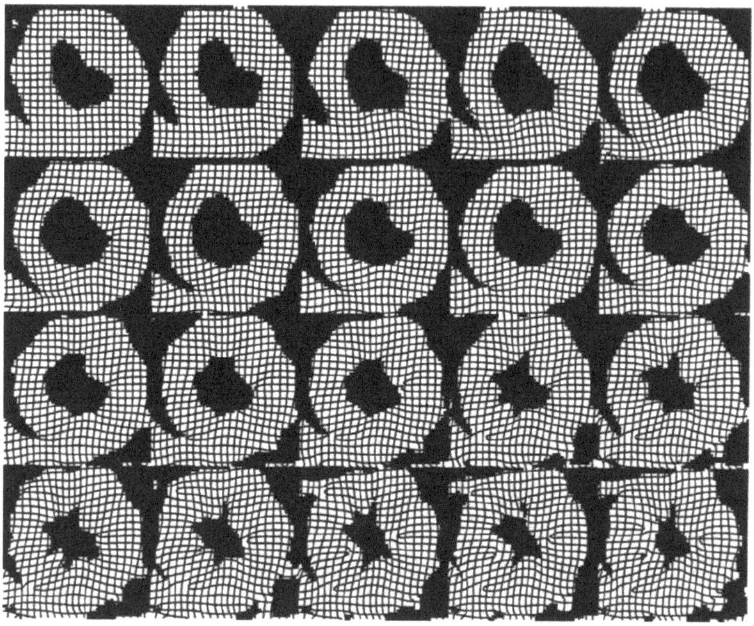

Figure 6.10: A sequence of motion grids ordered the same way as in Figure 6.2.

monic phase image $|a_l|$. Then if the target phase for an isocontour algorithm is $\pi/2$, two curves per period will be produced, evenly spaced at end-diastole, and there will be no additional curve generated at the discontinuities (because the discontinuities are removed by the absolute value operator). This procedure can be extended to generate more curves per tag period. The second stage would subtract $\pi/2$ from $|a_l|$, take another absolute value, and choose $\pi/4$ as the isocontour threshold. This procedure can be repeated again and again to get what amounts to arbitrarily close tag lines which are evenly spaced at end-diastole. To generate motion grids this algorithm is applied to both the horizontal and vertical harmonic phase images and the resulting isocontours are superposed.

Figure 6.10 shows a sequence of motion grids computed using two isocontours per period. The grid is masked by a segmentation of the myocardium created using HARP magnitude images. It is observed that the overall pattern of contraction evident in Figure 6.2 is still present, but the apparent resolution has increased by a factor of two.

6.5.2 Radial and Circumferential Eulerian Strain

Eulerian strain and Lagrangian strain are the same quantity except that they have different frames of reference. For example, in our work Lagrangian strain is referenced to the time of the first image frame, typically 15–30 ms after end-diastole.

Eulerian strain, on the other hand, is referenced to the moment that the tags were applied, typically end-diastole itself. Because of the difference in these reference times, Lagrangian strain is zero by definition in the first image, while Eulerian strain is generally not zero in this image. Another difference in the frames of reference occurs in the definition of the radial (hence, circumferential) direction. Lagrangian strain takes this direction from the systolic frame (where the myocardium is more nearly circular) and tracks this direction backward in time through the other frames. Eulerian strain, however, must define the radial direction in spatial coordinates from frame-to-frame.

Unlike Lagrangian strain, Eulerian strain is calculated using spatial rather than material derivatives. In this case, the deformation gradient is the spatial tensor given by

$$F = [\nabla \mathbf{q}(\mathbf{y}, t)]^{-1}, \tag{6.21}$$

From Equation (6.7) and since $\nabla \phi \approx \nabla^* \mathbf{a}$, it follows that

$$F \approx (\nabla^* \mathbf{a})^{-1} \Omega^{\mathrm{T}}, \tag{6.22}$$

Finite strain is best characterized using the right and left Cauchy-Green strain tensors, given by $C = F^{\mathrm{T}} F$ and $B = F F^{\mathrm{T}}$, respectively [19]. One can calculate simple and shear strains, as well as principle strains and related quantities from these tensors. We have found, as is conventional in the literature, that circumferential and radial strains are the most useful measures of heart wall strain from short-axis tagged MR images. Given a reference direction $\mathbf{e}$ — a unit normal vector taken to be either the radial or the circumferential direction — the *unit elongation* can be calculated using either Cauchy-Green strain tensor. If $\mathbf{e}$ is intended to reflect a direction in material coordinates (the reference time), then the appropriate calculation is

$$\epsilon_C = \sqrt{\mathbf{e}^{\mathrm{T}} C \mathbf{e}} - 1 \approx \|(\nabla^* \mathbf{a})^{-1} \Omega^{\mathrm{T}} \mathbf{e}\| - 1. \tag{6.23}$$

On the other hand, if $\mathbf{e}$ reflects a direction in spatial coordinates (deformed state) then the appropriate calculation is

$$\epsilon_B = \sqrt{\mathbf{e}^{\mathrm{T}} B \mathbf{e}} - 1 \approx \|\Omega (\nabla^* \mathbf{a})^{-\mathrm{T}} \mathbf{e}\| - 1. \tag{6.24}$$

Here, we define the radial and circumferential directions in spatial coordinates and therefore use (6.24) to calculate strain. A time sequence of computed radial strains in the paced canine data set is shown in Figure 6.11. The third image from the top-left corner reveals early thickening in the 5 o'clock position, the location of the pacing lead, persisting for several frames. The darker region in the septum, visible in the third time frame and later, indicates thinning in the myocardial wall which persists well in the systolic phase. This indicates a significant delay of the onset of contraction because the conduction does not travel through the normal

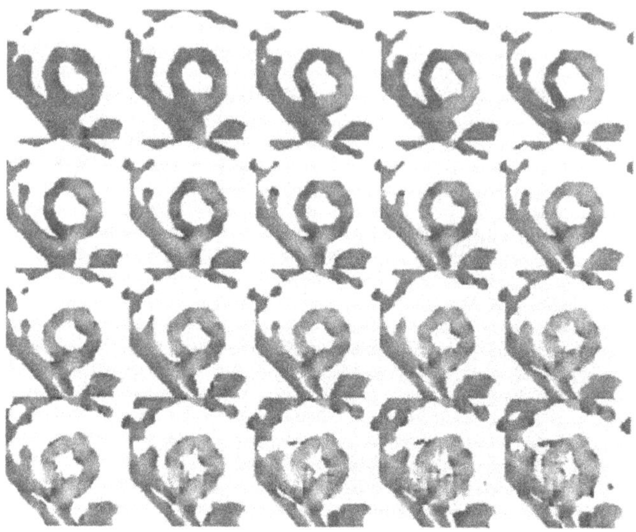

Figure 6.11: Radial strain in a short-axis image of a paced canine LV. The gray scale indicates the strain value, varying from the darkest level with 15% thinning to the lightest with 25% thickening.

pathways of the heart. Many of the basic conclusions presented in the 3D analysis in [11] are evident in our results obtained in a fast, completely automatic fashion.

A similar conclusion to that of the radial strain can be seen in the circumferential strain, shown in Figure 6.12. The third image in this sequence reveals early activation (circumferential contraction) in the 5 o'clock position, the location of the pacing lead, which persists for several frames. The lighter region in the septum also visible in the third frame indicates a prestretch of the myocardial fibers which persists well into the systolic phase. This indicates a significant delay of the onset of shortening because the conduction does not travel through the normal pathways of the heart. The computed strain also agrees with the 3D analysis in [11]. Moreover, we can see the contraction in a part of the right ventricle towards end-systole. In the third row from the top, we can see the lack of contraction at the location pacing lead, caused by the fatigue of local muscle, and in the other region where the prestretching occurred.

6.5.3 Minimum and Maximum Eulerian Strain

Radial and circumferential strain computations require a reference direction (in either material or spatial coordinates), and this currently requires manual intervention to identify the long axis of the left ventricle. The minimum and maximum strain values, however, can be computed directly from the strain tensor without the requirement of a reference direction. Let λ_{max} and λ_{min} be the maximum and

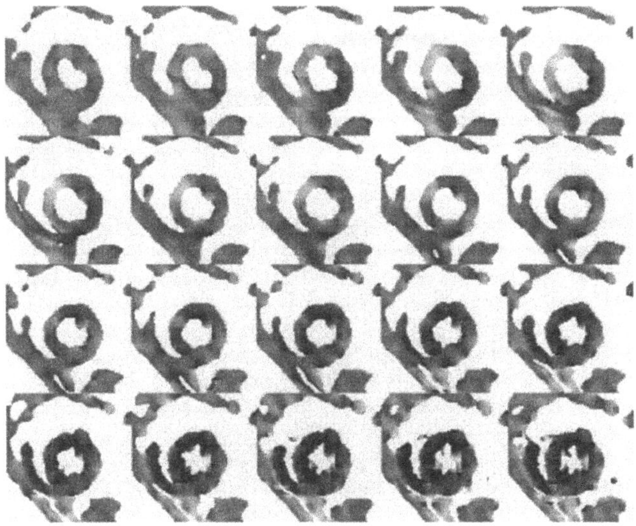

Figure 6.12: Circumferential strain in a short-axis image of a paced canine LV. The gray scale indicates the strain value, varying from the darkest level with 15% shortening to the lightest with 15% stretching.

minimum eigenvalues of B, respectively.[1] The maximum thickening strain ϵ_{max} and the maximum shortening strain ϵ_{min} are computed as follows.

$$\epsilon_{max} = \sqrt{\lambda_{max}} - 1\,, \tag{6.25}$$

$$\epsilon_{min} = \sqrt{\lambda_{min}} - 1\,. \tag{6.26}$$

These strains are associated with orthogonal directions in either the spatial or material coordinate systems corresponding to the directions of maximum and minimum unit elongation.

Figures 6.13 and 6.14 show the maximum stretching and minimum thinning, respectively. Unfortunately, the abnormal strain patterns that are evident in both the radial and circumferential strain maps are not apparent in the maximum and minimum strain maps. This is because the antero-septal stretch has fairly substantial thickening and thinning strains — they are just oriented differently than one expects in a normal contraction. So maximum and minimum strain maps are not likely to lead to differentiation of abnormal pacing patterns, or to the identification of ischemic heart muscle, which undergoes stretching similar to the late-activated tissue in this pacing model. Instead, these measures should be valuable in identifying and quantifying old infarction, where the muscle undergoes very little strain at all. They might also be useful in motion-based segmentation of the heart, should the location of the LV long axis not be known.

1 - The matrix C can be used also since it has the same eigenvalues as B.

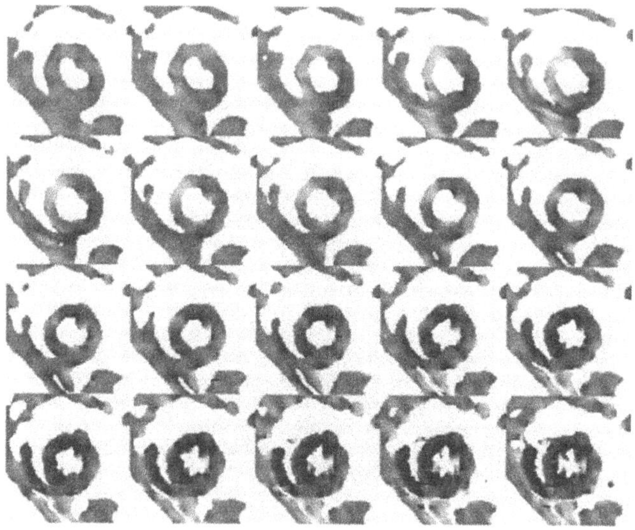

Figure 6.13: The maximum thickening map of a short-axis image of a paced canine LV. The gray scale indicates the strain value, varying from the darkest level with 15% shortening to the lightest with 25% stretching.

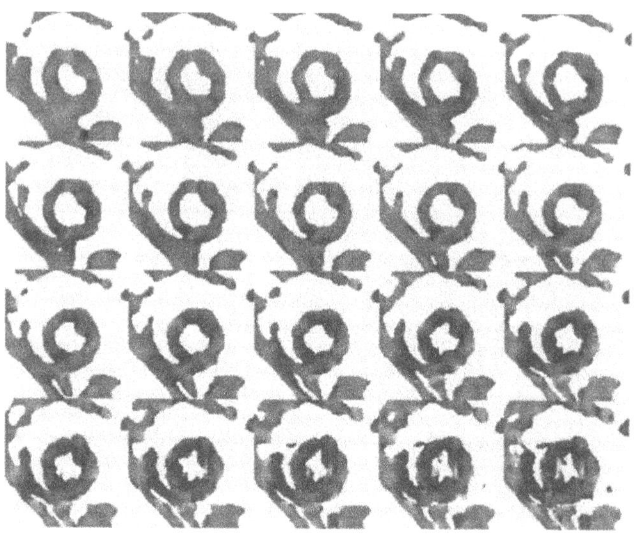

Figure 6.14: The maximum thinning map of a short-axis image of a paced canine LV. The gray scale indicates the strain value, varying from the darkest level with 15% shortening to the lightest with 15% stretching.

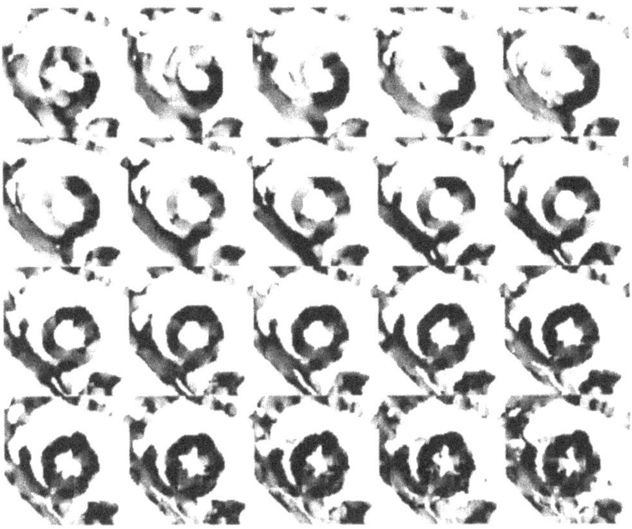

Figure 6.15: Contraction angle for the paced canine data set. Black indicates zero degrees and white indicates 90-degrees.

6.5.4 Contraction Angle

The orientation of maximum thickening has been shown to be a sensitive indicator of LV myocardial performance [20]. To quantify what is meant by orientation, the *contraction angle* β is defined to be the angle between the direction of maximum thickening and the radial direction. Let $\mathbf{v}_1$ denote the (unit) eigenvector of B corresponding to its largest eigenvalue. Then the contraction angle is given by

$$\beta = \arccos\left(\mathbf{v}_1 \cdot \mathbf{e}_R\right). \tag{6.27}$$

In a normal myocardium, the contraction angle is typically small (around 12-degrees) at end-systole, but is often much larger when there are local motion abnormalities [20].

We computed the contraction angle for the paced canine data set, and the results are shown in Figure 6.15. In early times, the motion is very small over most of the LV wall, so there is a fairly random pattern of angle. Near the start of activation, however, the angle approaches zero near the pacing site (5 o'clock) and 90-degrees on the opposite wall. One can observe a "wave" around the wall originating at the pacing site as the muscle contracts and the orientation of maximum thickening aligns with the radial direction. In mid-systole, the pacing site undergoes some stretching as the muscle relaxes, and toward end-systole all LV myocardium shows nearly zero contraction angle.

6.6 Combining CHARP and SHARP Methods

CHARP methods require a temporal sequence of tagged image pairs, use tracking, and can produce Lagrangian quantities references to any time-frame in the sequence, typically the first. SHARP methods, on the other hand, require only one tagged image pair taken at any time in the cardiac cycle, cannot track material points, but can produce Eulerian quantities referenced to the time of tag placement. If a tagged sequence exists, these methods can be combined for mutual benefit, as we now describe.

With tracking, it is possible to display *any* calculated quantity, material or spatial, in a Lagrangian sense — that is, by following the material point. As an example, we calculated the left Cauchy-Green strain tensor B at each pixel within each tagged image pair. We then tracked the circular grid pattern of Figure 6.5 through the entire image sequence. The circular grid automatically defined the radial and circumferential directions throughout the time sequence, from which the radial and circumferential elongations were computed at 48 points on the grid.

The temporal evolutions of Eulerian radial and circumferential strains, averaged over each octant, are depicted in Figure 6.16. Although these plots look superficially similar to those of Figure 6.6, which depicts Lagrangian strains, there is one significant difference. In particular, the Eulerian circumferential strain in the first time frame of Octant 5 is not zero, while the corresponding Lagrangian strain is identically zero. The reason for this difference is that the Eulerian strain is referenced to the time the tags were applied, not the first image time as in Lagrangian strain. This shows that in the first 10 ms or so, the heart muscle has already undergone a small amount of contraction due to the electrical excitation at the pacing lead.

We use contraction angle as a second demonstration of the potential of combined CHARP and SHARP. Using the same tracked grid as above, we averaged contraction angle over each quadrant. The resulting temporal evolution of contraction angle is shown in Figure 6.17. In a normal heart, all plots would approach zero together and stay small throughout systole. In this example, only Octants 4–6 rapidly approach zero. Octants 8, 1, and 2 — on the opposite wall — turn orthogonal to the desired orientation due to their inactivity. Later, Octant 5 demonstrates a relaxation in which the angle deviates again from normal. Finally, all regions are active and contracting in unison, which is shown by all contraction angles going toward zero. We expect that infarcts and ischemic tissues would have their own contraction angle "signatures" that could be recognized for diagnosis.

6.7 Summary and Conclusion

Harmonic phase MRI is a new approach to processing tagged MR images. It is based on the relationship between tissue motion and the phase of sinusoidally-tagged MR images, which can be extracted from standard tagged MR images.

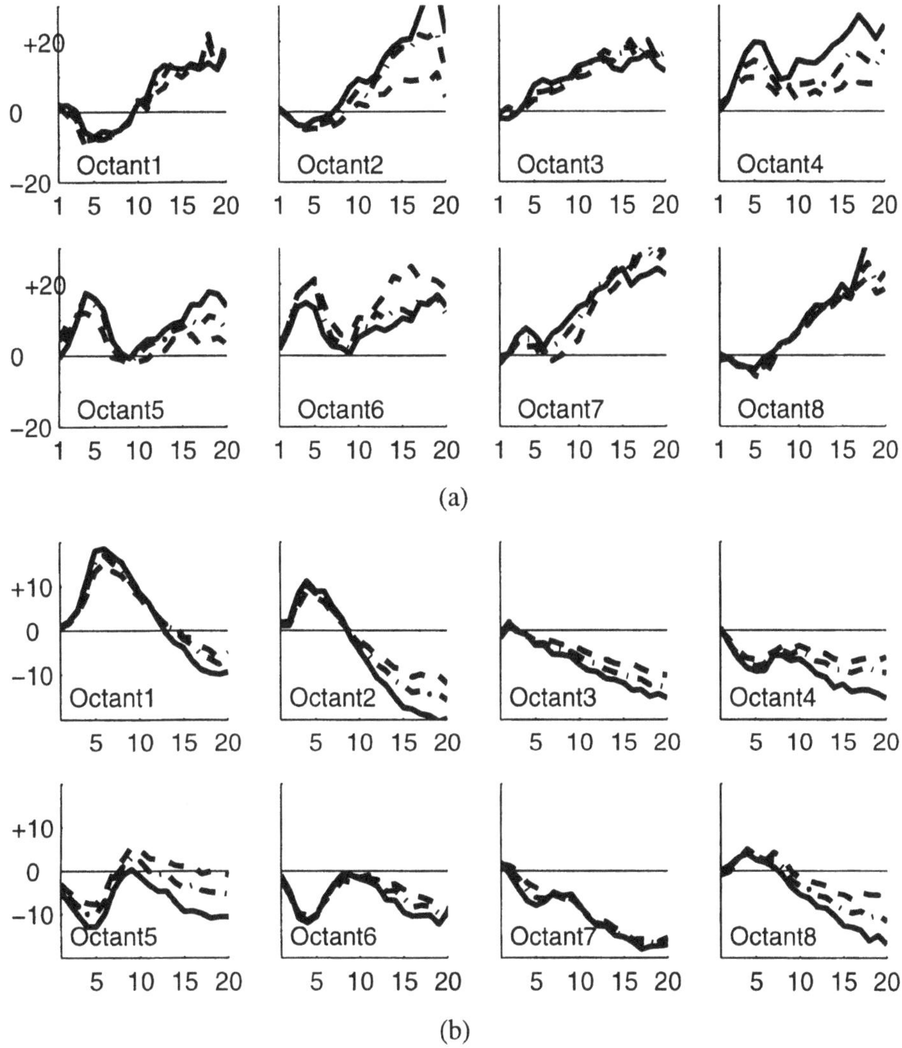

Figure 6.16: Time evolution of **(a)** radial and **(b)** circumferential Eulerian strain. The solid, dashed-dotted, and dashed lines represent the sub-endocardium, midwall, and sub-epicardium, respectively. The entire time course has 20 image frames with 14 ms between each frame. The vertical axes represent percent strain.

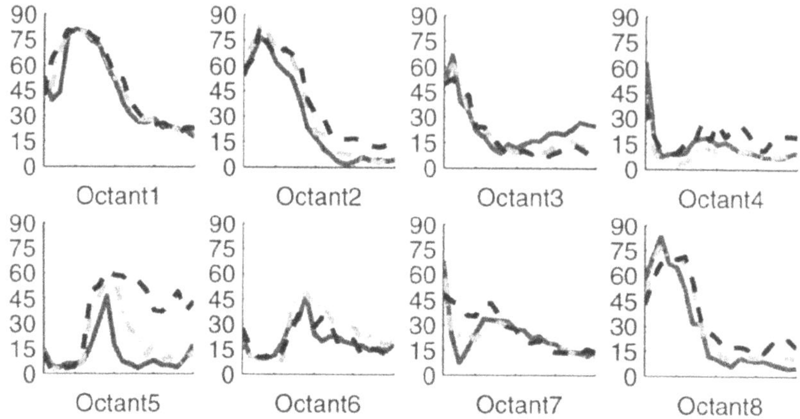

Figure 6.17: The temporal evolution of contraction angle in different octants for the paced canine data set. The solid, dashed-dotted, and dashed lines represent the sub-endocardium, midwall, and sub-epicardium, respectively. The entire time course has 20 frames with 14 ms between frames. The vertical axes are in degrees.

The general computational approaches in HARP are split into those involving sequences of tagged image pairs (CINE-HARP or CHARP) and those involving just a single image pair (Single Shot HARP or SHARP). Strain at the pixel resolution can be calculated in either the Lagrangian or Eulerian sense.

Nearly all of HARP is automated, with the exceptions being the specification of the long-axis of the LV and the definition of a circular grid in one image. HARP calculations are straightforward and fast; real-time calculations should be possible with optimized computer code. Because a relatively small amount of k-space is required for HARP calculations, special MR pulse-sequences can be developed to speed up acquisition time. This would enable either faster updating of 2-D HARP data or faster scanning of the three-dimensional heart volume. We refer to the combination of special scanning in combination with HARP processing as HARP-MRI.

HARP has undergone preliminary validation in human stress tests and canine infarction models [4, 5]. In these studies, HARP was shown to reliably reproduce the results of conventional tag analysis in a small fraction of the time. Potential for routine use in the clinical environment has been clearly demonstrated.

Acknowledgment

We thank Dr. Elliot McVeigh for providing us with the paced canine tagged MR images. This work was supported by NIH grant R01-HL47405.

References

[1] N. F. Osman, W. S. Kerwin, E. R. McVeigh, and J. L. Prince. Cardiac motion tracking using CINE harmonic phase (HARP) magnetic resonance imaging. Magn. Reson. Med., 42(6):1048–1060, 1999.

[2] N. F. Osman and J. L. Prince. Visualizing myocardial function using HARP MRI. Phys. in Med. and Bio., 45(6):1665–1682, 2000.

[3] N. F. Osman, E. R. McVeigh, and J. L. Prince. Imaging heart motion using harmonic phase MRI. IEEE Trans. Med. Imag., 19(3):186–202, 2000.

[4] J. Garot, D. Bluemke, N. F. Osman, C. Rochitte, E. R. McVeigh, E. Zerhouni, J. Prince, and J. Lima. Fast determination of regional myocardial strain fields from tagged cardiac images using harmonic phase (HARP) magnetic resonance imaging. Circulation, 101:981–988, 2000.

[5] J. Garot, D. Bluemke, N. F. Osman, C. Rochitte, E. R. McVeigh, E. Zerhouni, J. L. Prince, and J. A. Lima. Transmural contractile reserve after reperfused myocardial infarction in the dog. Journal of American College of Cardiology. to appear.

[6] N. F. Osman, S. Sampath, and J. L. Prince. Measuring 3d myocardial strain in a thin slice using harmonic phase MRI. In Proceedings of SPIE, Medical Imaging 2000: Physiology and Function from Multidimensional Images, San Diego, CA, February 12-17, 2000.

[7] J. L. Barron, D. J. Fleet, and S. S. Beauchemin. Performance of optical flow techniques. International Journal of Computer Vision, 12(1):43–77, 1994.

[8] N. F. Osman and J. L. Prince. Direct calculation of 2D components of myocardial strain using sinusoidal MR tagging. In Proc. SPIE Medical Imaging: Image Processing Conference, February 1998.

[9] N. F. Osman and J. L. Prince. Motion estimation from tagged MR images using angle images. In Proc. Int. Conf. Imag. Proc. volume 1, pages 704–708. Comp. Soc. Press, 1998. Chicago.

[10] N. F. Osman and J. L. Prince. On the design of the bandpass filters in harmonic phase MRI. Int. Conf. Imag. Proc. 2000 (ICIP00).

[11] E. R. McVeigh, F.W. Prinzen, B.T. Wyman, J.E. Tsitlik, H.P. Halperin, and W.C. Hunter. Imaging asynchronous mechanical activation of the paced heart with tagged MRI. Magn. Reson. Med., 39(4):507–513, April 1998.

[12] N. J. Pelc, R.J. Herfkens, A. Shimakawa, and D. Enzmann. Phase contrast cine magnetic resonance imaging. Magn. Reson. Quarterly, 7(4):229–254, 1991.

[13] N. J. Pelc, M. Drangova, L. R. Pelc, Y. Zhu, D. C. Noll, B. S. Bowman, and R. J. Herfkens. Tracking of cyclic motion with phase-contrast cine MR velocity data. J. Magn. Reson. Imaging, 5:339–345, 1995.

[14] R. T. Constable, K. M. Rath, A. J. Sinusas, and J. C. Gore. Development and evaluation of tracking algorithms for cardiac wall motion analysis using phase velocity MR imaging. Magn. Res. Med., 32:33–42, 1994.

[15] D. J. Fleet and A. D. Jepson. Computation of component image velocity from local phase information. Int. Jour. of Comp. Vision, 5(1):77–104, 1990.

[16] G. M. Beache, V. J. Wedeen, R. M. Weisskoff, P. T. O'Gara, B. P. Poncelet, D. A. Chesler, T. J. Brady, B. R. Rosen, and R. E. Dinsmore. Intramural mechanics in hypertrophic cardiomyopathy: Functional mapping with strain-rate MR imaging. Radiology, 197:117–124, 1995.

[17] V. J. Wedeen. Magnetic resonance imaging of myocardial kinematics. technique to detect, localize, and quantify the strain rates of the active human myocardium. Magn. Reson. Med., 27:52–67, 1992.

[18] V. J. Wedeen, R. M. Weisskoff, T. G. Reese, G. M. Beache, B. P. Poncelet, B. R. Rosen, and R. E. Dinsmore. Motionless movies of myocardial strain-rates using stimulated echoes. Magn. Res. Med., 33(3):401–8, 1995.

[19] M. E. Gurtin. An Introduction to Continuum Mechanics. Academic Press, Inc., San Diego, CA, 1981.

[20] J.T. Marcus, M.J.W. Gotte, A.C. Van Rossum, J.P.A. Kuijer, R.M. Heethaar, L. Axel, and C.A. Visser. Myocardial function in infarcted and remote regions early after infarction in man: Assessment by magnetic resonance tagging and strain analysis. Magn. Reson. Med., 38:803–810, 1997.

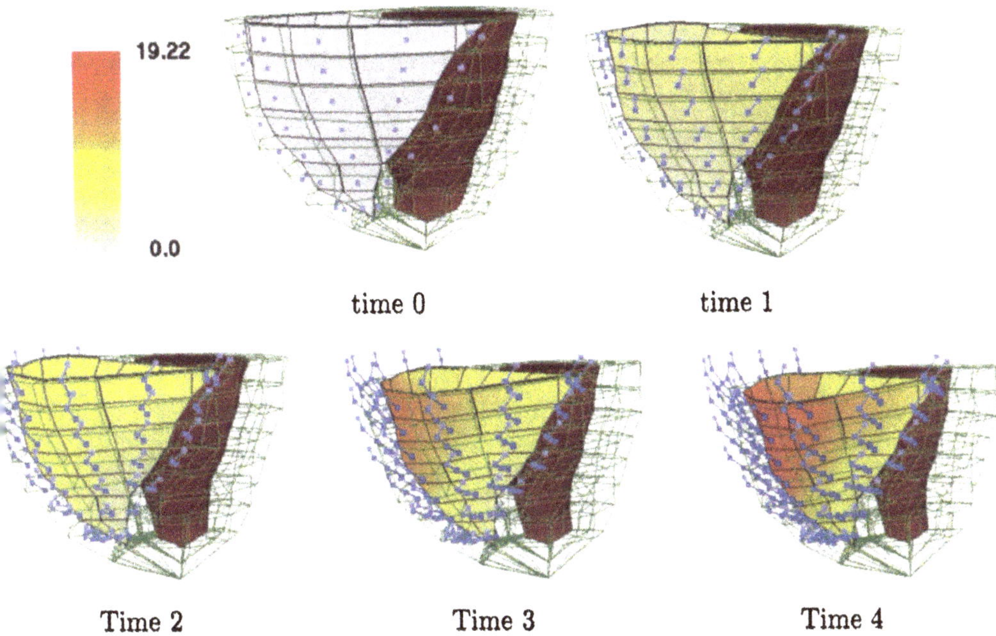

Plate 1: **[Figure 4.16]** Normal heart displacement through systole: Plot of displacement on the RV endocardial free wall. The paths of points located in the centers of the elements are shown from end-diastole (light blue) to end-systole (dark blue).

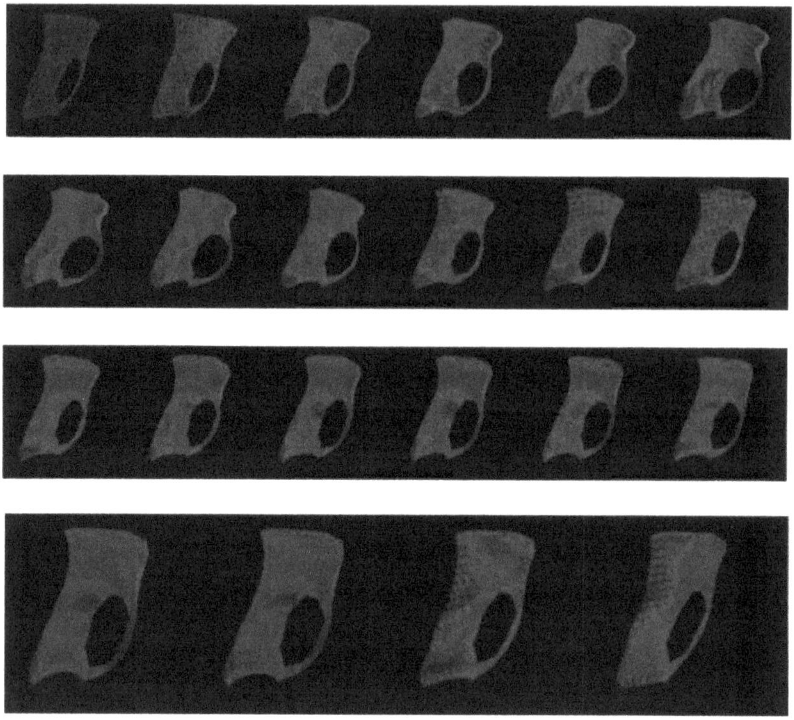

Plate 2: **[Figure 5.11]** **(Top Row)** Right atrial anterior section's motion during ventricular systole. **(Second Row)** Early diastole. **(Third Row)** Mid diastole. **(Bottom Row)** Atrial systole. In Plates 2[Figure 5.11] and 3[Figure 5.12], for all images, the surface color-coding represents the total Euclidean displacement from the initial time frame. The lines are trajectories of the points from the start of each row. The last image of the previous row is the same as the first image of the subsequent row.

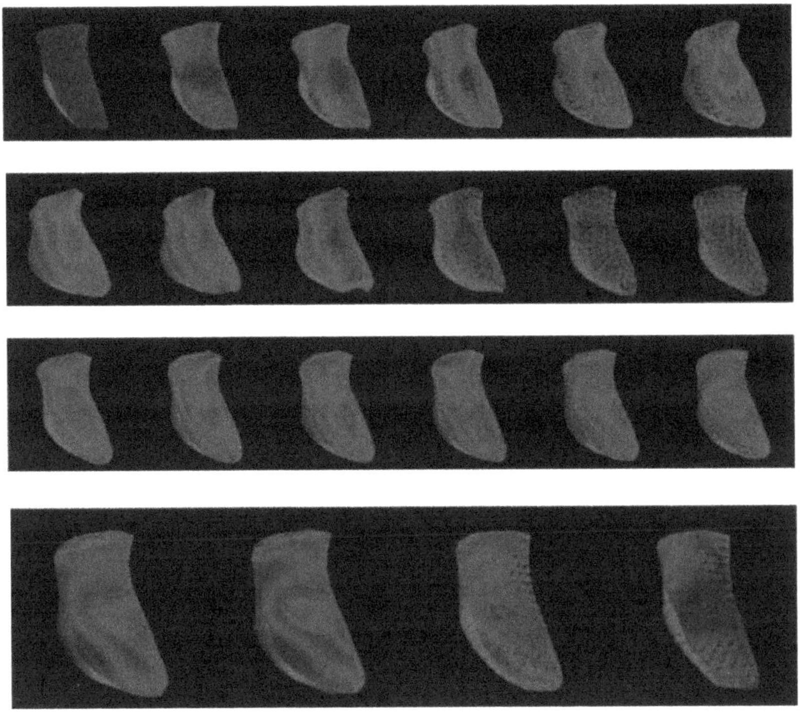

Plate 3: **[Figure 5.12]** **(Top Row)** Right Atrium Posterior Section's motion during ventricular systole. **(Second Row)** Early diastole. **(Third Row)** Mid diastole. **(Bottom Row)** Atrial systole. For further information see the caption of Plate 2[Figure 5.11].

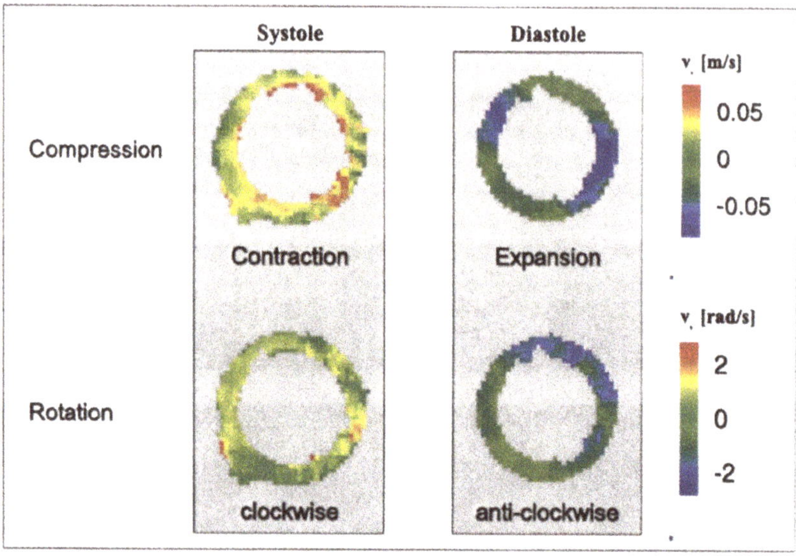

Plate 4: **[Figure 9.14]** Color coded velocities for a healthy volunteer. Positive values correspond to inward and clockwise, and negative values to outward and anti-clockwise motion respectively. The range of the velocities is indicated by the color bars.

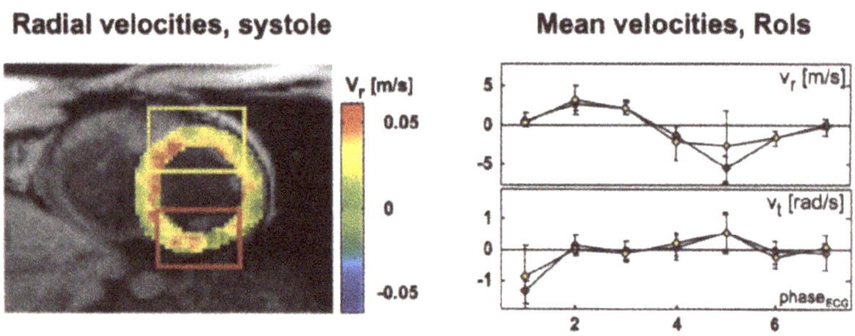

Plate 5: **[Figure 9.15]** Averaged compression ($\bar{\nu}_r$) and tangential ($\bar{\nu}_\phi$) velocities in two selected ROIs in a normal volunteer. Radial velocities of a systolic phase are displayed as color coded image, which is superimposed on the corresponding magnitude image. Time evolution of the average velocity components over the cardiac cycle inside the ROIs is displayed in the plots (red = posterior wall, yellow = anterior wall) on the right. The motion parameters exhibit coincident temporal evolution for both velocity components.

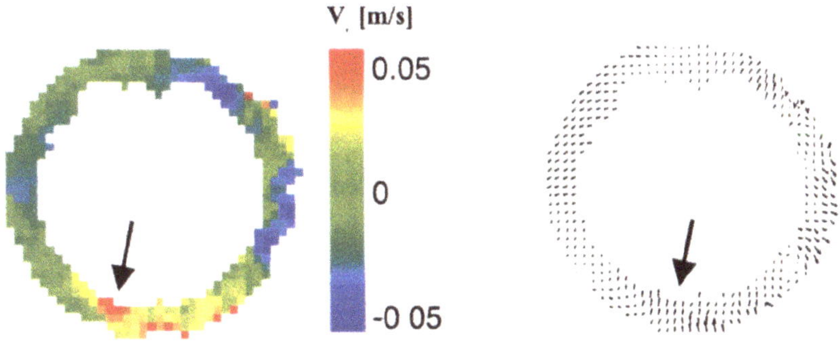

Plate 6: **[Figure 9.20]** Color coded image (left) and arrow plot (right) in a diastolic phase of a patient with posterior infarction. The arrows point towards the regions, which demonstrate dyskinetic motion in the infarcted region.

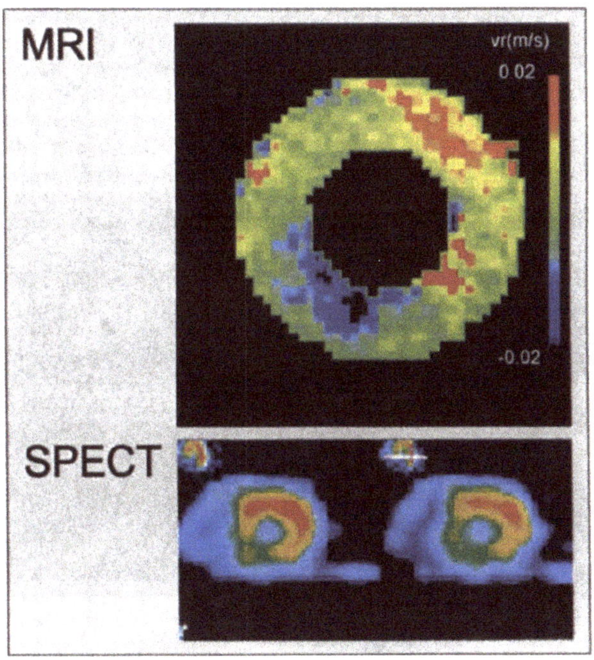

Plate 7: **[Figure 9.21]** Color-coded image of v_r in a slice 3 cm from the base of the left ventricle in a patient with a posterior infarction acquired at $t_{ecg} = 90$ ms (top) compared to a TI-201-SPECT examination (bottom). The scintigrams represent two parallel sections during a time frame in systole. A comparison of the velocity scale with Figure 9.14 shows the much higher variation of v_r over the myocardium. The infarcted region is akinetic or even dyskinetic (outward motion = blue).

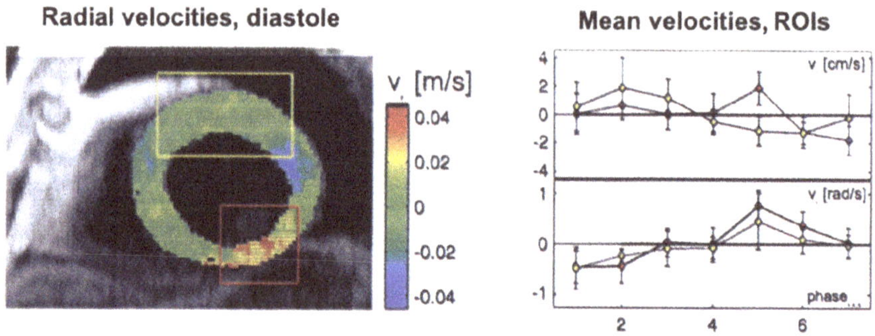

Plate 8: **[Figure 9.22]** Averaged compression ν_r and tangential ν_t velocities in two selected ROIs in a patient with posterior infarction. Temporal evolution of the average velocity components over the cardiac cycle inside the ROIs is displayed in the plots (red = postero-lateral wall, yellow = anterior wall). The radial velocities of the infarcted region show an opposite motion pattern compared to the lateral wall.

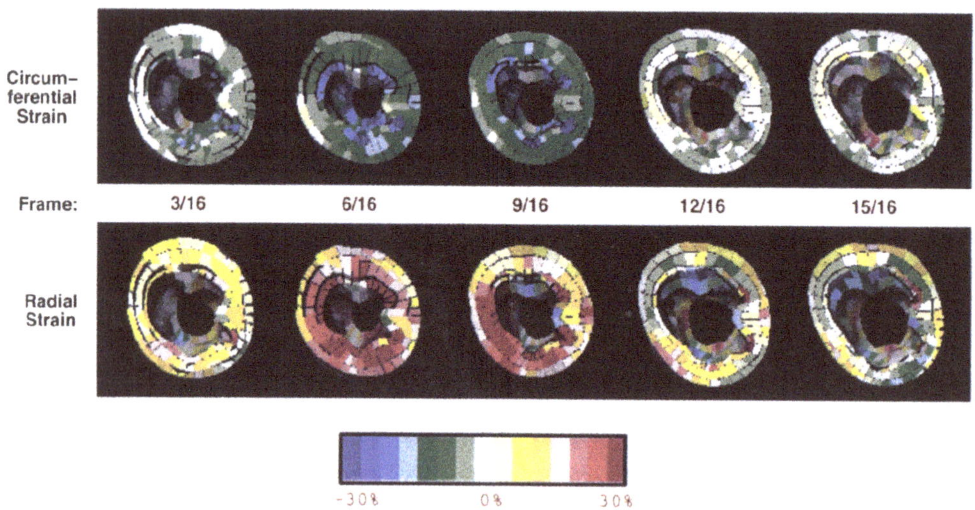

Plate 9: **[Figure 11.5]** Strain Development in Baseline Canine LV derived from cine-MRI. In this figure we show results from every third frame for circumferential (top) and radial (bottom) strain development in a normal canine LV.

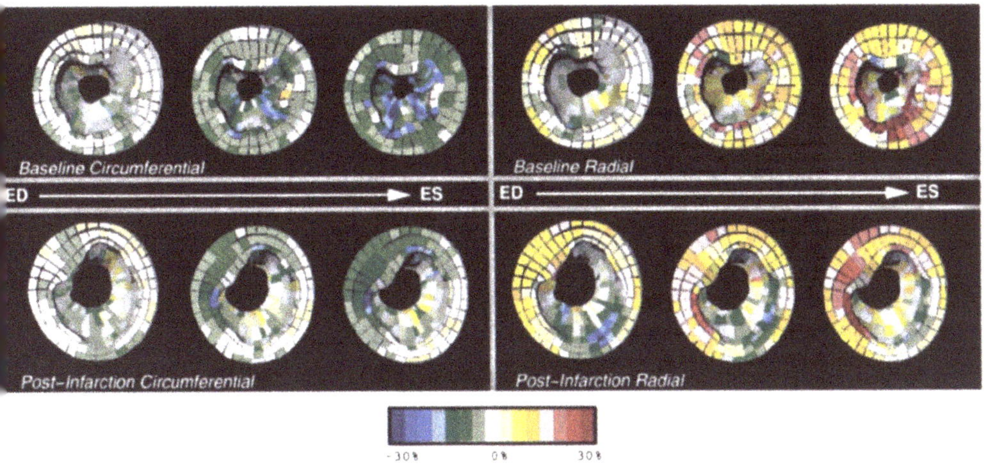

Plate 10: **[Figure 11.6]** Strain Development in Post-Infarction (and vs. Baseline) Canine LV derived from cine-MRI. Left side: mid-ventricle cut-away views through the 3D reconstructed volume show the strain patterns that develop at 1/3, 2/3 and 3/3 of the time between ED and ES. The leftmost displays illustrate the circumferential (CC) strains (normal ED-ES shortening is in the blue-green region). The displays just to the right show the radial (RR) strains (normal ED-ES thickening in yellow-red region).

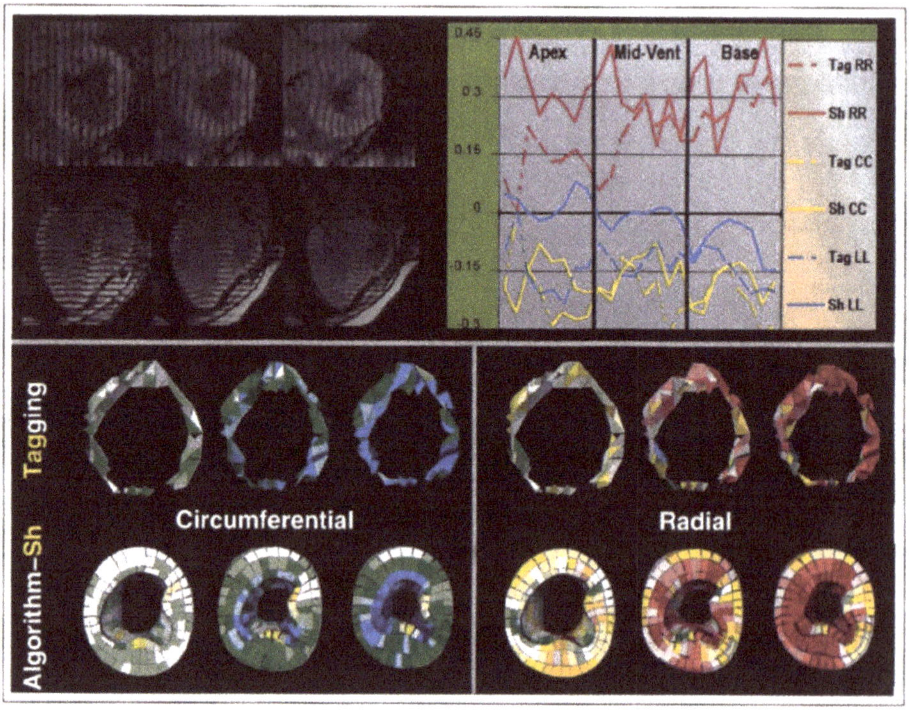

Plate 11: **[Figure 11.7]** MR Tagging-derived strains vs. strains from cine-MRI, derived using our algorithm using shape-based displacements. Top-left: Image slices shown with MR line tags in 2 (out of 3) orthogonal views at three time points. Bottom-left: MR tagging-derived (upper) and our-algorithm-derived (lower) circumferential strains at times 1/3, 2/3 and 3/3 from ED to ES. Refer to color scale in Plate 10. Bottom-right: MR tagging-derived (upper) and our -algorithm-derived (lower) radial strains at same times. For MR tag displays, tetrahedra connect only the tracked points. Top-right: Comparison of circumferential (CC,yellow), radial (RR,red) and longitudinal (LL,blue) ED-ES strains in a helical path from apex to base of LV derived using MR-tagging (Tag, dotted lines) and our-algorithm (Sh, solid lines).

Chapter 7

Automated Tag Detection

Thomas S. Denney Jr.
Department of Electrical and Computer Engineering,
Auburn University,
Auburn, AL
tdenney@eng.auburn.edu

7.1 Introduction

Tagged MRI [4, 30] is an excellent technique for measuring tissue deformations. For the deformation to be quantified, however, the tags must be identified and tracked through the image sequence. Tag identification and tracking is the most time consuming step in the analysis of tagged MR images because most techniques require that the myocardium is segmented from the background before the tags are identified and tracked. This segmentation requires user interaction in each image in the study.

While user-supervised tag tracking is currently the gold standard technique for tagged image analysis in research labs, a significant amount of automation in the tag tracking process is needed before quantitative analysis of tagged MRI can be viable in a clinical setting. In this chapter, we will describe some techniques for automated tag identification and tracking. The primary difference between our automated tag identification and tracking algorithms and existing user-supervised methods [1, 14, 16, 19, 29] is that our automated algorithms do not require a user-defined segmentation of the myocardium. In user-supervised processing, the user defines, with a semi-automated algorithm such as [14], the inner and outer contours of the myocardium which are used to construct a segmentation of the myocardium. As a result, tag detection becomes more tractable, since the tags are known to be in the myocardium. In our automated tag identification algorithms, the region of interest (ROI) contains both tagged and untagged tissue. Hence, we need to detect the presence of a tag line and estimate the location of its center.

Our approach, which we call the ML/MAP method, is based on classical signal parameter estimation and detection techniques. The ML/MAP method is composed

A.A. Amini and J.L. Prince (eds.),
Measurement of Cardiac Deformations from MRI: Physical and Mathematical Models, 151–181.

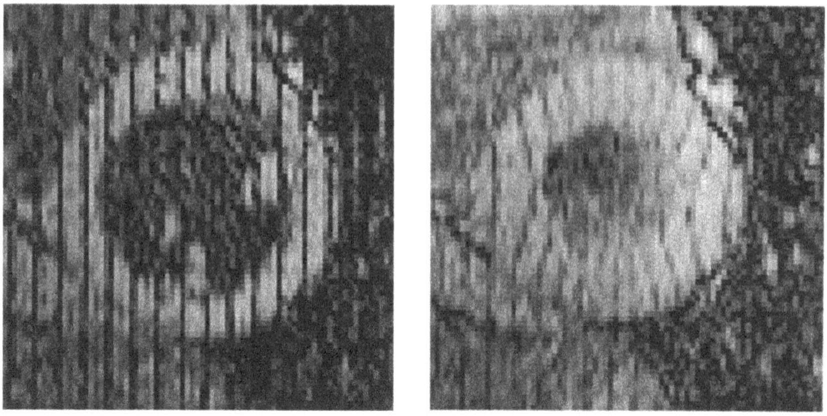

47ms 340ms

Figure 7.1: Tagged images of the left ventricle of a normal human volunteer at early systole (47 ms after the R wave) and end-systole (340 ms after the R wave).

of three stages. First a set of candidate tag line centers are estimated across the entire region-of-interest (ROI) with a snake algorithm [6, 18]. The image forces applied to each snake point are derived from a maximum-likelihood (ML) estimate of the tag center. A *maximum a posteriori* (MAP) hypothesis test is then used to construct a rough liberal segmentation of the myocardium. Spatial continuity of the snakes is not enforced across the segmentation boundaries. In the second stage, another, more conservative, MAP hypothesis test is used to detect the candidate tag centers that are actually part of a tag line. The third stage consists of a pruning algorithm that removes any detected tag centers that do not meet a spatio-temporal continuity criterion.

We develop the ML/MAP algorithm in the context of planar (or parallel) tagged, black blood cardiac images [10, 21] as shown in Figure 7.1. We then describe how the algorithm can be modified for planar tagged, white blood images. We present experiments on in vivo human data that demonstrate the ML/MAP algorithm for both of these imaging protocols.

7.2 Signal Models

In this section we derive a set of stochastic signal models for a neighborhood of pixels in a black blood, planar tagged image oriented perpendicular to the undeformed tag lines as shown in Figure 7.1. For the case of parallel vertical tag lines, the neighborhood would be oriented along an image row. For horizontal tag lines, the neighborhood would be oriented along the image columns. These signal models will be used in the sequel to derive a tag center estimator and spatially dependent thresholds for detecting tag lines. While a neighborhood can contain many different tissue types and combinations of tissue types, we only consider the

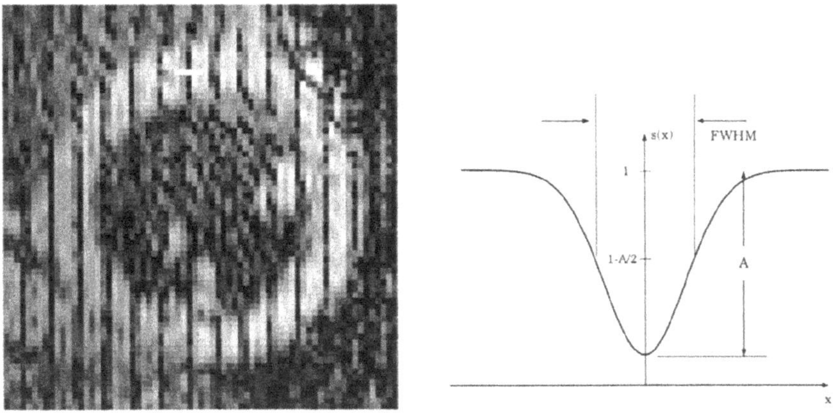

(a) (b)

Figure 7.2: **(a)** Tag line point neighborhood. **(b)** Ideal intensity profile of tag line in the neighborhood.

following three mutually exclusive hypotheses:

Hypothesis T: The neighborhood contains tagged myocardium.

Hypothesis M: The neighborhood contains untagged bright tissue (presumably, but not necessarily myocardium).

Hypothesis B: The neighborhood contains untagged dark tissue such as saturated blood (in black blood images) and air.

7.2.1 Tagged Myocardium

Under Hypothesis T, the MR image intensity in a neighborhood is a function of the tag pattern, proton density, T_1, T_2, the imaging protocol, and noise. For precise mathematical models see [7, 11, 23]. For the purposes of tag estimation and detection, however, we use a simplified model that approximates the intensity profile in the neighborhood of a single tag line as the intensity of the untagged myocardium $m_{\mathrm{M}}(x)$, which includes T_1, T_2, and other effects, multiplied by the tag profile $s(x)$ plus noise [3]

$$w(x) = m_{\mathrm{M}}(x)s(x-\mu) + n(x)\,, \tag{7.1}$$

where μ is the position of the tag center, which changes from time frame to time frame in a cine sequence due to the motion of the myocardium. For the tag profile $s(x)$, we use an inverted Gaussian model (Figure 7.2b) similar to the one used in template-matching algorithms [2, 14]:

$$s(x) = 1 - A(t)e^{-(4\ln 2)x^2/\mathrm{FWHM}^2}\,, \tag{7.2}$$

where $0 \leq A(t) \leq 1$ is the tag amplitude, and FWHM is the full width at half maximum of the tag. The tag pattern amplitude decays with time due to T_1 relaxation [30], which we model as

$$A(t) = e^{-t/T_{1_{\text{nom}}}},$$

where $T_{1_{\text{nom}}}$ is the nominal T_1 of the myocardium (we use $T_{1_{\text{nom}}} = 500$msec.). Since the myocardium deforms and, in later frames, the neighborhood is no longer strictly perpendicular to the tag line, the exact value of the FWHM is not known. In principal, a FWHM could be estimated for each candidate tag center, but we prefer to use the fixed nominal value for FWHM from the image protocol because it helps in the detection phase to distinguish between true tag lines and false tags due either to noise (with a narrower FWHM) or non-tag dark lines in the ROI such as the pericardial sac (with a wider FWHM).

We now consider a neighborhood of N_s pixels (we use $N_s = 5$) as shown in Figure 7.2a. These pixels can be stacked into an N_s-vector $\mathbf{w}$. Since these image pixels are samples of the intensity profile in Equation (7.1),

$$\mathbf{w} = \mathbf{S}(\mu)\mathbf{m}_{\text{M}} + \mathbf{n}, \tag{7.3}$$

where $\mathbf{m}_{\text{M}}$ and $\mathbf{n}$ are N_s-vectors of samples of the myocardium and noise signals respectively, and

$$\mathbf{S}(\mu) = \begin{bmatrix} s(-\mu) & & & \\ & s(\Delta - \mu) & & \\ & & \ddots & \\ & & & s((N_s - 1)\Delta - \mu) \end{bmatrix},$$

where Δ is the image pixel spacing. The vector $\mathbf{m}_{\text{M}}$ contains the local myocardial signal intensity in the vicinity of the tag line. The myocardial signal intensity can vary with spatial position in a given slice, so we model $\mathbf{m}_{\text{M}}$ as a Gaussian random vector [13, 20, 27] with mean $\overline{\mathbf{m}}_{\text{M}} = \overline{m}_{\text{M}}\mathbf{1}$, where $\mathbf{1}$ is an N_s-vector of ones, and covariance matrix $\mathbf{C}_{\text{M}}(i,j) = \sigma_{\text{M}}^2\, \rho_{\text{M}}^{|i-j|}$. This model allows the local myocardial signal to vary smoothly within the vector $\mathbf{w}$ and to vary with each tag center in the image. The parameter ρ_{M} describes the amount of spatial correlation between the myocardial signal samples in $\mathbf{m}_{\text{M}}$. A value of $\rho_{\text{M}} = 0$ means that the samples are uncorrelated (white noise), while a value of ρ_{M} close to one means that the signal varies smoothly with spatial position. The value of ρ_{M} could in principle be estimated from the image data, but for the sake of computational simplicity, we use a single value of $\rho_{\text{M}} = 0.9$.

The noise in MRI is signal dependent [17] and is described by a Rician density [24]. The Rician density approaches a Rayleigh density as the signal-to-noise-ration (SNR) approaches zero and a Gaussian density as the SNR increases [17]. Since the myocardium has fairly high SNR, we model the noise vector $\mathbf{n}$ as a zero mean white Gaussian vector with covariance $\sigma_n^2\mathbf{I}$.

The myocardial signal and image noise statistics vary from subject to subject, from scan to scan, and even from time frame to time frame. Therefore, values for $\overline{m}_{\mathrm{M}}$, σ_{M}^2, and σ_n^2 are estimated from the image data for each time frame in a cine sequence (see Section 7.5.1).

Given the above models for the myocardial signal, tag line, and noise, the observation vector $\mathbf{w}$ is a Gaussian random vector whose probability density function (PDF) is parameterized by μ. The PDF of the observation vector is given by [25]

$$\begin{aligned} f(\mathbf{w};\mu) &= \frac{1}{(2\pi)^{N_s/2}\sqrt{|\mathbf{C}_{\mathrm{T}}(\mu)|}} \times \\ &\quad \exp\left(-\frac{1}{2}[\mathbf{w}-\mathbf{m}_{\mathrm{T}}(\mu)]^T \mathbf{C}_{\mathrm{T}}^{-1}(\mu)[\mathbf{w}-\mathbf{m}_{\mathrm{T}}(\mu)]\right), \end{aligned} \tag{7.4}$$

where$|\cdot|$ denotes determinant, $\mathbf{m}_{\mathrm{T}}(\mu)$ is the mean of $\mathbf{w}$ given by

$$\mathbf{m}_{\mathrm{T}}(\mu) = \mathbf{S}(\mu)\overline{\mathbf{m}}_{\mathrm{M}},$$

and $\mathbf{C}_{\mathrm{T}}(\mu)$ is the covariance matrix of $\mathbf{w}$ given by

$$\mathbf{C}_{\mathrm{T}}(\mu) = \mathbf{S}(\mu)\mathbf{C}_{\mathrm{M}}\mathbf{S}(\mu) + \sigma_n^2\mathbf{I}.$$

7.2.2 Untagged Tissue

For the two untagged hypotheses (Hypothesis M and Hypothesis B), there is no modulation by the tag profile, so the signal model reduces to

$$\mathbf{w} = \mathbf{m}_* + \mathbf{n}, \tag{7.5}$$

where $* =$ M or B, $\mathbf{m}_*$ is an N_s-vector of signal samples and $\mathbf{n}$ is the noise vector. $\mathbf{m}_{\mathrm{M}}$ is described in Section 7.2.1. Similarly, the vector $\mathbf{m}_{\mathrm{B}}$ is modeled as a random vector with mean $\overline{\mathbf{m}}_{\mathrm{B}} = \overline{m}_{\mathrm{B}}\mathbf{1}$ and covariance matrix $\mathbf{C}_{\mathrm{B}}(i,j) = \sigma_{\mathrm{B}}^2\,\rho_{\mathrm{B}}^{|i-j|}$. Values for $\overline{m}_{\mathrm{M}}$, σ_{M}^2, $\overline{m}_{\mathrm{B}}$, σ_{B}^2 are estimated from the image data for each time frame in the sequence (see Section 7.5.1).

We use a Gaussian model for the noise vector $\mathbf{n}$ for both the myocardium and dark tissue hypotheses. Air and blood (in black blood images) have low SNR, and the Gaussian approximation for the noise density is less accurate than it is in the myocardium (high SNR) hypothesis. We have found, however, that the Gaussian noise assumption still works well in practice for the purposes of differentiating between tagged and untagged tissue.

The PDF of the observation vector under Hypotheses M or B is given by [25]

$$\begin{aligned} f(\mathbf{w}|H_*) &= \frac{1}{(2\pi)^{N_s/2}\sqrt{|\mathbf{C}_*|}} \times \\ &\quad \exp\left(-\frac{1}{2}[\mathbf{w}-\overline{\mathbf{m}}_*]^T \mathbf{C}_*^{-1}[\mathbf{w}-\overline{\mathbf{m}}_*]\right), \end{aligned} \tag{7.6}$$

where $\mathbf{C}_*$ is the covariance matrix of $\mathbf{w}$ under Hypothesis M or B and is given by

$$\mathbf{C}_* = \mathbf{C}_* + \sigma_n^2\mathbf{I}.$$

7.3 Tag Center Estimation

In this section we derive an algorithm for estimating the location of a connected line of tag points. Note when estimating tag lines, we always assume Hypothesis T (tagged myocardium) regardless of where we are in the image, since the other hypotheses do not contain this parameter. The estimated tag center will be used later along with the neighborhood pixel data in a Bayesian hypothesis test to determine if the tagged myocardium hypothesis is indeed true. Also we first consider estimation of a single tag center, then later incorporate the single tag estimator in an active contour (snake) estimation framework to track a connected set of tag points.

7.3.1 Single Tag Center Estimation

We first consider estimating the position of a single tag center μ from a neighborhood of N_s pixels along a line perpendicular to a tag line using the maximum likelihood estimation framework. Given neighborhood of image pixels $\mathbf{w}$, the maximum likelihood estimate of μ is the one that maximizes the PDF $f(\mathbf{w};\mu)$ defined in Equation (7.4). To simplify matters, we take the natural logarithm of $f(\mathbf{w};\mu)$ and delete constant terms, which yields the following expression for the maximum likelihood estimate of the tag center $\hat{\mu}$

$$\hat{\mu} = \arg\min_{\mu} L(\mu;\mathbf{w}), \tag{7.7}$$

where

$$L(\mu;\mathbf{w}) = \frac{1}{2}[\mathbf{w} - \overline{\mathbf{m}}_{\mathrm{T}}(\mu)]^T \mathbf{C}_{\mathrm{T}}^{-1}(\mu)[\mathbf{w} - \overline{\mathbf{m}}_{\mathrm{T}}(\mu)] + \frac{1}{2}\ln|\mathbf{C}_{\mathrm{T}}(\mu)|, \tag{7.8}$$

where $\ln(\cdot)$ denotes natural logarithm. A plot of $L(\mu;\mathbf{w})$ for a 5-pixel neighborhood of a tag line in an *in vivo* heart image is shown in Figure 7.3. Note than in actual images, it is possible that $\mathbf{w}$ will contain portions of profiles from neighboring tags. Minimizing $L(\mu;\mathbf{w})$ will still result in the true tag center provided the optimization algorithm is started sufficiently close to the true tag center. The issues of optimizing $L(\mu;\mathbf{w})$ and initialization are addressed in Section 7.3.2.

The log likelihood function in Equation (7.8) is similar in spirit to the tag energy functions on other model-based tag tracking methods [2, 14, 15, 22]. In the log likelihood function, however, the inverse covariance matrix $\mathbf{C}_{\mathrm{T}}^{-1}(\mu)$ provides a set of weights for comparing the data and tag template based on the physics of the tagging process and image statistics. If the myocardial signal is assumed to be constant with unit intensity (i.e. $\overline{m}_{\mathrm{myo}} = 1$, $\sigma^2_{\mathrm{myo}} = 0$) and the noise is assumed to have unit variance, $L(\mu;\mathbf{w})$ reduces to a discrete template match cost function similar to the one proposed by Guttman, et al. [14, 15]

$$L(\mu;\mathbf{w}) = \frac{1}{2}[\mathbf{w} - \mathbf{s}(\mu)]^T[\mathbf{w} - \mathbf{s}(\mu)], \tag{7.9}$$

where $\mathbf{s}(\mu) = \mathbf{S}(\mu)\mathbf{1}$ is the tag template. If the inner product in (7.9) is expanded and terms $\frac{1}{2}\mathbf{w}^T\mathbf{w}$ and $\frac{1}{2}\mathbf{s}^T(\mu)\mathbf{s}(\mu)$ are removed0This assumes that the power in the

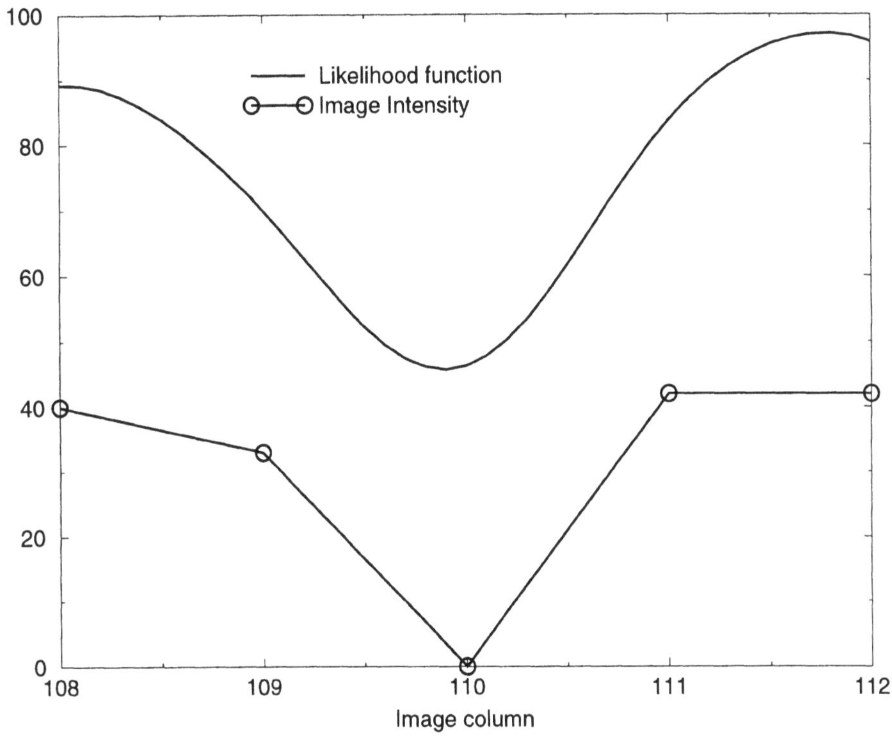

Figure 7.3: A plot of the tag center log likelihood function $L(\mu; \mathbf{w})$ versus position (image column) for a 5-pixel neighborhood of a tag line in an in vivo heart image. The image pixel intensities are denoted by circles. The position where $L(\mu; \mathbf{w})$ is minimum is the maximum likelihood estimate of the tag center.

tag template, $\mathbf{s}^T(\mu)\mathbf{s}(\mu)$, is constant with respect to a shift. For the tag templates used in this paper, this is approximately true for small shifts ($|\mu| \leq$ FWHM/2)., $L(\mu; \mathbf{w})$ reduces to a correlation function similar to the one proposed by Amini, et al. [2, 22]

$$L(\mu; \mathbf{w}) \approx -\sum_{k=0}^{k=N_s-1} w(k\Delta)s(k\Delta - \mu)\,. \tag{7.10}$$

The template match cost function in [14, 15] and the correlation function in [2, 22] both have normalization terms that adjust for amplitude differences between the tag template and the data. In the log likelihood function in Equation (7.8), this adjustment is accomplished by the mean myocardial signal intensity $\overline{m}_{\mathrm{M}}$ and a spatially varying normalization term, ζ_{ij}, in the snake algorithm described in the next section.

7.3.2 Tag Line Estimation

In principle, a tag line could be estimated by applying Equation (7.7) independently to a set of neighborhoods perpendicular to each tag line. Imaging artifacts and noise spikes, however, can cause large estimation errors, and since each tag line is estimated independently, there is nothing to prevent two tag lines from occupying the same physical position. For these reasons, we optimize Equation (7.8) for each tag center subject to spatial continuity constraints and a constraint on tag separation [15].

We denote the vector of candidate tag centers for the jth tag line as $\boldsymbol{\mu}_j = [\mu_{0\,j}\ \mu_{1\,j}\ \cdots\ \mu_{N_c-1\,j}]^T$, where each $\mu_{i\,j}$ is a real valued position on the ith image row. We define the optimal tag line as the tag line that minimizes the following energy function

$$\begin{aligned} E(\boldsymbol{\mu}_j) &= \sum_{i=0}^{N_c-1} [\zeta_{i\,j} L(\mu_{i\,j}, \mathbf{w}_{i\,j}) + \gamma_{i\,j} E_{\text{sep}}(\mu_{i\,j+1} - \mu_{i\,j}) \\ &\quad + \gamma_{i\,j} E_{\text{sep}}(\mu_{i\,j} - \mu_{i\,j-1})] + E_{\text{stretch}}(\mathbf{v}_j) + E_{\text{bend}}(\mathbf{v}_j)\,, \end{aligned} \tag{7.11}$$

where N_c is the number of centers in each tag line and $\mathbf{v}_j$ is the displacement of the tag line $\boldsymbol{\mu}_j$ from its initial (undeformed) position0 The initial position of each snake is specified by the user (see Section 7.4.1). $\mathbf{p}_j$ such that $\boldsymbol{\mu}_j = \mathbf{p}_j + \mathbf{v}_j$. $L(\mu_{i\,j}, \mathbf{w}_{i\,j})$ is the likelihood function defined in (7.8) for the ith center on the jth tag line and $\zeta_{i\,j}$ is a normalizing factor to be defined later.

E_{sep} is a tag separation constraint given by

$$E_{\text{sep}}(x) = \begin{cases} 0 & \text{for } x \geq d_{\text{sep}}, \\ \frac{1}{2}(d_{\text{sep}} - x)^2 & \text{for } x < d_{\text{sep}}, \end{cases}$$

where d_{sep} is the minimum distance between tag points. γ_{ij} is a user-specified parameter that controls the degree to which the separation constraint is enforced and is set to zero if μ_{ij} is outside the myocardium (see Section 7.4.1).

E_{stretch} and E_{bend} are constraints on the stretch and bending of the tag displacements [6, 18, 29] given by

$$\begin{aligned} E_{\text{stretch}}(\mathbf{v}_j) &= \frac{1}{2}\sum_{i=1}^{N_c-1} \frac{\alpha_{ij}}{h}|v_{ij} - v_{i-1\,j}|^2 , \\ E_{\text{bend}}(\mathbf{v}_j) &= \frac{1}{2}\sum_{i=1}^{N_c-2} \frac{\beta_{ij}}{h^2}|v_{i+1\,j} - 2v_{ij} + v_{i-1\,j}|^2 , \end{aligned} \tag{7.12}$$

where h is spacing between candidate tag centers, which for the case of a candidate center for each row is the MR image pixel spacing. The weights α_{ij} and β_{ij} vary with each tag center depending on whether or not the center and its neighbors are determined to be inside the myocardium. Specifically, $\alpha_{ij} = \alpha$ if μ_{ij} and $\mu_{i-1\,j}$ are inside the myocardium and set to zero otherwise. Similarly, $\beta_{ij} = \beta$ if $\mu_{i+1\,j}$, μ_{ij}, and $\mu_{i\,j-1}$ are inside the myocardium and set to zero otherwise. α and β are user-specified parameters. Setting the weights to zero in this manner ensures that tag centers outside the myocardium cannot influence the position of tag centers inside the myocardium through the smoothing constraints.

The energy function in Equation (7.11) is optimized using the method proposed by Kass, et al. [18]. First Equation (7.11) is differentiated with respect to $\mathbf{v}_j$, which results in

$$\mathbf{A}_j\mathbf{v}_j - \mathbf{q}_j(\boldsymbol{\mu}_{j-1}, \boldsymbol{\mu}_j + \boldsymbol{\mu}_{j+1}) = \mathbf{0} , \tag{7.13}$$

where $\mathbf{A}_j$ is an $N_c \times N_c$ pentadiagonal matrix obtained from differentiating the the internal energy terms in Equation (7.14) with respect to v_{ij} (see [6] for details) . The vector $\mathbf{q}_j$ contains force terms, which will be defined in the sequel. Following [6, 18] the right-hand side of (7.13) is set equal to the negative time derivative of $\mathbf{v}_j$, which yields the following iteration for the jth optimal tag line displacement

$$(\mathbf{I} + \tau\mathbf{A}_j^k)\mathbf{v}_j^k = \mathbf{v}_j^{k-1} + \tau\mathbf{q}_j(\boldsymbol{\mu}_{j-1}^{k-1}, \boldsymbol{\mu}_j^{k-1} + \boldsymbol{\mu}_{j+1}^{k-1}) , \tag{7.14}$$

where k is the iteration index, and τ is a step size. There is an Equation (7.14) for each tag line in the ROI, and these equations are solved simultaneously using a banded system solver [12]. After each iteration of Equation (7.14), each tag center is tested to see if it is inside or outside the myocardium. If the status of a tag center changes, then a new $\mathbf{A}_j^k$ is computed. The initial snake displacement $\mathbf{v}_j^0$ is computed by linearly extrapolating its displacement from its displacement in the previous two time frames. In the first time frame, the initial snake position is the initial tag position and $v_{ij}^0 = 0$. In the second time frame, the initial snake displacement is the final snake displacement from the first time frame.

The vector $\mathbf{q}_j$ contains "force" terms derived from the log likelihood function and the tag separation constraint. The ith component of $\mathbf{q}_j$ is

$$\begin{aligned} q_{j\,i}(\mu_{j-1}, \mu_j, \mu_{j+1}) &= -\zeta_{i\,j} \frac{d}{d\mu} L(\mu_{i\,j}; \mathbf{w}_{i\,j}) \\ &\quad + \gamma_{i\,j}[(d_{\text{sep}} - \mu_{i\,j} + \mu_{i\,j-1}) u(d_{\text{sep}} - \mu_{i\,j} + \mu_{i\,j-1}) \\ &\quad - (d_{\text{sep}} - \mu_{i\,j+1} + \mu_{i\,j}) u(d_{\text{sep}} - \mu_{i\,j+1} + \mu_{i\,j})], \quad (7.15) \end{aligned}$$

where $u(x) = 1$ for $x \geq 0$ and $u(x) = 0$ otherwise. The derivative of the likelihood function $L(\mu_{i\,j}; \mathbf{w}_{i\,j})$ is derived in the appendix. $\zeta_{i\,j}$ is a normalizing factor defined as

$$\zeta_{i\,j} = \frac{1}{\max_{i \in \left[i - \frac{N_s}{2}, i + \frac{N_s}{2}\right]} \left| \frac{d}{d\mu} L(\mu_{i\,j}; \mathbf{w}_{i\,j}) \right|}$$

if $\mu_{i\,j}$ is in the myocardium and zero otherwise. This normalization stabilizes the snake algorithm by keeping the forces acting on the snake from being too large relative to the iteration step size [6].

Equation (7.14) leaves the position of candidate centers outside the myocardium unchanged. After the iteration in Equation (7.14) is complete, the position of candidate centers outside the myocardium is computed by using a smoothing spline to interpolate between the positions of candidate centers inside the myocardium [see Figure 7.8(a)]. This smoothing spline minimizes the stretching and bending energies described in Equation (7.12), with the exception that the smoothness constraints are applied to candidate centers outside the myocardium. Connecting centers outside the myocardium in this manner makes it easier for a candidate center to move inside the myocardium in the next time frame. The positions of candidate centers inside and outside the myocardium are computed separately to ensure that the position of centers inside the myocardium influence the position of centers outside the myocardium, but not vice versa.

7.4 Hypothesis Testing

The tag center estimation algorithm described in the previous section applies different smoothing constraints and image forces to a candidate tag center depending on if the center is in the myocardium or not. Ideally, once the estimation algorithm is complete, any candidate tag center considered to be inside the myocardium would be on a tag line. Because of estimation errors, however, it is possible for a candidate tag center to be in the myocardium but not on a tag line. So to ensure that only candidate tag centers on tag lines are considered valid, we apply a more conservative test to each tag center to determine if it is part of a tag line. In this section, two maximum *a posteriori* (MAP) hypothesis tests [25] are developed based on the signal model derived in Section 7.2. The first test determines if a candidate center is inside the myocardium, the second test determines if a candidate center is part of a tag line.

We assume that the probability of each of the three hypotheses is known and denote P_{T}, P_{M}, P_{B}, $\left(P_{\text{T}} + P_{\text{M}} + P_{\text{B}} = 1\right)$ as the probabilities of Hypotheses T, M, and B respectively.

7.4.1 Myocardium Detection

A candidate tag center $\hat{\mu}$ is considered to be inside the myocardium if it is more likely to be either part of a tag line (H_{T}) or in untagged myocardium tissue (H_{M}) than in the background tissue (H_{B}). In terms of the PDF's defined in Equations (7.4) and (7.6) and the known probabilities P_{B}, P_{M}, and P_{T}, the MAP decision rule is that $\hat{\mu}$ is inside the myocardium if [25]

$$\frac{f(\mathbf{w}|H_{\text{T}})}{f(\mathbf{w}|H_{\text{B}})} > \frac{P_{\text{B}}}{P_{\text{T}}} \quad \text{or} \quad \frac{f(\mathbf{w}|H_{\text{M}})}{f(\mathbf{w}|H_{\text{B}})} > \frac{P_{\text{B}}}{P_{\text{M}}} \,. \tag{7.16}$$

Taking the natural logarithm of both sides of the inequalities in (7.16) and canceling terms results in the rule that an estimated tag center $\hat{\mu}$ is inside the myocardium if

$$\max[L(\hat{\mu};\mathbf{w}), \eta_{\text{M}}(\mathbf{w})] < \eta_{\text{B}}(\mathbf{w}), \tag{7.17}$$

where $\eta_{\text{M}}(\mathbf{w})$ and $\eta_{\text{B}}(\mathbf{w})$ are given by

$$\begin{aligned} \eta_{\text{M}}(\mathbf{w}) &= \frac{1}{2}[\mathbf{w} - \overline{\mathbf{m}}_{\text{myo}}]^T \mathbf{C}_{\text{M}}^{-1}[\mathbf{w} - \overline{\mathbf{m}}_{\text{myo}}] + \frac{1}{2}\ln|\mathbf{C}_{\text{M}}| - \ln(P_{\text{M}}/P_{\text{T}}), \\ \eta_{\text{B}}(\mathbf{w}) &= \frac{1}{2}[\mathbf{w} - \overline{\mathbf{m}}_{\text{back}}]^T \mathbf{C}_{\text{B}}^{-1}[\mathbf{w} - \overline{\mathbf{m}}_{\text{back}}] + \frac{1}{2}\ln|\mathbf{C}_{\text{B}}| - \ln(P_{\text{B}}/P_{\text{T}}). \end{aligned}$$

Note that the prior probabilities P_{B}, P_{M}, and P_{T} effectively bias the decision rule in favor of one hypothesis or another. We use $P_{\text{B}} = P_{\text{M}} = P_{\text{T}} = 1/3$, which means that all three hypotheses are equally likely. In this case, $\ln(P_{\text{M}}/P_{\text{T}}) = \ln(P_{\text{B}}/P_{\text{T}}) = 0$. Results of the myocardium detector in Equation (7.17) applied to the images in Figure 7.1 are shown in Figure 7.4.

7.4.2 Tag Line Detection

In principle, once the tag center estimation algorithm has converged, any candidate tag center inside the myocardium should be the center of an actual tag line. The myocardium detector, however, is not perfect and sometimes non-myocardium tissue is classified as part of the myocardium. For this reason, it is necessary to explicitly test each candidate tag center to determine if it is part of an actual tag line. A candidate center $\hat{\mu}$ is considered to be part of a tag line if it is more likely to be part of a tag line (H_{T}) than either untagged myocardium (H_{M}) or background tissue (H_{B}). The MAP decision rule based on the PDF's defined in Equations (7.4) and (7.6) and the known probabilities P_{B}, P_{M}, and P_{T} is to choose H_{T} if [25]

$$\frac{f(\mathbf{w}|H_{\text{T}})}{f(\mathbf{w}|H_{\text{M}})} > \frac{P_{\text{M}}}{P_{\text{T}}} \quad \text{and} \quad \frac{f(\mathbf{w}|H_{\text{T}})}{f(\mathbf{w}|H_{\text{B}})} > \frac{P_{\text{B}}}{P_{\text{T}}} \,. \tag{7.18}$$

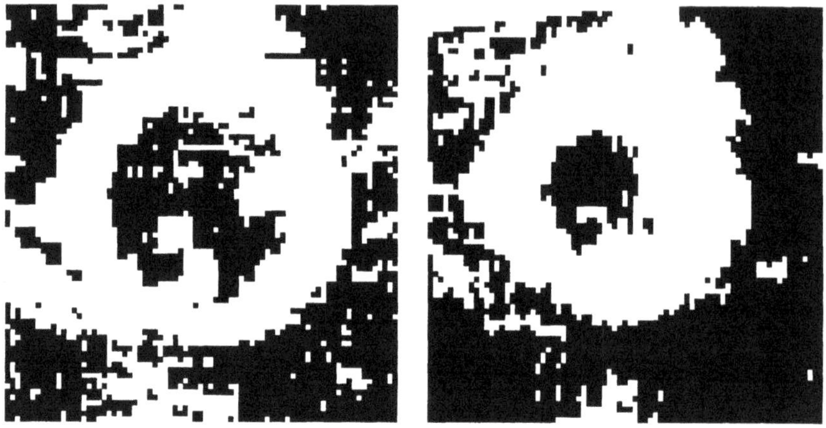

Figure 7.4: The results of the MAP myocardium detector applied to each pixel in the images in Figure 7.1.

Taking the natural logarithm of both sides of the inequalities in (7.18) and canceling terms results in the rule that an estimated tag center $\hat{\mu}$ is part of a tag line if

$$L(\hat{\mu}; \mathbf{w}) < \min[\eta_{\mathrm{M}}(\mathbf{w}) \, , \eta_{\mathrm{B}}(\mathbf{w})] \, . \tag{7.19}$$

7.4.3 Removal of False Tag Points

With real image data, the tag detector in Equation (7.19) sometimes detects a false tag. These false tag detections usually occur in small, isolated clusters that spontaneously appear and disappear in time. As a result after the tag lines have been estimated and detected, we use a pruning algorithm, which consists of two subroutines. The first, called `removeShortRuns()` deletes all tag points that appear in contiguous groups of less than N_{min} in size. We use $N_{\text{min}} = 3$, which removes isolated tag points and isolated pairs of tag points. The second, called `applyTemporalContinuity()`, deletes all tag points that do not have a neighboring tag point in the same tag line within $\pm N_{\text{nbhd}}$ points in either the previous or next time frame. This allows the tag line to either grow or shrink by N_{nbhd} points due to the expansion or contraction of the myocardium between time frames. The value of N_{nbhd} should be roughly proportional to the temporal resolution. For a temporal resolution of 32.5ms, we use $N_{\text{nbhd}} = 1$. After the tags have been estimated and detected, these subroutines are called for each time frame in the following order:

1. `removeShortRuns()`
2. `applyTemporalContinuity()`
3. `removeShortRuns()`

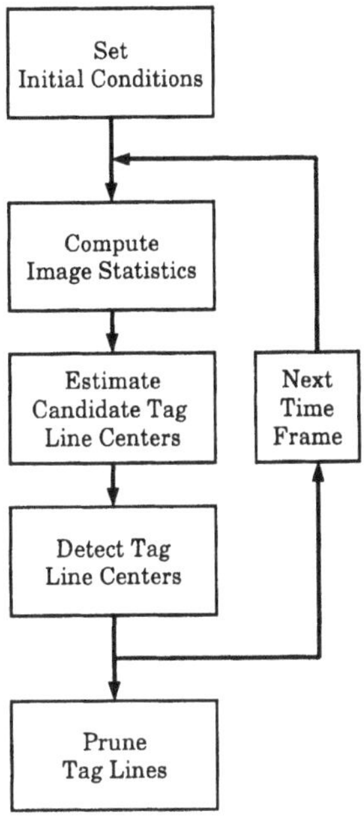

Figure 7.5: ML/MAP algorithm flow chart.

The first call to `removeShortRuns()` deletes isolated tags and isolated tag pairs in each image, which are usually the result of imaging noise creating a dark pixel between two relatively bright pixels in untagged regions such as the blood pool. The call to `applyTemporalContinuity()` deletes tag points in regions of the image that are not persistently tagged. This procedure sometimes creates new groups of isolated tag points, which are removed by the second call to `removeShortRuns()`.

7.5 Algorithm Implementation

7.5.1 Black Blood Images

Figure 7.5 summarizes how the tag estimation, detection, and pruning algorithms are implemented. First the user specifies a rectangular region of interest (ROI) and a rectangular region over which the image noise statistics were computed (see below). These regions are shown in Figure 7.6a. The same regions are used for each time frame in a given slice. The user also specifies the initial position of the tag lines as shown in Figure 7.6b. The spacing between undeformed tag planes is known from the imaging protocol, so only a single user-specified offset is needed to set the initial position of all tags in the ROI. The same set of initial conditions (two rectangular regions and the initial position) are used for each slice in a stack of short-axis images with the same tag plane orientation. For long-axis images, the initial conditions are set separately for each individual slice because of the

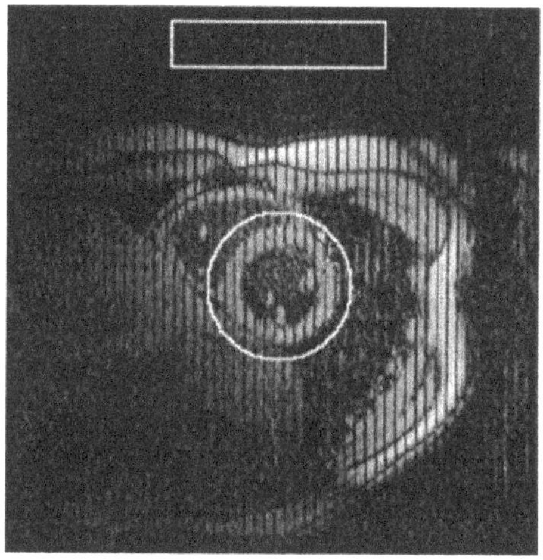

(a)

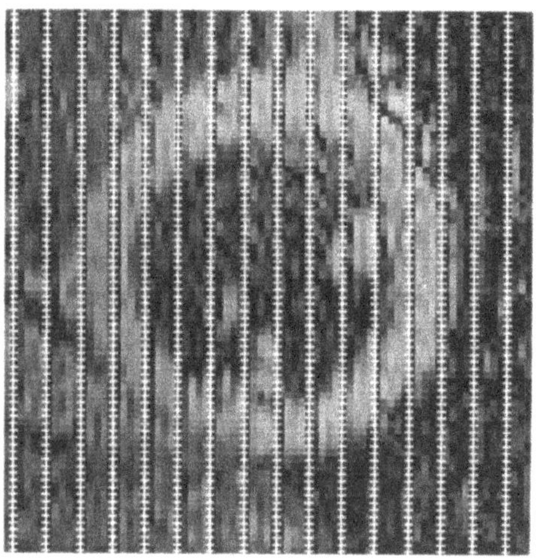

(b)

Figure 7.6: **(a)** Region of interest (ROI) for both noise computation (upper box) and tag tracking (lower box). **(b)** Initial tag position.

differences in orientation of the image planes. These initial conditions are the only user intervention used by the algorithm. At this point for each imaged phase (time frame) of the cardiac cycle, the algorithm first computes the image statistics (see below) and runs the tag estimation algorithm [Equation (7.14)]. The snake iteration in Equation (7.14) is performed for each tag line until either the maximum change in tag position is less than 0.01 or 150 iterations are completed. Next the tag detection routine [Equation (7.19)] is applied to each time frame. Finally after all time frames are processed, the tag pruning algorithm [Section 7.4.3] is run over all time frames.

Choice of Algorithm Parameters

We use the tag full width at half maximum (FWHM) determined from the imaging protocol [21], and the tag center neighborhood size (N_s) is set to the smallest odd integer larger than twice the FWHM. The minimum tag separation d_{sep} is chosen based on a visual inspection of an end-systolic short-axis image. The prior probabilities P_{T}, P_M, and P_{B} must sum to one as described in Section 7.4, and are chosen such that all probabilities were equal. This choice reflects an assumption that a candidate center is as likely to be on a tag line as it is to be in untagged myocardium or background. The remaining parameters are chosen experimentally.

Computation of Image Statistics

In order to run the tag estimation and detection algorithms, an estimate of the noise variance σ_n^2 and the mean and variance of the myocardium pixels ($\overline{m}_{\text{M}}$, σ_{M}^2) and background pixels ($\overline{m}_{\text{B}}$, σ_{B}^2) must be computed for each image in the sequence. There are several possible techniques for estimating these parameters [13,20,26,27] including the tissue classification algorithm we use in Section 7.5.2 for white blood images. We only need a rough estimate, however, and, in black blood images, the myocardium is bright (with the exception of the tag lines) and saturated blood and air are dark. We have found that the following computationally simple approach works well in practice. The noise variance is computed using the pixels enclosed by the rectangular region specified by the user as a sample. We assume that the enclosed pixel intensities represent the absolute value of a zero mean white noise process, and set the noise variance equal to the mean-square value of the enclosed pixel intensities. The myocardium and background statistics are computed by first performing a morphological closing operation over the ROI to remove the tag lines as described in [14]. The resulting pixel intensities are then sorted. $\overline{m}_{\text{M}}$ and σ_{M}^2 were set equal to the sample mean and variance of the brightest 50% of the pixel intensities. $\overline{m}_{\text{B}}$ and σ_{B}^2 were set equal to the sample mean and variance of the darkest 50% of the pixel intensities.

7.5.2 White Blood Images

In white blood images, the intensity of the blood pool in the LV can range from slightly darker than the myocardium to significantly brighter. Consequently, the method described above for computing image statistics is not valid, since the brightest pixels in the ROI contain both myocardium and blood. The rough myocardium segmentation described in Section 7.4.1 is also not valid for white blood images, since it depends on an estimate of the image statistics. In this section we present a technique for computing image statistics and a rough myocardium segmentation for white blood, planar tagged images.

White Blood Image Segmentation

To obtain a rough segmentation of the myocardium, we use a template match to identify pixels in the ROI that are likely to be part of a tag line, then morphologically dilate the tagged pixels. The template match test, however, is only reliable in high SNR regions, so first we identify high SNR regions in the ROI.

We use a Bayesian approach to segment high SNR regions in the ROI. The probability density of a pixel in MR images is Rician, which for low SNR can be approximated by a Rayleigh density. For high SNR, the Rician density is approximately Gaussian. Therefore, we consider a pixel p_i to be in a high SNR region if

$$f_{\text{Rayleigh}}(p_i) > f_{\text{Gaussian}}(p_i)\,, \tag{7.20}$$

where

$$f_{\text{Rayleigh}}(p) = \frac{p}{\sigma_R^2} e^{-p^2/2\sigma_R^2}\,, \tag{7.21}$$

$$f_{\text{Gaussian}}(p) = \frac{1}{\sqrt{2\pi}\sigma_G} e^{-(p-\mu_G)^2/2\sigma_G^2}\,, \tag{7.22}$$

and the mean and variances are computed locally from a 3×3 neighborhood of p_i as follows:

$$\sigma_R^2 = \frac{1}{18} \sum p_j^2\,, \tag{7.23}$$

$$\mu_G = \frac{1}{9} \sum p_j\,, \tag{7.24}$$

$$\sigma_G^2 = \frac{1}{8} \left(\sum p_j^2 - 9\mu_G^2 \right)\,. \tag{7.25}$$

We promote connectivity in the segmentation by modeling the segmentation as a Markov random field. We assume the segmentation has the following Gibbs density:

$$f(\mathbf{p}) = \frac{1}{Z} \exp\left(-\beta U(\mathbf{p})\right)\,, \tag{7.26}$$

where Z is the partition function, β is an empirically determined parameter (we use $\beta = 10$), and $U(\mathbf{p})$ is the energy function

$$U(\mathbf{p}) = \sum_j \left[\sum_{i \in N_i} \delta(p_i - p_j) + \frac{1}{\sqrt{2}} \sum_{i \in \tilde{N}_i} \delta(p_i - p_j) \right] , \tag{7.27}$$

where N_i and $\tilde{N}_i$ are respectively the sets of four nearest neighbors and four nearest diagonal neighbors of the pixel i, and $\delta(\cdot)$ is the Kronecker delta function.

The MAP estimate of the segmentation using iterated conditional modes (ICM) optimization [5] yields the following iteration. A pixel p_i is marked as high SNR if

$$\ln(f_{\text{Rayleigh}}(p_i)) + \beta N_R(p_i) \leq \ln(f_{\text{Gaussian}}(p_i)) + \beta N_G(p_i) , \tag{7.28}$$

where $N_R(p_i)$ and $N_G(p_i)$ are respectively the number of neighboring pixels classified as Rayleigh (low SNR) and Gaussian (high SNR). We run this iteration until the segmentation is unchanged or 30 iterations have been reached. Note we do not consider the case of intermediate SNR, which would primarily be edge pixels. Instead, we rely on the above iteration to segregate low and high SNR regions by promoting regional connectivity.

Next we distinguish between bright tagged and bright untagged regions in the ROI. We cannot use the MAP hypothesis tests developed in Section 7.4.1 in this step because we do not have an estimate of the intensity statistics for the myocardium and blood pool. Instead, we distinguish between these two tissue types with a template match. We use two templates — one for tagged tissue and one for untagged tissue. For tagged tissue, we use a 3×FWHM tag template, where each row of the template is identical and equal to the tag template ($\mu = 0$) in Equation (7.2). For untagged tissue, we use a constant template the same size as the tagged tissue template. We classify a pixel as tagged tissue if

$$(\mathbf{w} - \mathbf{t}_{\text{tag}})^T (\mathbf{w} - \mathbf{t}_{\text{tag}}) \leq (\mathbf{w} - \mathbf{t}_{\text{untag}})^T (\mathbf{w} - \mathbf{t}_{\text{untag}}) , \tag{7.29}$$

where $\mathbf{t}_{\text{tag}}$ and $\mathbf{t}_{\text{untag}}$ are the tagged and untagged tissue templates respectively. This test only identifies pixels that are in the center of a tag line. We want to include the surrounding tissue as well, so we compute the final myocardium segmentation by morphologically dilating the tagged tissue image with a structuring element the size of the templates. The final result is shown in Figure 7.7. A pixel is classified as blood if it is in the high SNR segmentation but not in the myocardium segmentation.

White Blood Image Statistics

Estimates of the means and variances of the dark tissue, myocardium, and blood pool are obtained by first the ROI is morphologically closed in the same way as

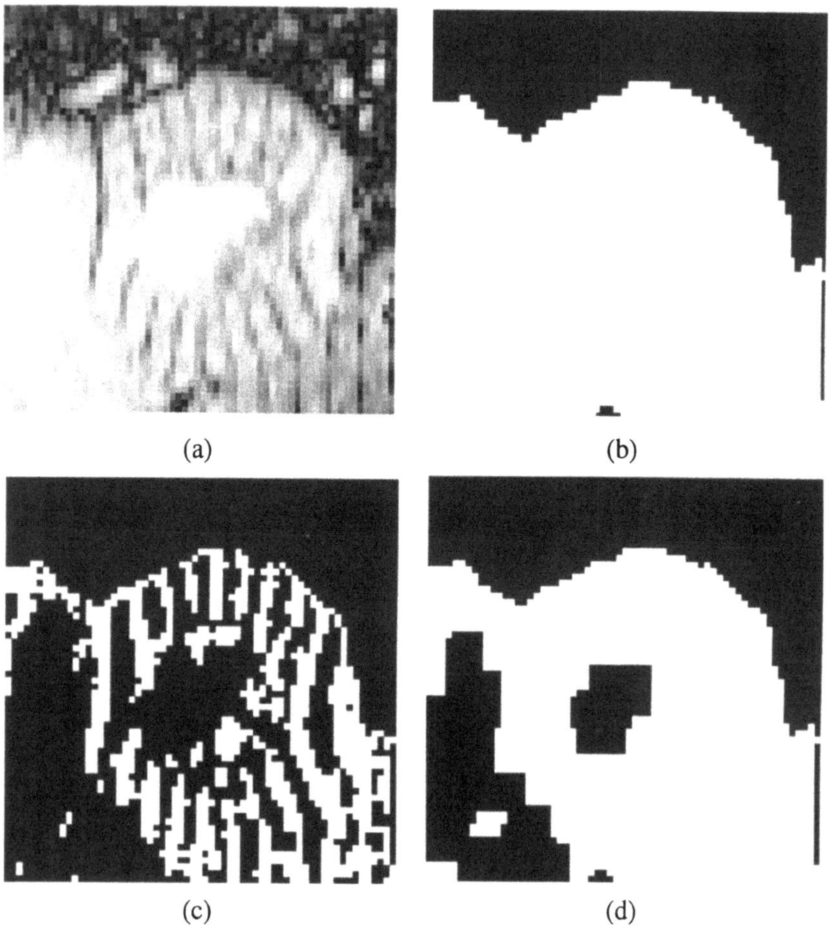

Figure 7.7: Segmenting the myocardium in white blood images: **(a)** white blood image **(b)** segmentation of high-SNR region **(c)** tag line segmentation **(d)** final segmentation after morphological dilation.

black blood images. The myocardium mean and variance is then estimated from pixels in the closed image that are classified as myocardium in the segmentation described in the previous section. The dark tissue mean and variance are estimated from pixels in the closed image that are classified as dark tissue. A similar procedure is used for blood.

7.6 In Vivo Experiments

7.6.1 Imaging Protocol

The LV of a normal human volunteer and a volunteer with coronary artery disease were imaged using a cine, black blood, breath-hold parallel planar tag imaging protocol [21]. Another normal human volunteer and another volunteer with coronary artery disease were imaged using a cine, white blood, breath-hold parallel planar tag imaging protocol [21]. Two short-axis sequences and one long-axis image sequence were acquired. The short-axis image sequences consisted of six parallel 8mm thick slices with no separation between slices. Each short-axis slice was imaged with tag plane orientations of 0 and 90 degrees. Different tag plane orientations were acquired by keeping the tag lines in a vertical orientation and rotating the slice prescription by the appropriate angle [21]. The long-axis image sequence consisted of six 8mm thick slices radially oriented around the long-axis of the LV with an angular separation of 30 degrees. Each long-axis slice was imaged once with tag planes oriented parallel to the short-axis image planes. The resulting images are 256×256 with a 36cm $\times$ 36cm field of view. The tag planes were separated in the reference state (end-diastole) by 7mm. Ten cardiac phases were imaged spaced 32.5ms apart through systole for a total of 180 images acquired during the study.

7.6.2 Black Blood Images

The ML/MAP algorithm summarized in Figure 7.5 was run on both the normal and abnormal black blood studies. The same parameters were used in images of both studies. Figure 7.8a shows a mid-ventricular short-axis image from the normal study overlaid with the results of the tag estimation algorithm. Note that the continuity of each snake is broken near the boundaries of the myocardium and that the tag separation constraint keeps the tags from crossing one another. The results of the tag detection algorithm are shown in Figure 7.8b. Most of the tag points inside the myocardium are preserved, and the false tag points occur in small, isolated clusters. The tag pruning algorithm results are shown in Figure 7.8c. Most of the the false tag centers are removed while preserving the tag centers inside the myocardium. Note that the third tag line from the left is attracted to a dark pixel in Figure 7.8a, but the erroneous tag centers are removed by the tag detection (Figure 7.8b) and pruning (Figure 7.8c) stages.

The final results of the ML/MAP tag tracking algorithm for a a mid-ventricular

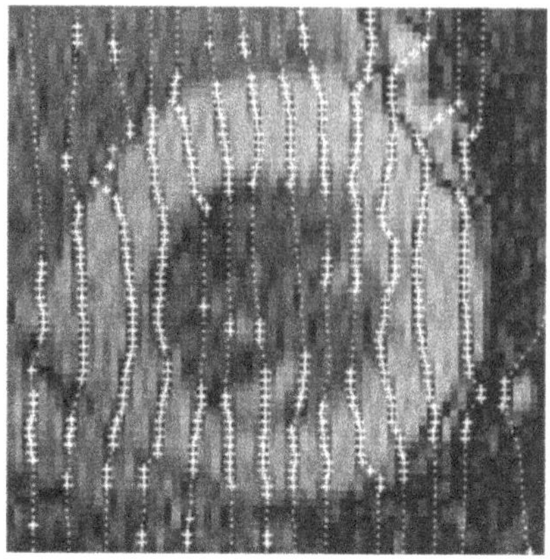

(a)

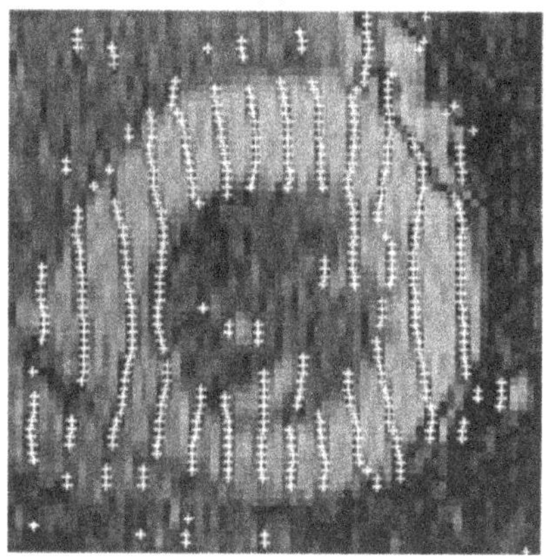

(b)

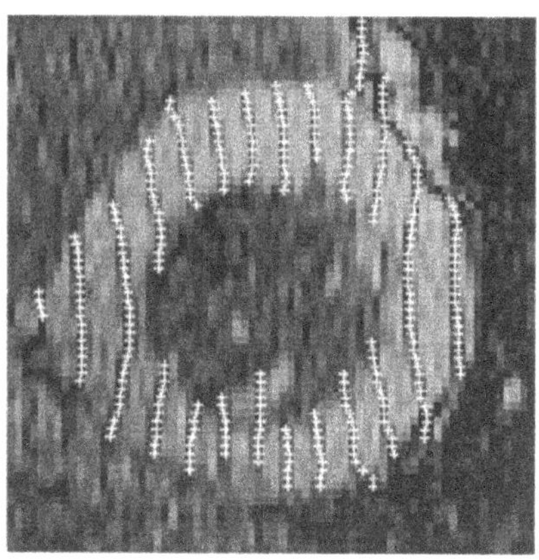

(c)

Figure 7.8: Intermediate results in ML/MAP tag tracking algorithm: **(a)** Result of the snake tag estimation algorithm. Candidate tag centers considered to be inside the myocardium are shown with +'s, and centers outside the myocardium are shown by ·'s. **(b)** Result of the MAP tag detector. **(c)** Final result after the spatio-temporal pruning algorithm.

short-axis slice and a long-axis slice of the normal study are shown in Figure 7.9. Only the portion of the image contained in the ROI is shown. The 90 degree tag plane angle images are acquired by keeping the tag lines in a vertical orientation and rotating the slice prescription +90 degrees [21]. The 90 degree images in Figure 7.9 have been rotated -90 degrees so that the heart is in the same orientation in both the 0 and 90 degree tag orientation images. Note that the algorithm will preserve tag centers in any persistently tagged tissue as seen on the right hand column of Figure 7.9. In the long-axis images, the contrast between the myocardium and the blood pool is much lower than in the short-axis images, which violates the assumption in Section 7.5.1 that the myocardium pixels are the brightest 50% of the pixels in the ROI. In spite of this violation, the ML/MAP algorithm still does a good job of tag line identification.

The ML/MAP tag tracking results for the abnormal study are shown in Figure 7.10. The contrast-to-noise-ratio (CNR) in this study is lower than in the normal study. The ML/MAP algorithm still does a good job of tag identification with the exception of the anterior wall (short-axis images) and free-wall near the base (long-axis image) where the tags are washed out.

7.6.3 White Blood Images

The ML/MAP algorithm summarized in Figure 7.5 was run on both the normal and abnormal white blood studies with the myocardium segmentation and statistics described in Section 7.5.2 used in the short-axis images. The long-axis images were imaged using the same protocol as in the black blood studies. The same parameters used in the black blood studies were used in the white blood studies.

The ML/MAP tag tracking results for the normal and abnormal white blood studies are shown in Figures 7.11 and 7.12. The tag identification in the normal study is excellent with few false positives outside the myocardium. As with the black blood studies, the CNR of the abnormal study is lower than the normal study. As a result, the detection rate is not as high as in the normal study. The tags that are identified, however, are in their correct position, and there are few false positives.

7.7 Discussion

In this chapter we presented an automated technique for tracking and identifying tag lines in planar tagged cardiac MR images called the ML/MAP algorithm. The ML/MAP algorithm is based on classical signal parameter estimation and detection techniques and is composed of three stages. First a set of candidate tag line centers are estimated across the entire region-of-interest (ROI) with a snake algorithm. The image forces applied to each snake point are derived from a maximum-likelihood (ML) estimate of the tag center. A *maximum a posteriori* (MAP) hypothesis test is then used to construct a rough liberal segmentation of the myocardium. Spatial continuity of the snakes is not enforced across the segmentation boundaries. In the second stage, another, more conservative, MAP hypothesis test is used to detect the

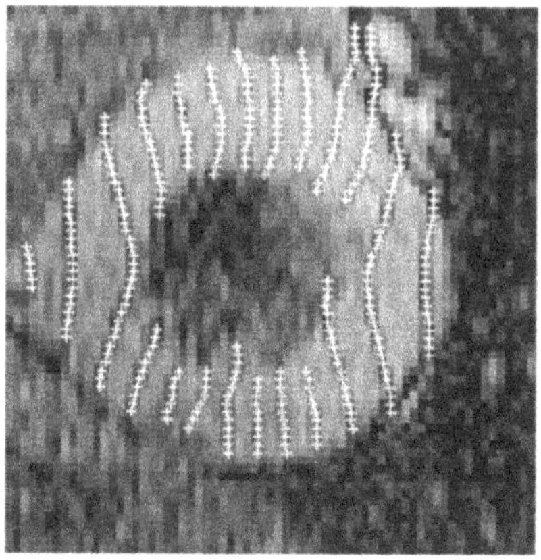

(a)

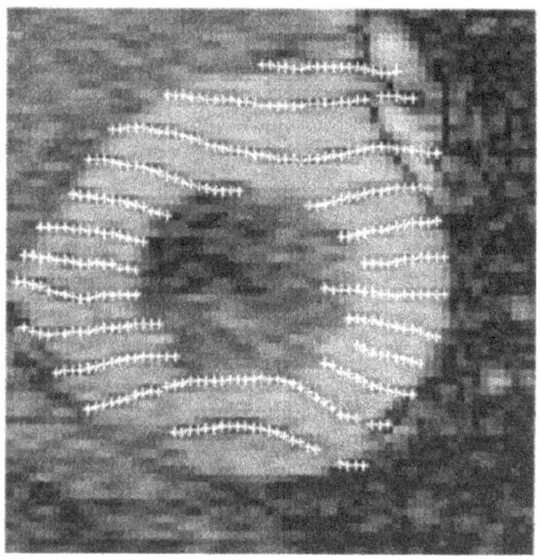

(b)

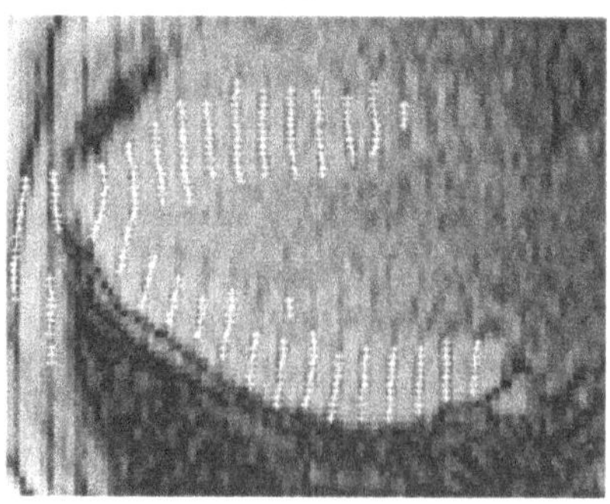

(c)

Figure 7.9: ML/MAP tag tracking for a normal human volunteer near end-systole: **(a)**,**(b)** mid-ventricular short-axis slice **(c)** long-axis slice. (Black blood case.)

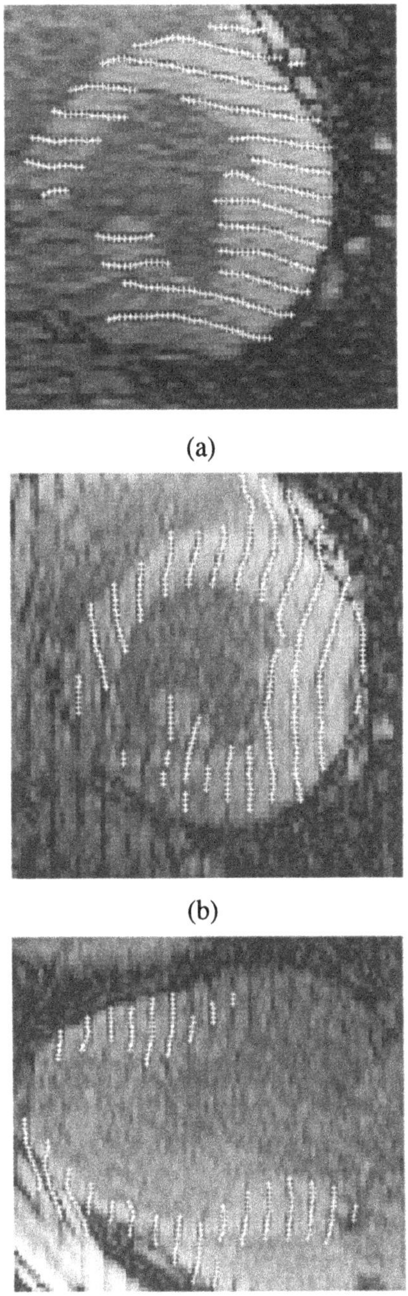

(a)

(b)

(c)

Figure 7.10: ML/MAP tag tracking for an abnormal human volunteer near end-systole: **(a)**,**(b)** mid-ventricular short-axis slice **(c)** long-axis slice. (Black blood case.)

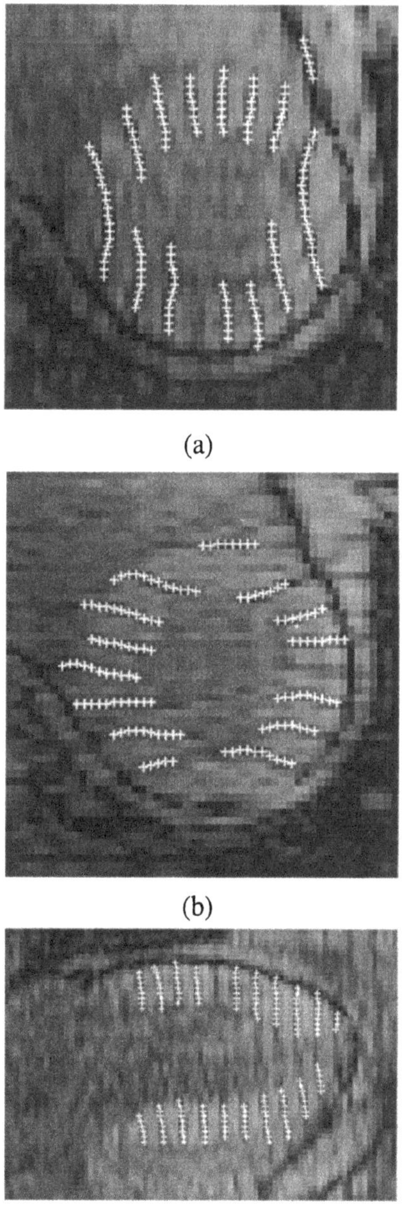

(a) (b) (c)

Figure 7.11: ML/MAP tag tracking for a normal human volunteer near end-systole: **(a)**,**(b)** mid-ventricular short-axis slice **(c)** long-axis slice. (White blood case.)

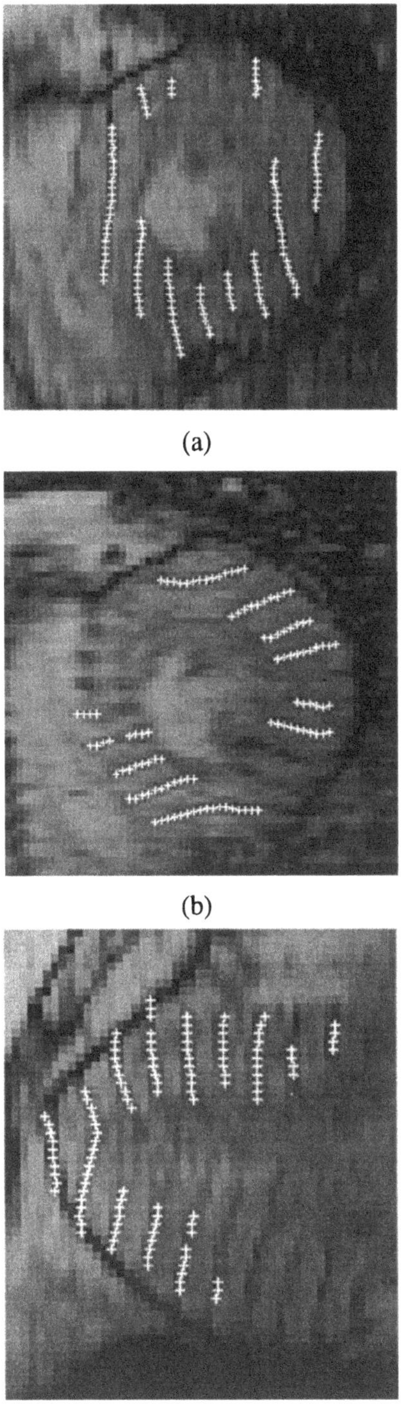

(a)

(b)

(c)

Figure 7.12: ML/MAP tag tracking for a normal human volunteer near end-systole: **(a)**,**(b)** mid-ventricular short-axis slice **(c)** long-axis slice. (White blood case.)

candidate tag centers that are actually part of a tag line. The third stage consists of a pruning algorithm that removes any detected tag centers that do not meet a spatio-temporal continuity criterion. The only user interaction required for the algorithm is an ROI and initial tag alignment. Since both initial conditions need only be specified once per stack of image slices, a typical study with two short-axis stack and one long-axis stack only needs three ROI's and three initial alignments.

We presented algorithms for both black blood and white blood images. White blood images are problematic because the blood pool intensity can range from slightly darker than the myocardium to significantly brighter. We presented a technique for distinguishing between myocardium and blood based on a deterministic template match test for tag lines, which we used to obtain a rough myocardium segmentation and to compute image statistics.

We demonstrated the ML/MAP algorithm on *in vivo* tagged image data from both normal volunteers and volunteers with coronary artery disease using both black blood and white blood imaging protocols. The same set of algorithm parameters was used in all cases. A study of the ML/MAP algorithm's accuracy and precision for normal human black blood studies as well as a parameter robustness study can be found in [8]. The only exception was a different algorithm was used for segmenting the myocardium and estimating image statistics for white blood short-axis images. The ML/MAP algorithm accurately estimated the positions of tag lines inside the myocardium with only a few false positives detected outside the myocardium. False negatives can occur inside the myocardium in regions with low CNR.

Because the ML/MAP does not use any prior knowledge of the myocardial contours, some tag points are detected outside the myocardium, particularly in tagged non-myocardium tissue. While these tag points could be removed with user supervised processing, this approach would not be practical in a clinical environment. Since non-myocardium tag points tend to move differently than myocardium tag points, however, a more interesting alternative is use an algorithm that identifies the myocardial contours based on differences in the spatio-temporal motion of both myocardium and non-myocardium tag points. A reconstruction algorithm based on this approach is currently under development. Preliminary versions of this algorithm are described in [9, 28].

As with other tag identification algorithms, ML/MAP tags can sometimes be attracted to a non-tag feature in the ROI. When this situation occurs, the tag line must be manually edited using a graphical user interface such as the one described in [16]. Methods for reducing or eliminating this type of error by exploiting tag continuity between slices and between tag plane orientations are currently under investigation. Also, particularly in early time frames of long axis sequences, it is possible that tags can move more than one half tag spacing between time frames and cause a tag identification algorithm to skip a tag line in the image data. In the ML/MAP algorithm, tag line correspondences are not explicitly constrained, but a temporal prediction model is used to extrapolate the initial position of each tag line from the previous two time frames. Methods for explicitly constraining tag line correspondences are a topic of future research.

The ML/MAP algorithm contains a tag center estimation algorithm that uses a Gaussian tag profile to generate image forces for a snake algorithm. This approach is similar in spirit to snake-based tag estimation algorithms proposed by other researchers [2, 15, 19, 29]. The ML/MAP algorithm, however, differs from these other snake-based algorithms in the following ways. First, the maximum likelihood (ML) estimation framework provides a set of spatially varying weights for comparing the image data with the Gaussian tag template based on the physics of the tagging process and signal intensity and noise statistics computed from the image data. In previous tag tracking methods, the points used to compare the image data with the tag template are equally weighted. Second, the myocardium is automatically segmented in the ROI by using a maximum *a posteriori* (MAP) hypothesis test. Previous tag tracking algorithms require user-defined contours to segment the myocardium.

At present, the algorithm assumes a parallel tag pattern like the one shown in Figure 7.4a, but the methods presented in this paper can be extended for use in radial [30] or grid [4] tag patterns. In tag patterns such as radial tags [30], where the undeformed tag lines are at an oblique angle relative to the slice and read gradient directions, the tag profile samples would still be taken perpendicular to the initial (undeformed) tag line position. The tag line normal would no longer be an image row but an oblique line, and tag center displacements would be computed in the direction of the tag line normal.

In summary the ML/MAP algorithm presented in this paper is capable of identifying tag lines without user-defined myocardial contours and has the potential to remove some of the technological roadblocks keeping MR cardiac tagging techniques from routine clinical use.

Acknowledgments

The author would like to thank Elliot R. McVeigh, PhD for making the *in vivo* human data available to him and for helpful discussions on MR tagging and tag identification. This work is supported by Biomedical Engineering Research Grant from The Whitaker Foundation and grant HL6134301 from the National Heart, Lung, and Blood Institute of the National Institutes of Health.

Appendix: Likelihood Function Derivative

In this appendix we derive the derivative of the likelihood function $L(\mu; \mathbf{w})$ defined in Equation (7.8) with respect to the tag center μ.

We begin by repeating Equation (7.8).

$$L(\mu; \mathbf{w}) = \frac{1}{2}[\mathbf{w} - \overline{\mathbf{m}}_{\mathrm{T}}(\mu)]^T \mathbf{C}_{\mathrm{T}}^{-1}(\mu)[\mathbf{w} - \mathbf{m}_{\mathrm{T}}(\mu)] + \frac{1}{2}\ln|\mathbf{C}_{\mathrm{T}}(\mu)|\,.$$

Taking the derivative with respect to μ and noting that $\mathbf{C}_{\mathrm{T}}^{-1}(\mu)$ is symmetric yields

$$\begin{aligned}
\frac{d}{d\mu}L(\mu) &= -\frac{d}{d\mu}\overline{\mathbf{m}}_{\mathrm{T}}(\mu)^T \mathbf{C}_{\mathrm{T}}^{-1}(\mu)[\mathbf{w} - \overline{\mathbf{m}}_{\mathrm{T}}(\mu)] \\
&\quad -\frac{1}{2}[\mathbf{w} - \overline{\mathbf{m}}_{\mathrm{T}}(\mu)]^T \mathbf{C}_{\mathrm{T}}^{-1}(\mu)\frac{d}{d\mu}\mathbf{C}_{\mathrm{T}}(\mu)\mathbf{C}_{\mathrm{T}}^{-1}(\mu)[\mathbf{w} - \overline{\mathbf{m}}_{\mathrm{T}}(\mu)] \\
&\quad +\frac{1}{2}\frac{1}{|\mathbf{C}_{\mathrm{T}}(\mu)|}\frac{d}{d\mu}|\mathbf{C}_{\mathrm{T}}(\mu)|\,,
\end{aligned}$$

where we used the matrix identity

$$\frac{d}{d\mu}\mathbf{A}^{-1}(\mu) = -\mathbf{A}^{-1}(\mu)\frac{d}{d\mu}\mathbf{A}(\mu)\mathbf{A}^{-1}(\mu)\,.$$

For notational convenience, we define the following function

$$\dot{s}(x-\mu) = \frac{d}{d\mu}s(x-\mu) = -\frac{8\ln 2A(t)}{\mathrm{FWHM}^2}(x-\mu)e^{-4\ln 2(x-\mu)^2/\mathrm{FWHM}^2}\,,$$

and define the matrix $\dot{\mathbf{S}}(\mu)$ as the same as $\mathbf{S}(\mu)$ except with samples of $\dot{s}(x-\mu)$ along its diagonal. We can now express the following derivatives with respect to μ as

$$\frac{d}{d\mu}\mathbf{m}_{\mathrm{T}}(\mu) = \dot{\mathbf{S}}(\mu)\mathbf{m}_{\mathrm{T}}\,, \tag{7.30}$$

and

$$\begin{aligned}
\frac{d}{d\mu}\mathbf{C}_{\mathrm{T}}(\mu) &= \frac{d}{d\mu}[\mathbf{S}(\mu)\mathbf{C}_{\mathrm{T}}\mathbf{S}(\mu)]\,, \\
&= \dot{\mathbf{S}}(\mu)\mathbf{C}_{\mathrm{T}}\mathbf{S}(\mu) + \mathbf{S}(\mu)\mathbf{C}_{\mathrm{T}}\dot{\mathbf{S}}(\mu)\,.
\end{aligned}$$

The derivative of the determinant term is given by

$$\frac{d}{d\mu}|\mathbf{C}_{\mathrm{T}}(\mu)| = \sum_{k=1}^{N_s}|\mathbf{C}_{\mathrm{T}}^{(k)}(\mu)|\,,$$

where $\mathbf{C}_{\mathrm{T}}^{(k)}(\mu)$ is the matrix $\mathbf{C}_{\mathrm{T}}(\mu)$ with the kth row replaced by the kth row of $d/d\mu\mathbf{C}_{\mathrm{T}}(\mu)$.

References

[1] Amini, A., Chen, Y., Curwen, R., Mani, V., and Sun, J. (1998). Coupled B-snake grids and constrained thin-plate splines for analysis of 2-D tissue deformations from tagged MRI. IEEE Transactions on Medical Imaging, 17(3):344–356.

[2] Amini, A., Curwen, R., Constable, R., and Gore, J. (1994). MR physics-based snake tracking and dense deformation from tagged cardiac images. In American Association for Artificial Intelligence (AAAI) Spring Symposium Series. Applications of Computer Vision in Medical Image Processing, pages 126–129. The AAAI Press.

[3] Atalar, E. and McVeigh, E. (1994). Optimization of tag thickness for measuring position with magnetic resonance imaging. IEEE Transactions on Medical Imaging, 13(1):152–160.

[4] Axel, L. and Dougherty, L. (1989). MR imaging of motion with spatial modulation of magnetization. Radiology, 171:841–845.

[5] Besag, J. (1986). On the statistical analysis of dirty pictures. J. Royal Stat. Soc. B, 48:259–302.

[6] Cohen, L. (1991). Note on active contour models and balloons. CVGIP: Image Understanding, 53(2):211–218.

[7] Crum, W., Berry, E., Ridgeway, J., Sivananthan, U., Tan, L.-B., and Smith, M. (1997). Simulation of two-dimensional tagged MRI. Journal of Magnetic Resonance Imaging, 7(2):416–24.

[8] Denney, T. (1999). Estimation and detection of myocardial tags in MR images without user-defined myocardial contours. IEEE Transactions on Medical Imaging, 18(4):330–344.

[9] Denney, T. and Yan, L. (2000). Unsupervised reconstruction of left ventricular strain from tagged cardiac MR images. In 8th Meeting of the International Society for Magnetic Resonance in Medicine, Denver, CO.

[10] Edelman, R., Chien, D., and Kim, D. (1991). Fast selective black blood MR imaging. Radiology, 181(3):655–60.

[11] Fischer, S., McKinnon, G., Maier, S., and Boesiger, P. (1993). Improved myocardial tagging contrast. Magnetic Resonance in Medicine, 30(2):191–200.

[12] Golub, G. H. and Loan, C. F. V. (1989). Matrix Computations. Johns Hopkins University Press, Baltimore, 2nd ed. edition.

[13] Guillemaud, R. and Brady, M. (1997). Estimating the bias field of MR images. IEEE Transactions on Medical Imaging, 16(3):238–251.

[14] Guttman, M., Prince, J., and McVeigh, E. (1994). Tag and contour detection in tagged MR images of the left ventricle. IEEE Transactions on Medical Imaging, 13(1):74–88.

[15] Guttman, M., Zerhouni, E., and McVeigh, E. (1995). Fast, contourless tag segmentation and displacement estimation for analysis of myocardial motion. In Proc. SMR/ESMRMB, volume 1, page 41, Nice. SMR.

[16] Guttman, M., Zerhouni, E., and McVeigh, E. (1997). Analysis and visualization of cardiac function from MR images. IEEE Computer Graphics and Applications, 17(1):30–38.

[17] Henkelman, R. (1985). Measurement of signal intensities in the presence of noise in MR images. Medical Physics, 12(2):232–233.

[18] Kass, M., Witkin, A., and Terzopoulos, D. (1988). Snakes: active contour models. International Journal of Computer Vision, 1:321–331.

[19] Kumar, S. and Goldgof, D. (1994). Automatic tracking of SPAMM grid and the estimation of deformation parameters from cardiac MR images. IEEE Transactions on Medical Imaging, 13(1):122–132.

[20] Laidlaw, D., Fleischer, K., and Barr, A. (1998). Partial-volume Bayesian classification of material mixtures in MR volume data using voxel histograms. IEEE Transactions on Medical Imaging, 17(1):74–86.

[21] McVeigh, E. and Atalar, E. (1992). Cardiac tagging with breath-hold cine MRI. Magnetic Resonance in Medicine, 28:318–327.

[22] Radeva, P., Amini, A., Huang, J., and Marti, E. (1996). Deformable B-solids and implicit snakes for localization and tracking of MRI-SPAMM data. In IEEE Workshop on Mathematical Models in Biomedical Image Analysis, San Francisco, CA.

[23] Reeder, S. and McVeigh, E. (1994). Tag contrast in breath-hold CINE cardiac MRI. Magnetic Resonance in Medicine, 31(5):521–5.

[24] Rice, S. (1948). Statistical properties of a sine-wave plus random noise. Bell Sys. Tech. J., 27:109–157.

[25] Shanmugan, K. and Breipohl, A. (1988). Random signals: detection, estimation and data analysis. John Wiley and Sons, Inc.

[26] Singleton, H. and Pohost, G. (1997). Automatic cardiac MR image segmentation using edge detection by tissue classification in pixel neighborhoods. Magnetic Resonance in Medicine, 37(3):418–24.

[27] W.M. Wells, I., Grimson, W., Kikinis, R., and Jolesz, F. (1996). Adaptive segmentation of MRI data. IEEE Transactions on Medical Imaging, 15(4):429–442.

[28] Yan, L. and Denney, T. (1998). Joint reconstruction of 2-D left ventricular displacement and contours from tagged magnetic resonance images using Markov random field edge prior. In Proceedings of the 1998 IEEE Workshop on Biomedical Image Analysis, San Diego, CA.

[29] Young, A., Kraitchman, D., Dougherty, L., and Axel, L. (1995). Tracking and finite element analysis of stripe deformation in magnetic resonance tagging. IEEE Transactions on Medical Imaging, 14(3):413–421.

[30] Zerhouni, E., Parish, D., Rogers, W., Yangand, A., and Shapiro, E. (1988). Human heart: tagging with MR imaging — a method for noninvasive assessment of myocardial motion. Radiology, 169:59–63.

Chapter 8

Analysis of Tagged MR Cardiac Images with B-spline Models

Yasheng Chen
CVIA Laboratory,
Box 8086, 660 S. Euclid Ave.,
Washington University School of Medicine,
St. Louis, MO 63110
yc3@cec.wustl.edu

Yu-Ping Wang
The Advanced Digital Imaging Research, LLC.,
2525 South Shore Blvd., #100,
League City, TX 77573
wyp@adires.com

Amir A. Amini
CVIA Laboratory,
Box 8086, 660 S. Euclid Ave.,
Washington University School of Medicine,
St. Louis, MO 63110
amini@cauchy.wustl.edu

8.1 Introduction

Noninvasive imaging techniques for assessing the dynamic behavior of the human heart are invaluable in the diagnosis of myocardial diseases. MRI is a noninvasive imaging technique that provides superb anatomic information with excellent spatial resolution and soft tissue contrast. Conventional MR studies of the heart provide accurate measures of global and regional myocardial function, chamber volumes, and ejection fractions. In MR tagging, the magnetization property of selective material points are altered in order to create tagged patterns within a deforming body such as the heart muscle. The resulting pattern defines a time-varying

A.A. Amini and J.L. Prince (eds.),
Measurement of Cardiac Deformations from MRI: Physical and Mathematical Models, 183–217.

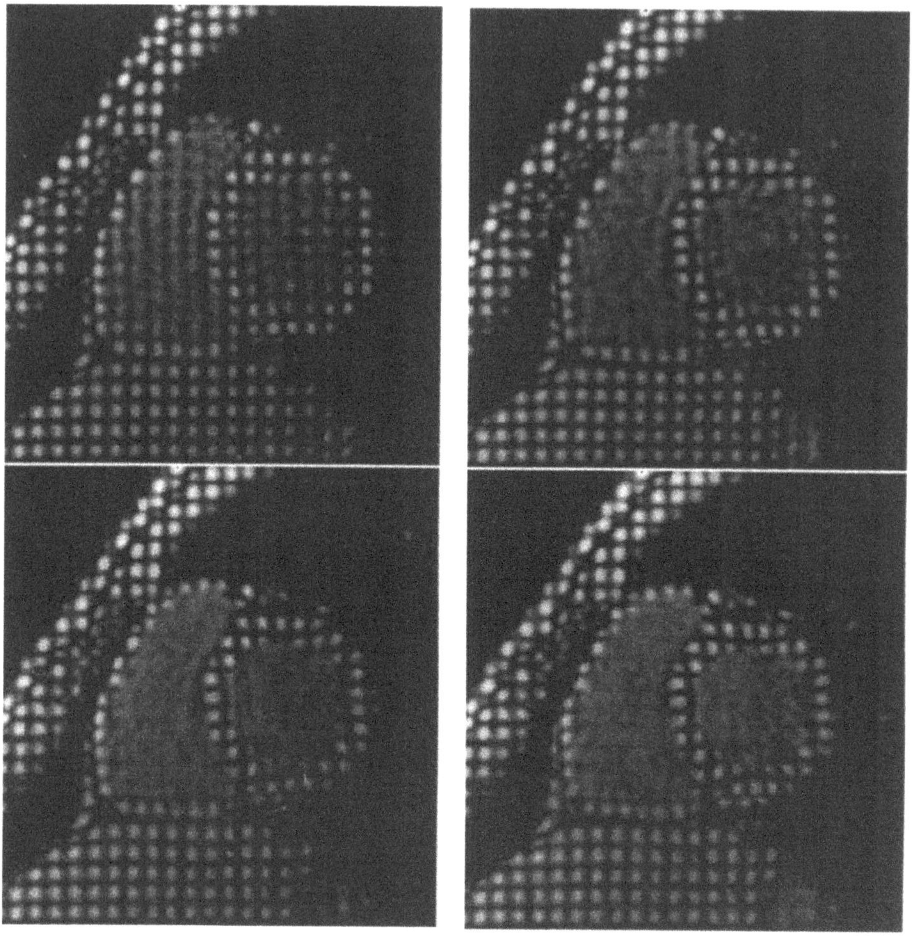

Figure 8.1: A sequence of systolic SPAMM tagged images in the middle of the LV for a healthy human volunteer. The dark tag lines in the data are intersections of spin tag planes with image slices.

curvilinear coordinate system on the underlying tissue. During tissue contractions, the grid patterns move, allowing for visual tracking of the grid intersections over time. The intrinsic high spatial and temporal resolutions of such myocardial analysis schemes provide unsurpassed information about local contraction and deformation in the myocardium which can be used to derive local strain and deformation indices from different regions.

Several techniques for acquiring tagged images (see Chapters 2-7 and references therein) have been reported in recent years. SPAMM [7] is a technique based on binomial pulses for producing a regular grid of spin tag planes in the tissue. The intersection of the resulting planes with image slices produce tag grid line patterns on cine images as shown in Figure 8.1.

The various tagged MR image acquisition methods including SPAMM, provide the means for encoding of tag patterns within the myocardial tissue. However, methods are needed for quantitative analysis and extraction of the tag patterns in acquired images in order to measure the motion of tag lines in 2D and more generally, tag surfaces in 3D. There has been a flurry of activity in this area. In [25], an analysis system based on snakes was adopted and the stripe displacements were fitted by a 3D Finite Element Model (FEM). The work described in [17] considers geometric primitives which are generalization of volumetric ellipsoids. Use of parametric functions in this context allows for spatial adjustment of aspect ratios of the model to fit the LV. The models are further generalized to parameterize twisting motion of the LV as a function of distance along the long axis as well as the radial direction.

In [16], the authors perform least squares fitting of a truncated power series in the prolate spheroidal coordinate system on the whole of the myocardium in order to measure dense deformations. One difficulty with this approach is that the interpolation is not local. An alternate approach to motion reconstruction developed in [9] utilizes a multidimensional stochastic model for the true displacement field and the Fisher estimation framework to estimate displacement vectors in points on the lattice.

In [12], a 4D time-varying B-spline model is fitted to tag data to generate a B-solid which varies continuously over time. One important advantage of this approach is that 3D material point localization and 3D displacement field reconstruction are achieved simultaneously at any time instant in a single step. The displacements are obtained by taking the difference of fitted B-solids between two frames. In [18], a volumetric B-solid model was proposed to concurrently track tag lines in different image slices by implicitly defined B-spline surfaces which align themselves with tagged data. The solid is a 3D tensor product B-spline whose isoparametric curves deform under image forces towards tag lines in different image slices. In [13], tag surfaces were constructed using thin-plate splines, and subsequently intersection of the thin-plate spline surfaces were computed based on an alternating projection algorithm to yield displacements of myocardial points. In [5], machinery were provided for very fast computation of tag surfaces using parametric B-spline surfaces. Furthermore, since by design the surfaces are parametric, a naturally easy to implement algorithm was arrived at for computing displacement of myocardial points.

In [1, 2], tag lines were tracked with dynamic programming B-snakes and B-snake grids. In [1, 3], a constrained thin-plate spline reconstruction of the displacement field from points and lines was described. In [24], a shifted B-spline bases representation to the displacement field was proposed which improved on the computational speed in [3], resulting in reconstruction times on the order of one minute.

The organization of the chapter is as follows. Section 2 presents definitions and properties of B-splines used in the rest of the chapter. Section 3 presents coupled

B-snake grids for localization and tracking of tag grid lines from a cine sequence of images. Section 4 describes the constrained thin-plate spline model for estimation of heart wall deformations. The derived numerical techniques adopt shifted B-spline representation of the deformations. In Section 5, a SPAMM imaging protocol for non-invasive placement and tracking of myocardial beads with tagged MRI is described. Furthermore, in this section, efficient algorithms for reconstruction of tag surfaces and localization of beads with deformable B-spline surface models are discussed.

8.2 B-spline basics

B-splines are suitable for representing a variety of quantities including industrial and anatomical shapes [1, 10, 14, 15], scalar images [23], or vector data [24]. The advantages of B-spline representations are: (1) they are smooth and parametrically continuous, capable of representing open or closed shapes. Furthermore, due to parametric continuity, B-spline representations allow for sub-pixel accuracy; (2) geometric objects represented by B-splines are generally completely specified by a few control points; and (3) individual movement of control points will only affect the representation locally. In particular, local tissue deformations can easily be captured by movement of individual control points without affecting the static portions of the representation.

8.2.1 Definitions and Notations

The general forms of B-splines are given in [10]. In practice, the knots are usually equally placed, in which case, we have the uniform B-spline and the expressions are simplified significantly. We follow the convention of [23] and define the continuous uniform B-spline of order n by $\beta^n(x)$, which can be generated by repeated $n+1$ convolution of a B-spline of order 0,

$$\beta^n(x) = \beta^0 * \beta^{n-1}(x) = \overbrace{\beta^0 * \beta^0 * \cdots \beta^0}^{n+1}(x) \tag{8.1}$$

where the 0th-order B-spline $\beta^0(x)$ is the pulse function with support $[0, 1]$, that is, it is zero everywhere except for $[0, 1]$, where it is one. An alternative definition of these normalized B-spline functions is given by

$$\beta^n(x) = \sum_{j=0}^{n+1} \binom{n+1}{j} \frac{(-1)^j}{n!} (x-j)^n \mu(x-j) \tag{8.2}$$

where $\mu(x)$ is the step function

$$\mu(x) = \begin{cases} 1 & \text{for } x \geq 0 \\ 0 & \text{for } x < 0 \end{cases}$$

and where $\binom{n+1}{j}$ are the binomial coefficients.

The discrete sampled B-spline $b^n(k)$ of order n is obtained by directly sampling the n-th order continuous B-spline:

$$b^n(k) = \beta^n(k), \quad \forall k \in Z. \tag{8.3}$$

The continuous convolution of functions f and g is defined as

$$f * g(x) = \int_{-\infty}^{\infty} f(x-t)g(t)dt, \qquad x \in R \tag{8.4}$$

The discrete convolution between two sequences $\{a\}$ and $\{b\}$ is the sequence $\{a * b\}$:

$$b * a(k) = \sum_{l=-\infty}^{\infty} b_{k-l}a_l. \tag{8.5}$$

The above definition of 1-D B-splines can easily be extended to the 2-D case through the tensor product (as examples, see Equations (8.18) and (8.35)).

8.2.2 Properties

In the rest of this section, we discuss the B-spline properties used in the chapter. Some additional details on properties of B-splines may be found in [10], [20], and [23].

- The shifted B-spline bases constitute a stable and complete approximation of a square integrable function.

- The B-spline basis $\beta^n(x)$ has compact support $[0, n+1]$ and is symmetric with respect to the midpoint $(n+1)/2$; i.e.,

$$\beta^n(n+1-x) = \beta^n(x). \tag{8.6}$$

- If a curve is represented as a B-spline, one can increase the smoothness by increasing the order of the B-splines. The derivative of the n-th order of B-splines is the difference of lower order B-splines. For example, the first and second order derivatives of B-splines are:

$$\begin{aligned}(\beta^n)'(x) &= \beta^{n-1}(x) - \beta^{n-1}(x-1), \\ (\beta^n)''(x) &= \beta^{n-2}(x) - 2\beta^{n-2}(x-1) + \beta^{n-2}(x-2).\end{aligned} \tag{8.7}$$

- The convolutions of two B-splines bases are still B-splines:

$$\beta^n(x-l) * \beta^m(x-k) = \beta^{n+m+1}(x-k+l). \tag{8.8}$$

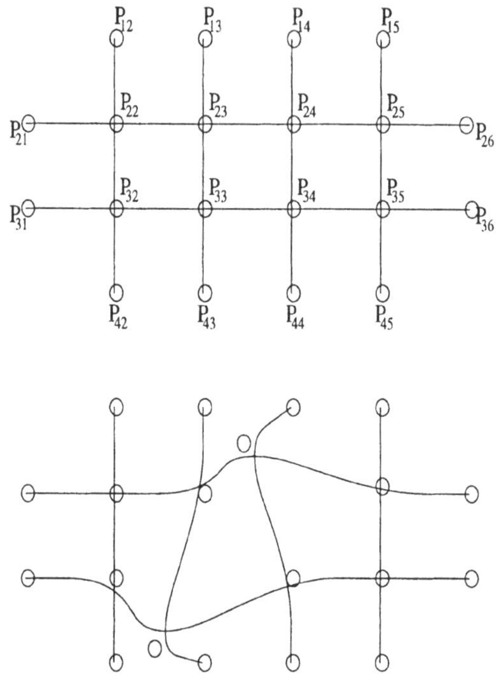

Figure 8.2: The spatial organization of control points for a coupled B-snake grid. Dependence of horizontal and vertical splines of deformable grids is captured by the shared control points.

8.3 Coupled B-snake Grids

A B-spline curve is expressed as

$$\alpha(u) = \sum_{i=0}^{N-1} \mathbf{p}_i \, \beta_i^k(u) \tag{8.9}$$

where $\beta_i^k(u) = \beta^k(u-i), (i \in Z)$ is the shifted B-spline of order k at location i, and $\mathbf{p}_i$ is the ith *control point* of the B-spline curve.

Coupled snake grids are a sequence of spatially ordered deformable curves represented by B-spline bases, which respond to image forces, and track non-rigid tissue deformations from SPAMM data. The spline grids are constructed by having the horizontal and vertical grid lines share control points. By moving a spline control point, the corresponding vertical and horizontal snakes deform. This representation is reasonable since the point of intersection of two tag lines is physically the same material point, the tissues are connected, and furthermore through shared control points, a more efficient representation is achieved.

We define a MN spline grid by $\{(M \times N) - 4\}$ control points which we represent

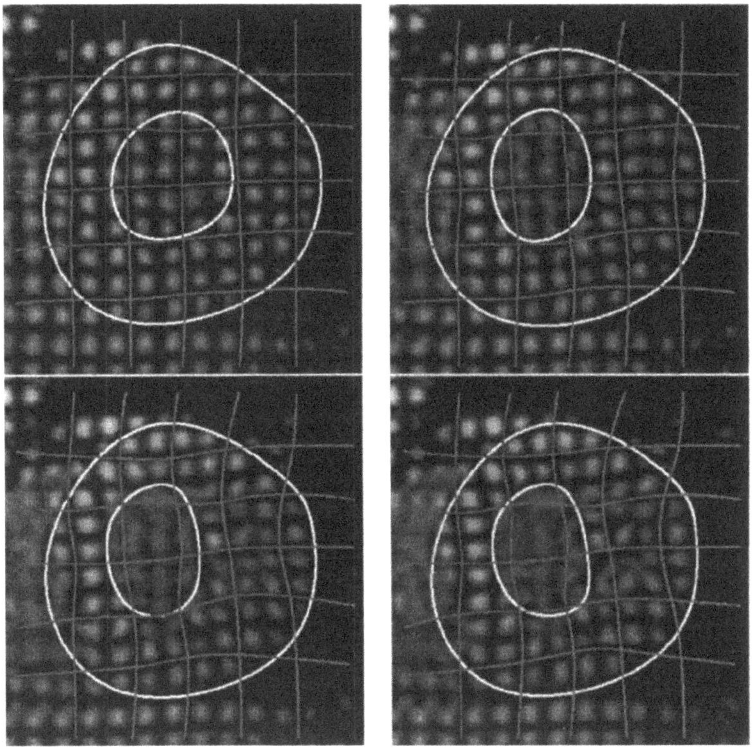

Figure 8.3: Results of tracking SPAMM images with deformable spline grids ($\eta_1 = 100$, $\eta_2 = 1$).

by the set

$$\{\{\mathbf{p}_{12}, \mathbf{p}_{13}, \cdots, \mathbf{p}_{1,N-1}\}, \{\mathbf{p}_{21}, \mathbf{p}_{22}, \cdots, \mathbf{p}_{2,N}\}, \cdots, \{\mathbf{p}_{M,2}, \mathbf{p}_{M,3}, \cdots, \mathbf{p}_{M,N-1}\}\} \quad (8.10)$$

where $\mathbf{p}_{ij}$ is the spline control point at row i and column j (Figure 8.2).

To detect and localize SPAMM tag lines, we optimize grid locations by finding the minimum intensity points in the image, as tag lines are darker than surrounding tissues. However, there is an additional energy term present in our formulation which takes account of the local 2D structure of image intensity values at tag intersections. Although we can not specify an exact correspondence for points along a tag line, we do know the exact correspondence for points at tag intersections–assuming 2D motion for the LV. This is the familiar statement of the aperture problem in image sequence analysis. The way to incorporate this familiar knowledge into our algorithm and therefore distinguish between 1D and 2D tagged points is to utilize the SSD (sum-of-squared-differences) function in the energy minimization

$$\mathcal{E}(\mathbf{p}_{12}, \mathbf{p}_{13}, \cdots, \mathbf{p}_{M,N-1}) = \eta_1 \sum_k \int I(\alpha_k(u))du + \eta_2 \sum_{ij} \mathrm{SSD}(\mathbf{r}_{ij}) \quad (8.11)$$

where I is the image intensity function, α_k is a horizontal or vertical spline, $\mathbf{r}_{ij}$ denotes the intersection point of 2 snake curves, and η_1 and η_2 are pre-set constants. The SSD function determines the sum-of-squared-differences of pixels in a window around point $\mathbf{r}_{ij}$ in the current frame (with intensity function I) with a window around the corresponding B-snake grid intersection in the previous frame (with intensity function J).[1] That is, when the location of the grid in I is sought

$$SSD(\mathbf{r}_{ij}) = \sum_{i=1}^{K} (I(q_i) - J(q_i'))^2 \tag{8.12}$$

for corresponding locations q_i and q_i' in an image window with K total pixels. In order to minimize the discrete version of $\mathcal{E}$, at each iterative step, we compute the gradient of $\mathcal{E}$ with respect to $\mathbf{p}_{ij}$, perform a line search in the $\nabla\mathcal{E}$ direction, move the control points to the minimum location (which will result in real values for $\mathbf{p}_{ij}$), and continue the procedure until the change in energy is less than a small number, defining convergence. Given $\mathbf{p}_{ij} = (x_{ij}, y_{ij})$, we approximate the components of $\nabla\mathcal{E}$ as

$$\begin{aligned}
\frac{\partial\mathcal{E}}{\partial x_{ij}} &\simeq \frac{\mathcal{E}(\mathbf{p}_{12}, \cdots, (x_{ij} + \Delta x, y_{ij}), \cdots, \mathbf{p}_{M,N-1})}{\Delta x} - \\
&\qquad \frac{\mathcal{E}(\mathbf{p}_{12}, \cdots, (x_{ij}, y_{ij}), \cdots, \mathbf{p}_{M,N-1})}{\Delta x} \\
\frac{\partial\mathcal{E}}{\partial y_{ij}} &\simeq \frac{\mathcal{E}(\mathbf{p}_{12}, \cdots, (x_{ij}, y_{ij} + \Delta y), \cdots, \mathbf{p}_{M,N-1})}{\Delta y} - \\
&\qquad \frac{\mathcal{E}(\mathbf{p}_{12}, \cdots, (x_{ij}, y_{ij}), \cdots, \mathbf{p}_{M,N-1})}{\Delta y}.
\end{aligned} \tag{8.13}$$

In practice, we have an additional constraint in computing the energy function: we only use the intersections and points on the snake grid that lie in the heart tissue. To track the grid over multiple frames, the localized grid for the current temporal frame becomes the initial grid for the next frame, which is then optimized on the new data. Initialization of the spline grid may be performed automatically based on the imaging protocol of section 8.5.1 which includes short-axis and long-axis slice acquisitions. An *in-vivo* result from localization and tracking of spline grids with gradient descent is shown in Figure 8.3. The endocardial and epicardial contours were each manually segmented through-out this sequence using a six control point B-spline representation. Further details on validation of the method may be found in [3].

8.4 Constrained Thin-Plate Spline Reconstruction

Tracking tissue deformations with SPAMM using coupled B-snake grids provides 2D displacement information at tag intersections and 1D displacement information along other 1D snake points [1], [3]. The displacement measurements

1 - We assume known location of the spline grid in frame 0 when the tags are undeformed.

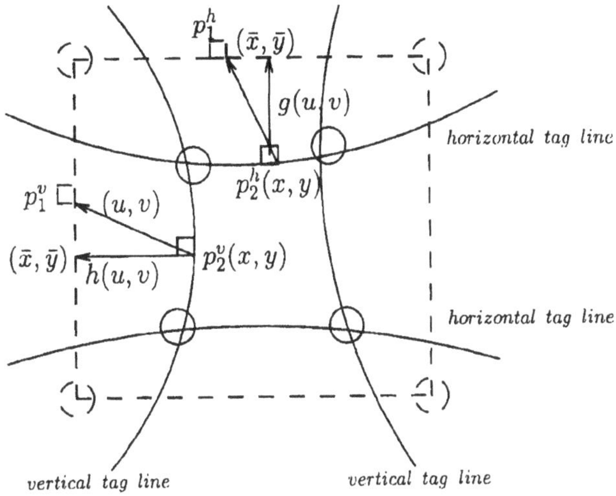

Figure 8.4: Deformed tag lines (solid lines) and their corresponding undeformed tag lines (dotted lines). The intersections, which serve as landmark points, are highlighted in the figure with circles. At intersections, we know both the x and y component of the displacements. But for other tag points we only know the y or x component of the displacements: $g(u, v)$ for p_2^h (along horizontal tag lines) and $h(u, v)$ for p_2^v (along vertical tag lines). We want to make use of all available information to estimate the dense displacement field.

from tag lines however are sparse; interpolation is required to reconstruct a dense displacement field from which strain, torsion, and other mechanical indices of function can be computed at all myocardial points. As shown in Figure 8.4, the reconstructed vector field should adhere to three properties:

1. The intersection points of deformed tag lines should be warped back to their corresponding intersection points in the undeformed state.

2. Points other than intersection points located along deformed tag lines should be warped back to lie on their corresponding undeformed tag lines.

3. For other points in the plane, where no information is available, a smooth vector field should be interpolated.

In this section, we describe an efficient solution to this displacement reconstruction problem, improving on previous methods discussed in [1,3] in the required computation time. We now state the three components of an energy function which once minimized achieves the three stated goals.

The intersections of two grids are "pulled" towards one another by minimizing

$$\Phi_1 = \sum_N (u - u^{int})^2 + (v - v^{int})^2, \tag{8.14}$$

where u and v are the x and y components of displacement vector field at a certain time frame relative to the initial undeformed frame. u^{int} and v^{int} are the x and y components of displacement at tag intersections as well as intersections of myocardial contours with tag lines. The summation in (8.14) is over all the tag intersection points N.

Assuming 2D tissue motion, a further physical constraint is necessary: any point on a deformed tag in frame n must be warped to lie on its corresponding undeformed tag in frame 0 of the sequence. As described in [4], for a vector field to perform such a warp, $h(u, v)$ and $g(u, v)$ of Figure 8.4 must be minimized. Let $p_2 = (x, y)$ be any point on the deformed tag line, and $p_1(x, y) = (x, y) + (u, v)$ be the corresponding point in the undeformed frame as in Figure 8.4. The following term is then summed over all deformed horizontal and vertical grid points:

$$\begin{aligned}\Phi_2 &= \sum_{N_y} h(u,v)^2 + \sum_{N_x} g(u,v)^2 \\ &= \sum_{N_y} ((p_1(u,v) - p_2) \cdot n_x)^2 + \sum_{N_x} ((p_1(u,v) - p_2) \cdot n_y)^2 \\ &= \sum_{N_y} (x + u - \bar{x})^2 + \sum_{N_x} (y + v - \bar{y})^2 \qquad (8.15)\end{aligned}$$

where n_x and n_y are the normal direction along x and y respectively. In the above equation, (x, y) are the coordinates of a point on the tag line in the current frame, and $(\bar{x}, \bar{y})$ is the closest point to $(x + u, y + v)$ on the corresponding tag line in the undeformed frame. The quantities $h(u, v)$ and $g(u, v)$ are the horizontal and vertical distance from the point (x, y) to the undeformed vertical and horizontal tag line respectively. Therefore, points on a deformed vertical tag line can be warped back to lie on its corresponding undeformed vertical tag line, following minimization of $\sum((h(u, v))^2$. Similarly, minimization of $\sum((g(u, v))^2$ will result in warping points on deformed horizontal tag lines to horizontal tag lines in frame 0. The summation is over N_y vertical tag points and N_x horizontal tag points, respectively.

The vector field continuity constraint is the bending energy of a thin-plate which is applied to the x and y component of the displacement field $(u(x, y), v(x, y))$:

$$\Phi_3 = \iint (u_{xx}^2 + 2u_{xy}^2 + u_{yy}^2)dxdy + \iint (v_{xx}^2 + 2v_{xy}^2 + v_{yy}^2)dxdy \qquad (8.16)$$

serving as the smoothness constraint on the reconstructed vector field, characterizing approximating thin-plate splines.

An energy function can be obtained by a linear combination of the three terms in (8.14), (8.15), and (8.16):

$$\Phi = \lambda_1\Phi_1 + \lambda_2\Phi_2 + \lambda_3\Phi_3. \qquad (8.17)$$

The characterization of the solution to this variational problem is described in [21], which is treated as an optimization problem in a reproducing kernel Hilbert space.

The interpolation of given specified landmarks is characterized by the thin-plate splines as investigated by Bookstein [8]. However, it is hard to get the explicit form of the solution to this general problem. Instead, an accurate solution can be found computationally by minimizing (8.17) in a certain finite-dimensional approximating subspace. We chose such a subspace as that spanned by the shifted B-spline bases. In other words, the vector field is represented as

$$\mathbf{U} = \sum_{i=1}^{M_x} \sum_{j=1}^{M_y} \mathbf{C}_{ij} \beta_{ij}^n(x,y), \quad \beta_{ij}^n(x,y) = \beta_i^n(x)\beta_j^n(y) \tag{8.18}$$

where $\mathbf{U} = (u,v)^T$ is the vector field, $\mathbf{C_{ij}} = (c_{ij}, d_{ij})^T$ is the control point matrix (representing in this case, the 2D deformation field), and $\beta_i^n(x) = \beta^n(x-i), (i \in Z)$, as before. M_x, M_y is the size of the control point matrix and is set by the user. Larger values for M_x and M_y will result in higher computational costs. In the experiments, we set the size to 256×256. Since we assume known locations of the epicardial and endocardial contours, only the displacement vectors in the region between them will be computed. Because the linear combinations of these shifted B-spline bases constitute a complete and stable approximation of $L^2(R)$, the representation in (8.18) is reasonable. In the next section we will describe how to get an efficient numerical solution by using this subspace approximation approach.

8.4.1 Solution Using Subspace Approximations

For the sake of simplicity in deriving the algorithm, in this section we assume the order of B-splines is 3. Additionally, we present here only details of derivation of optimal values for c_{mn}. Derivations for d_{mn} are very similar.

Through (8.14), (8.15), and (8.16), we know that (8.17) is a convex optimization problem. Therefore, a necessary and sufficient condition on the solution is that the gradient of (8.17) should be zero. Equivalently, we have the following normal equations:

$$\begin{gathered} \lambda_1 \frac{\partial \Phi_1}{\partial c_{mn}} + \lambda_2 \frac{\partial \Phi_2}{\partial c_{mn}} + \lambda_3 \frac{\partial \Phi_3}{\partial c_{mn}} = 0, \\ m = 1, 2, \cdots, M_x, n = 1, 2, \cdots, M_y. \end{gathered} \tag{8.19}$$

The gradients of these three energy functionals is derived in detail in [24]. Substituting (8.18) into (8.19), and taking derivatives, one obtains:

$$\begin{gathered} 2\lambda_1 \sum_{i=1}^{N} \Big(\sum_{k=1}^{M_x} \sum_{l=1}^{M_y} c_{kl} \beta_{kl}^3(x_i, y_i) - u_i^{int} \Big) \beta_{mn}^3(x_i, y_i) + \\ 2\lambda_2 \sum_{i=1}^{N_y} \Big(\sum_{k=1}^{M_x} \sum_{l=1}^{M_y} c_{kl} \beta_{kl}^3(x_i^{vert}, y_i^{vert}) - \Delta x_i \Big) \beta_{mn}^3(x_i^{vert}, y_i^{vert}) + \\ 2\lambda_3 \sum_{k=1}^{M_x} \sum_{l=1}^{M_y} c_{kl} \sigma_{kl;mn} = 0 \end{gathered} \tag{8.20}$$

where we denote $\sigma_{kl;mn} = \sigma^{(1)}_{kl;mn} + 2\sigma^{(2)}_{kl;mn} + \sigma^{(3)}_{kl;mn}$ and

$$\begin{aligned}\sigma^{(1)}_{kl;mn} &= \iint (\beta^3)''_k(x)\beta^3_l(y)(\beta^3)''_m(x)\beta^3_n(y)dxdy \\ &= \int (\beta^3)''_k(x)(\beta^3)''_m(x)dx \int \beta^3_l(y)\beta^3_n(y)dy, \end{aligned} \tag{8.21}$$

$$\begin{aligned}\sigma^{(2)}_{kl;mn} &= \iint (\beta^3)'_k(x)(\beta^3)'_l(y)(\beta^3)'_m(x)(\beta^3)'_n(y)dxdy \\ &= \int (\beta^3)'_k(x)(\beta^3)'_m(x)dx \int (\beta^3)'_l(y)(\beta^3)'_n(y)dy, \end{aligned} \tag{8.22}$$

$$\begin{aligned}\sigma^{(3)}_{kl;mn} &= \iint \beta^3_k(x)(\beta^3)''_l(y)\beta^3_m(x)(\beta^3)''_n(y)dxdy \\ &= \int \beta^3_k(x)\beta^3_m(x)dx \int (\beta^3)''_l(y)(\beta^3)''_n(y)dy. \end{aligned} \tag{8.23}$$

Note that from the local support $[0, 4]$ of cubic B-splines,

$$\sigma^{(1)}_{kl;mn} = \sigma^{(2)}_{kl;mn} = \sigma^{(3)}_{kl;mn} = 0, \quad \text{if } |k-m| > 4 \text{ or } |n-l| > 4. \tag{8.24}$$

Also, we only need to evaluate the values of B-splines of order 3, 5, and 7 at integers in order to compute (8.21), (8.22), and (8.23) [24]. One can find these values in Appendix C of [24]. Rearranging (8.20),

$$\begin{aligned} &\lambda_1 \sum_{i=1}^{N} \sum_{k=1}^{M_x} \sum_{l=1}^{M_y} \beta^3_k(x_i, y_i)\beta^3_m(x_i, y_i)c_{kl} + \\ &\lambda_2 \sum_{i=1}^{N_y} \sum_{k=1}^{M_x} \sum_{l=1}^{M_y} \beta^3_{kl}(x_i^{vert}, y_i^{vert})\beta^3_{mn}(x_i^{vert}, y_i^{vert})c_{kl} + \lambda_3 \sum_{k=1}^{M_x} \sum_{l=1}^{M_y} \sigma_{kl;mn}c_{kl} = \\ &\lambda_1 \sum_{i=1}^{N} u_i^{int}\beta^3_{mn}(x_i, y_i) + \lambda_2 \sum_{i=1}^{N_y} \Delta x_i \beta^3_{mn}(x_i^{vert}, y_i^{vert}) \end{aligned} \tag{8.25}$$

where $m = 1, 2, \cdots, M_x$ and $n = 1, 2, \cdots, M_y$.

For simplicity, if we denote $k' = kM_x + l$ and $m' = mM_x + n$, to order the matrix lexicographically, and $bb^3_{k'}(i) = \beta^3_{kl}(x_i, y_i)$ and $\tilde{bb}^3_{m'}(i) = \beta^3_{mn}(x_i^{vert}, y_i^{vert})$ to denote discrete bi-variate B-splines at points (x_i, y_i) and (x_i^{vert}, y_i^{vert}) respectively, the above equation can be simplified to

$$\begin{aligned} &\lambda_1 \sum_{i=1}^{N} \sum_{k'=1}^{M} bb^3_{k'}(i)bb^3_{m'}(i)c_{k'} + \lambda_2 \sum_{i=1}^{N_y} \sum_{k'=1}^{M} \tilde{bb}^3_{k'}(i)\tilde{bb}^3_{m'}(i)c_{k'} + \lambda_3 \sum_{k'=1}^{M} \sigma_{k'm'}c_{k'} \\ &= \lambda_1 \sum_{i=1}^{N} u_i^{int} bb^3_{m'}(i) + \lambda_2 \sum_{i=1}^{N_y} \delta x_i bb^3_{m'}(i), \quad m' = 1, 2 \cdots, M \end{aligned} \tag{8.26}$$

where $M = M_x \times M_y$. Alternatively, we can write the solution of coefficients column $C^T = (c_1, c_2, \cdots, c_M)^T$ in matrix form as:

$$(\lambda_1 BB^T + \lambda_2 B^{vert}(B^{vert})^T + \lambda_3 \Sigma)C = \lambda_1 BU^{int} + \lambda_2 (B^{vert})\Delta X \quad (8.27)$$

where the matrix $B = (bb_m^3(n))_{M\times N}$, $B^{vert} = (\tilde{bb}_m^3(n))_{M\times N_y}$ and $\Sigma_{M\times M}$ are given by

$$B = \begin{pmatrix} bb_1^3(1) & bb_1^3(2) & \cdots & bb_1^3(N) \\ bb_2^3(1) & bb_2^3(2) & \cdots & bb_2^3(N) \\ \vdots & \vdots & \ddots & \vdots \\ bb_M^3(1) & bb_M^3(2) & \cdots & bb_M^3(N) \end{pmatrix},$$

$$B^{vert} = \begin{pmatrix} \tilde{bb}_1^3(1) & \tilde{bb}_1^3(2) & \cdots & \tilde{bb}_1^3(N_y) \\ \tilde{bb}_2^3(1) & \tilde{bb}_2^3(2) & \cdots & \tilde{bb}_2^3(N_y) \\ \vdots & \vdots & \ddots & \vdots \\ \tilde{bb}_M^3(1) & \tilde{bb}_M^3(2) & \cdots & \tilde{bb}_M^3(N_y) \end{pmatrix},$$

and

$$\Sigma = \begin{pmatrix} \sigma_{11} & \sigma_{12} & \cdots & \sigma_{1M} \\ \sigma_{21} & \sigma_{22} & \cdots & \sigma_{2M} \\ \vdots & \vdots & \ddots & \vdots \\ \sigma_{M1} & \sigma_{M2} & \cdots & \sigma_{MM} \end{pmatrix}.$$

The column vector U^{int} and ΔX are given by

$$(U^{int})^T = (u_1^{int}, u_2^{int}, \cdots, u_N^{int}) \quad \text{and} \quad (\Delta X)^T = (\delta x_1, \delta x_2, \cdots, \delta x_{N_y}).$$

The element of BB^T is given by

$$e_{k'm'} = \sum_{i=1}^{N} bb_{k'}^3(i) bb_{m'}^3(i).$$

Due to the local property of B-spline bases, we can conclude that if the locations of two spline bases are far apart, i.e., if $|k' - m'| > p$ (for cubic spline, $p = 4M_x$), then $e_{k'm'} = 0$. In other words, the matrix BB^T is sparse and block-band diagonal since only a few elements are non-zeros. This also holds for $B^{vert}(B^{vert})^T$.

Due to (8.24), we know that Σ is also diagonal and band limited. Therefore, we can see that the matrix on the left of (8.27) is sparse, symmetric, and positive-definite and therefore we can employ a fast solver for this linear system of equations. We have adopted the sparse Cholesky Factorization technique [11] to solve (8.27) for C.

In the above derivation we have only discussed the solution for the $\{c_{ij}\}$ coefficients. Using a similar approach, we can also show that the solution of $\{d_{ij}\}$ satisfies

$$(\lambda_1 BB^T + \lambda_2 B^{hori}(B^{hori})^T + \lambda_3 \Sigma)D = \lambda_1 BV^{int} + \lambda_2 (B^{hori})\Delta Y \quad (8.28)$$

Table 8.1: The thirteen k-parameters of the kinematic model.

k_1	Radially dependent compression
k_2	Left ventricular torsion
k_3	Ellipticalization in long-axis (LA) planes
k_4	Ellipticalization in short-axis (SA) planes
k_5	Shear in x direction
k_6	Shear in y direction
k_7	Shear in z direction
k_8	Rotation about x-axis
k_9	Rotation about y-axis
k_{10}	Rotation about z-axis
k_{11}	Translation in x direction
k_{12}	Translation in y direction
k_{13}	Translation in z direction

where B^{hori} is the matrix of splines defined on the horizontal tag lines and

$$(V^{int})^T = (v_1^{int}, v_2^{int}, \cdots, v_N^{int}) \quad \text{and} \quad (\Delta Y)^T = (\delta y_1, \delta y_2, \cdots, \delta y_{N_y}).$$

Once we get the solution of $\{c\}$ and $\{d\}$, we can estimate the deformation of LV for any dense set of points using (8.18).

In summary, in this section, we have described details of an algorithm for computing a B-spline representation of the deformation field (Equation (8.18)) which warps an area in the plane such that two embedded snake grids obtained from two tagged frames (one from the undeformed reference state and another from a deformed state) are brought into registration, interpolating a dense displacement vector field. The vector field adheres to the known displacement information at the intersections, forces corresponding snakes to be warped into one another, and for all other points in the plane, where no information is available, a smooth vector field is interpolated.

8.4.2 Validations

Cardiac Simulator

An environment based on a 13 parameter kinematic model of Arts et al. [6] has been implemented for simulating a time sequence of tagged MR images at arbitrary orientation, as was described in [22]. Through the discretization of the space between 2 concentric shells and by varying the canonical parameters of the model, both a sequence of tagged MR images as well as a "ground truth" vector field of actual material point deformations are available.

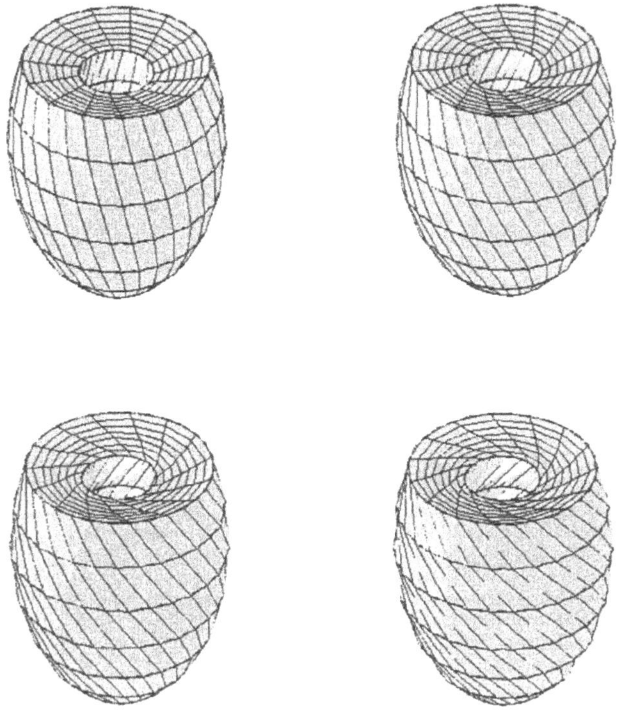

Figure 8.5: Deformed models of the LV resulting from change of k_2 from 0.2 (top left) to 0.8 (bottom right) in increments of 0.2.

A pair of prolate spheres represents the endocardial and epicardial LV surfaces, and provides a geometric model of the LV myocardium. The motion model involves application of a cascade of incompressible linear transformations describing rigid as well as non-rigid motions. The parameters of the motion model, referred to as k-parameters, and the transformations to which they correspond are stated in Table 8.1. Figure 8.5 displays a sequence of 3D deformed LV models resulting from change of k_2.

In order to simulate MR images, an imaging plane intersecting the geometric model is selected, and tagged spin-echo imaging equations are applied for simulating the *in-vivo* imaging process. Figure 8.6 shows the deformed tagged image slices, which intersect the deformed LV models in Figure 8.5. Also, this figure shows the detected tag lines using the coupled B-spline tracker of Section 8.3.

For the purposes of validating 2D deformation fields, we have used the parameters k_2, k_4, k_5, and k_{10} for generating 2D deformations of the geometric model, based on which images and in addition 2D displacement vector fields of *actual* material points are produced. The error norms used in comparing the ground truth

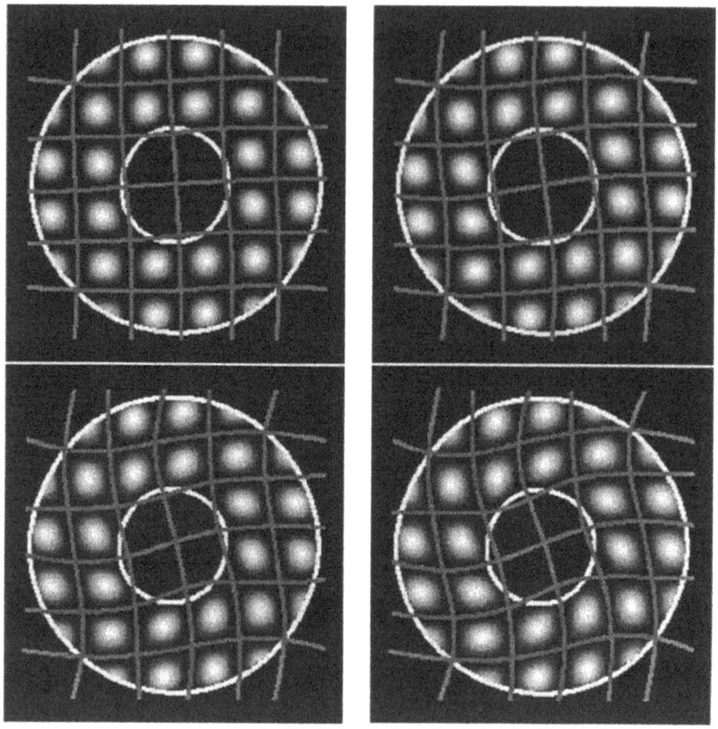

Figure 8.6: Results of coupled B-snake tracker on simulated data ($\eta_1 = 75$, $\eta_2 = 1$). From top-left ($k_2 = 0.2$) to bottom-right ($k_2 = 0.8$) in increments of 0.2. Temporal resolution is 20 ms.

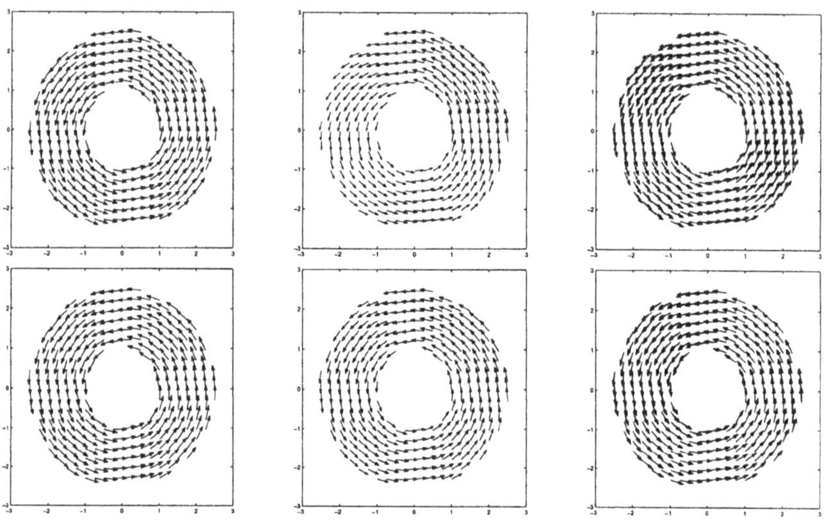

Figure 8.7: Comparison of true (left column) and computed (middle column) displacement vector fields corresponding to torsion ($k_2 = 0.03$ (top) and $k_2 = 0.15$ (bottom)). Third column is an overlap display.

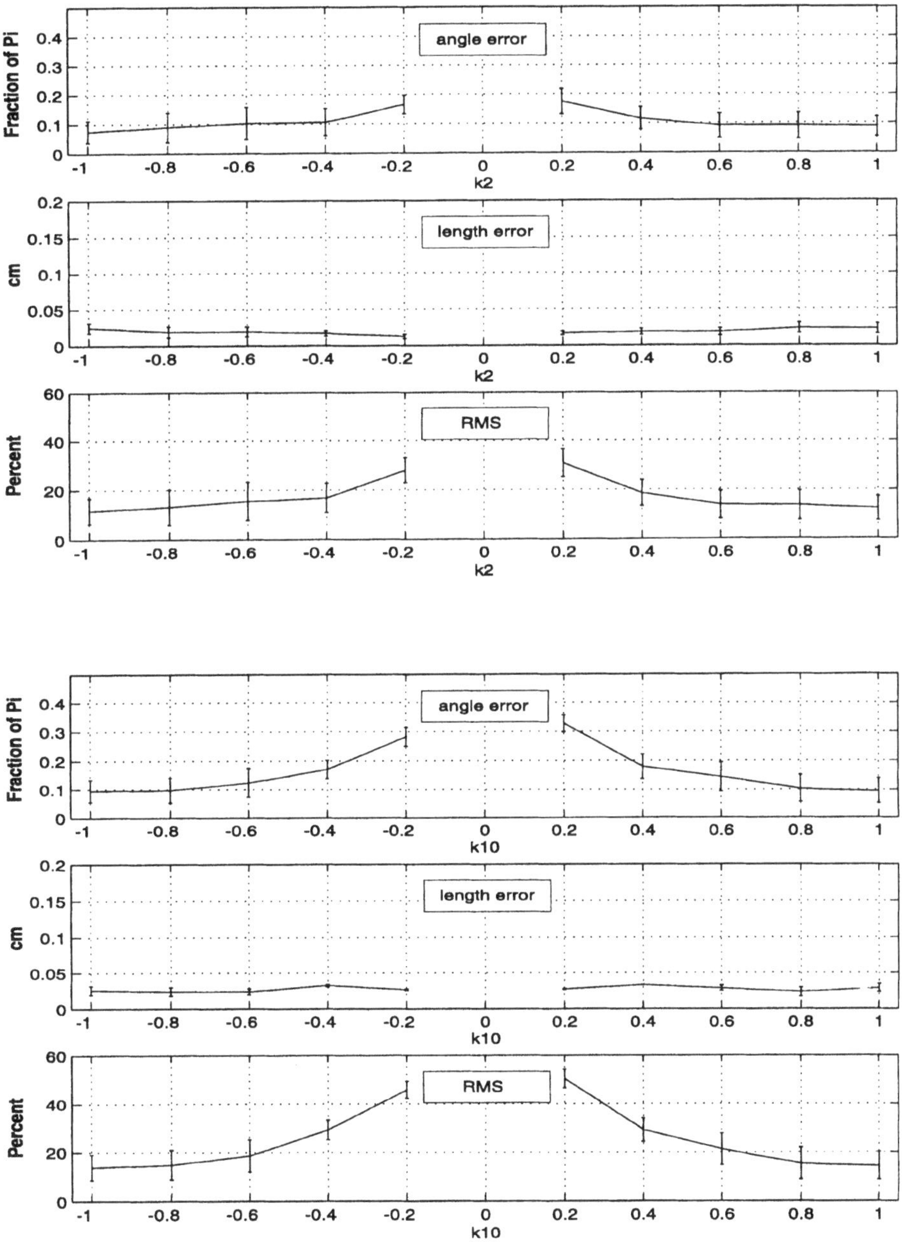

Figure 8.8: The statistical error plots for length, angle, and relative RMS errors for k_2 and k_{10}. Please see text for details.

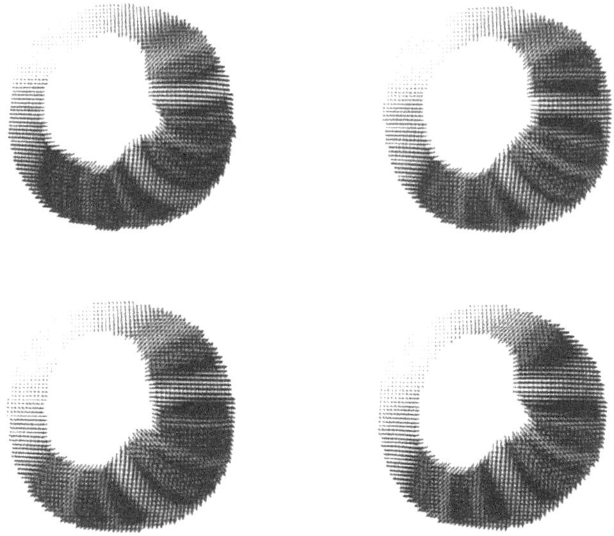

Figure 8.9: Four displacement vector fields from tagged images of a patient with antero-septal MI at $87, 116, 145$, and 174 ms after the ECG R wave. Each vector field warps the tag grid for the given time back to the undeformed tag grid at 0 ms. Segmental motion of all myocardial points can easily be quantified and visualized from the location, direction, and length of the displayed vectors. Notice in particular the small length of the vectors between the 10 and 1 o'clock positions indicative of akinesis. (The slices in this and following figures are ordered from left to right and top to bottom).

vector field ($\mathbf{V}_g$) with the vector field measured by our algorithm ($\mathbf{U}$) are:

$$\varepsilon_L = \frac{1}{N} \sum ||\mathbf{U}| - |\mathbf{V}_g|| \tag{8.29}$$

and

$$\varepsilon_\theta = \frac{1}{\sum |\mathbf{V}_g|} \sum |\mathbf{V}_g|. \arccos \frac{\mathbf{V}_g \cdot \mathbf{U}}{|\mathbf{V}_g||\mathbf{U}|} \tag{8.30}$$

where ε_L measures the average difference in length between $\mathbf{V}_g$ and $\mathbf{U}$, and ε_θ measures the deviation in angle between $\mathbf{V}_g$ and $\mathbf{U}$. As can be seen from (8.30), we weight individual angle deviations by the magnitude of the material point displacement vector; normalized by the sum of magnitude of all ground truth vectors. The reason for this is to emphasize angle deviation of points that have large displacements, and similarly, to de-emphasize the angle deviation of points which have a smaller displacement.

We also employ the relative root mean squared (RRMS) figure of merit to mea-

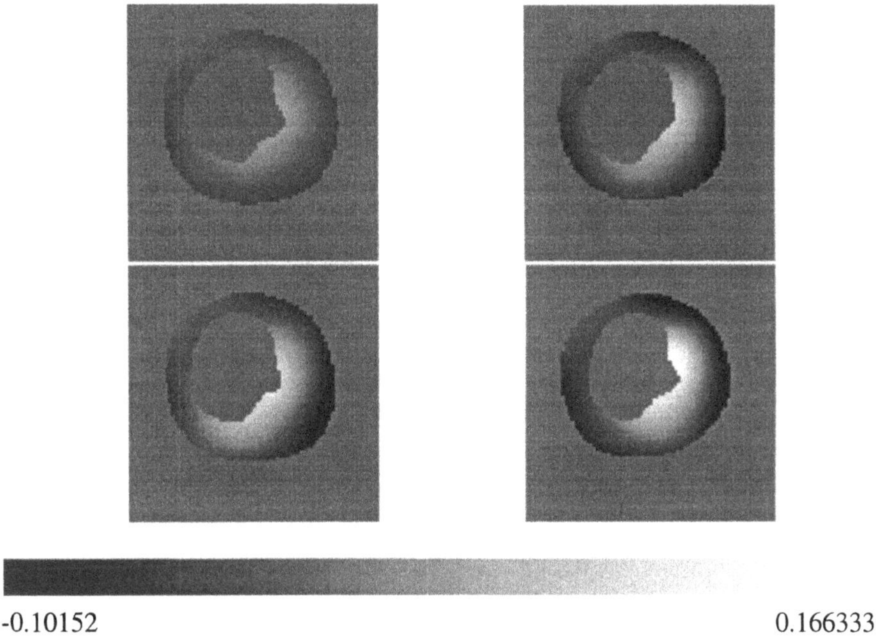

Figure 8.10: The figure shows the computed radial strains corresponding to the same time points as in Figure 8.9. The grey value of zero strain corresponds to that of the background value.

sure the accuracy of the computed motion fields:

$$\varepsilon_r = \frac{\sqrt{\frac{1}{N}\sum|\mathbf{U}-\mathbf{V}_g|^2}}{\frac{1}{N}\sum|\mathbf{V}_g|} \times 100\% \tag{8.31}$$

where N is the number of vectors in the field.

Results

In Figure 8.7 we compare the computed and ground truth displacement vector fields for the case of torsional deformation. One can visually appreciate the high accuracy of the reconstructions.

In order to measure the accuracy quantitatively, we plot the length errors, angle errors, as well as the relative RMS in Figure 8.8 by comparing $\mathbf{U}$ and $\mathbf{V}_g$ as a function of a range of values of k_2 and k_{10}, keeping the rest of the k parameters constant. Additionally, as part of the validations and in order to test the sensitivity of the algorithms to different values of algorithm coefficients λ_1, λ_2, and λ_3, we varied each of these coefficients individually in the range $\{0, 1, \cdots, 10\}$, and kept the other 2 coefficients at the constant value of 1 (excluding $\lambda_1 = 0$). The experiment is performed on 32 parameters, and the mean and variance are computed to test the influence of these parameters. The error bars in these plots show the 3

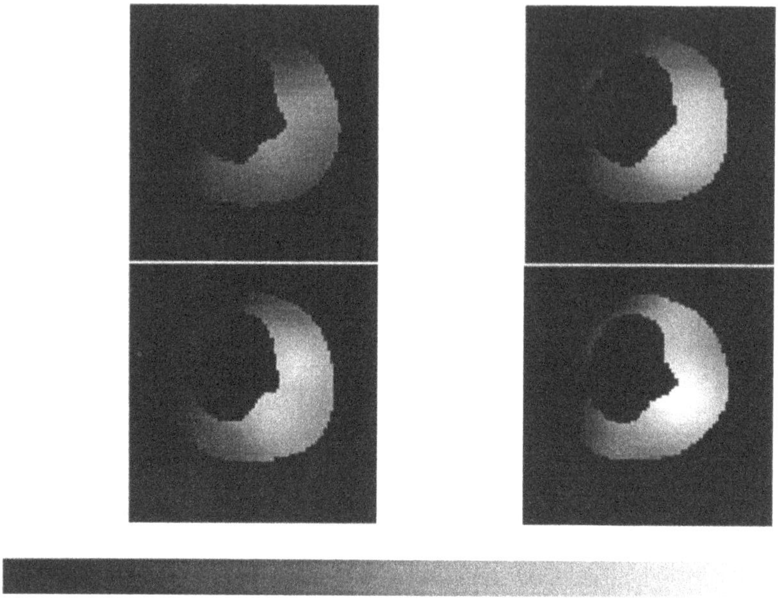

Figure 8.11: The figure shows the circumferential strains corresponding to the same time points as in Figure 8.9. The grey value of zero strain corresponds to that of the background value.

standard-deviation range on either side of the error mean for particular values of each k parameter.

As can be seen from the plots in Figure 8.8, to a large degree the displacement reconstruction algorithm is insensitive to the exact values of λ_i's. An additional remarkable point regarding the error plots is the fact that for smaller motions, the value of ε_θ is larger than that for bigger motions. The reason for this non-intuitive result can only be attributed to the larger percent inaccuracies in reconstruction of smaller displacements by the warping algorithm. Also, it should be noted that error plots in Figure 8.8 subsume the errors incurred in localization of tags and myocardial contours. Although the magnitude of errors are bound to be smaller if a more accurate location of contour and tag lines in the simulated images were to be used, our complete system for tracking and reconstruction of tag lines would not be tested, and furthermore since the exact location of tags and contours are not known in real images, phantom validation results would not be a good model of realistic situations.

In order to test the influence of the order of B-spline bases on the reconstructions, we studied the error norms introduced earlier in this section as a function of order of B-splines in the case of k_2 and k_{10}. It was found that increasing the B-spline order beyond 2 has negligible effect on the reconstruction accuracy.

The method also offers significant advantages in computational speed. The typi-

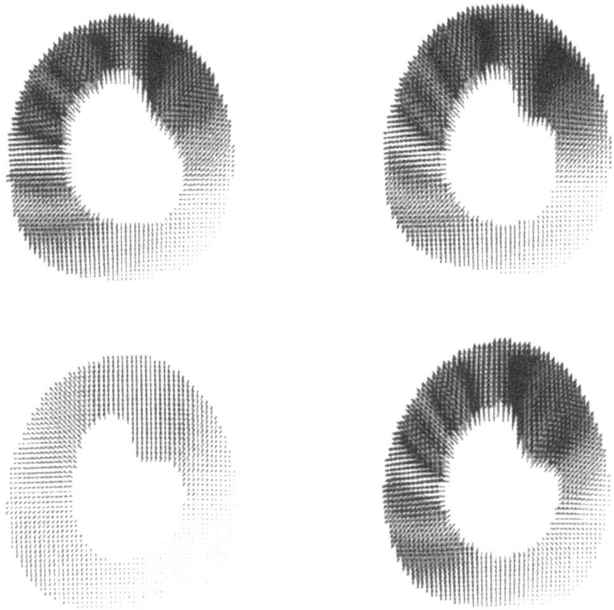

Figure 8.12: Four displacement vector fields for *in-vivo* tagged slices for a pig immediately after induction of a postero-lateral myocardial infarction. Notice the consistently small magnitude of the vector field in the infarct area (between 3 and 7 o'clock positions).

cal time for computing the deformation field between 2 frames is on the order of 1 minute on a Sun Ultra 30/300 MHz workstation.

8.4.3 Myocardial Strains

Starting at any time point during the cardiac cycle, as in [4], the heart's motion is viewed here in the Eulerian reference frame; i.e., a mapping which warps the *deformed* tag configuration ($\mathbf{x} = (x, y)$) into the *undeformed* configuration ($\mathbf{X} = (X, Y)$): $\mathbf{X} = \Gamma(\mathbf{x})$. Equivalently, with $\mathbf{X} = \mathbf{U}(\mathbf{x}) + \mathbf{x}$, the deformation gradient tensor can be written as $\mathbf{F} = \nabla\Gamma(\mathbf{x}) = \nabla\mathbf{U}(\mathbf{x}) + \nabla\mathbf{x}$ where $\mathbf{U}$ is the computed displacement vector field. Please note that the out-of-plane motion of the heart near the apex is small and the method could be directly applicable to the case of looking at motion fields in short axis slices near the apex without any loss of accuracy. Therefore, assuming little or no through-plane motion,

$$\mathbf{F} = \begin{pmatrix} u_x + 1 & u_y \\ v_x & v_y + 1 \end{pmatrix}. \tag{8.32}$$

The strain tensor can then be expressed as

$$\mathbf{E} = \frac{1}{2}(\mathbf{F}^T\mathbf{F} - \mathbf{I}). \tag{8.33}$$

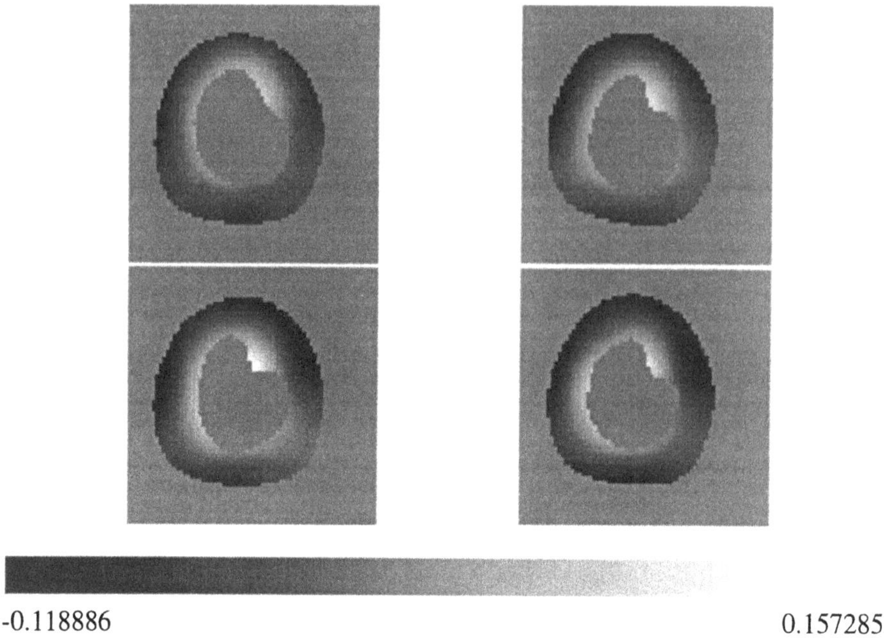

Figure 8.13: The figure shows the computed radial strains corresponding to the same time points as in Figure 8.12. The grey value of zero strain corresponds to that of the background value.

Once a displacement vector field is available, the strain of deformation can be computed at all myocardial points within a short-axis slice. Furthermore, the quantity $\mathbf{M}^T\mathbf{E}\mathbf{M}$ will give the value of strain for the direction $\mathbf{M}$. For example, $\mathbf{M}$ can be the radial or the circumferential directions.

Figures 8.9-8.11, and 8.12-8.14 show examples of the computation of deformation fields and corresponding strains in a patient with an old antero-septal myocardial infarction (MI), and a pig immediately after induction of a postero-lateral MI. Notice that the vector fields display small magnitudes in the infarct area (between 10 and 1 o'clock positions in figure 8.9 and between 3 and 7 o'clock positions in figure 8.12). Also, in comparison to normal myocardium, strain magnitudes (particularly the circumferential strains) are depressed in these areas.

8.5 Measurement of 3D Motion of Myocardial Beads

The procedure outlined in Section 8.4.1 provides a mechanism for tracking points within short-axis image slices. However, as shown in Figure 8.15, in MRI, the position of image slices are fixed relative to the magnet's coordinate system, and therefore this procedure can only yield 2D motion of material points within a short-axis-slice. To obtain information about the movements of points in the "out-of-plane" direction, a second sequence of images is acquired with slices parallel to the heart's long-axis and with the requirement that tag planes intersecting the new slices be in

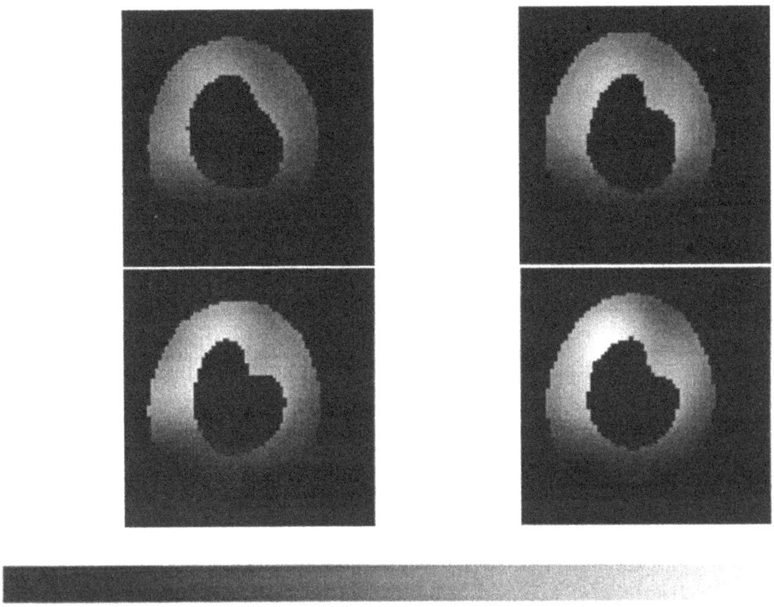

Figure 8.14: The figure shows the circumferential strains corresponding to the same time points as in Figure 8.12. The area between 3 and 7 o'clock positions exhibit small strain values indicative of akinesis. The grey value of zero strain corresponds to that of the background value.

parallel to short axis images.

8.5.1 Imaging Protocol

A breath-hold, segmented k-space, SPAMM pulse sequence was used to collect multiple images in both short-axis and long-axis views of the entire heart without gaps. Immediately after the ECG trigger, rf tagging pulses were applied in two orthogonal directions. The repetition time (TR) of the imaging sequence was approximately 7.1 ms, the echo time (TE) was 2.9 ms, the rf flip angle was 15 degrees, and the time extent of rf tag pulses was 22 ms. Echo sharing was used in collecting each time-varying image sequence for a given slice position. Five data lines were collected for any time frame during each heart cycle, but two data lines were overlapped between two consecutive cardiac frames, resulting in an effective temporal resolution of approximately 22 ms. Other imaging parameters were: field of view = 330 mm, data acquisition matrix size = 160×256 (phase-encoding by readout), in-plane resolution = $2.1 \times 1.3\text{mm}^2$, slice thickness = 7 mm, and tag spacing = 7 mm.

The image orientations for the short-axis and long-axis views of the heart were first determined by collecting multiple oblique angle scout images. For the short-axis images, one of the tagging planes was placed parallel to the long-axis imaging planes of the heart by manually setting the angles of the tagging plane in the coordinate system of the magnet to be the same as those of the long-axis view as determined from scout images. The coordinates of the center of the central tagging plane in the reference coordinates system (relative to the center of the magnet) were set to be the same as those of the center of one of the long- axis image planes to be acquired, again determined by the scout images. As a result, one set of tagging planes intersecting short-axis image slices coincided with long-axis images since both tag spacing and slice thickness were 7 mm center-to-center. The other short-axis tagging plane was placed orthogonal to the first tagging plane. Similarly, long-axis images were acquired with their tag planes coinciding with short-axis slice positions. It should be noted however that these requirements are not stringent.

Indeed, the method described in Section 8.5.3 will continue to apply as long as 3 sequences of intersecting tag planes are encoded within the LV myocardium. However, the fact that at end-diastole, long-axis tag planes coincide with short-axis image slice locations and one set of short-axis tag planes coincides with long-axis image slice locations leads to an interesting byproduct, namely, that location of myocardial tag lines on short-axis and long-axis images at end-diastole can simply be read off from image headers. To illustrate, Figure 8.16 displays position of the short-axis image slices on one long-axis image at end-diastole.

As a result of the imaging protocol outlined in this section, the tag intersections are the myocardial beads corresponding precisely to the intersection of three tag planes, and revealing for all time points in the cardiac cycle, 3D motion of these special points.

8.5.2 Reconstruction of Tag Planes

Given a spatial stack of m spline curves on m slices, each represented by n control points, a matrix of control points is constructed as follows:

$$\begin{pmatrix} \mathbf{p}_{11} & \cdots & \mathbf{p}_{1n} \\ & \cdots & \\ \mathbf{p}_{m1} & \cdots & \mathbf{p}_{mn} \end{pmatrix} \tag{8.34}$$

where the first index denotes ordering of control points across image slices and the second index denotes ordering of control points along the curve – within the image slice. The matrix immediately gives rise to the surface

$$\mathbf{S}(u,v) = \sum_i \sum_j \mathbf{p}_{ij} \beta_i^k(u) \beta_j^k(v) \tag{8.35}$$

where once again, we use $k = 3$ to ensure that there is the necessary flexibility in the parametrized shapes. Figure 8.17 illustrates the construction of intersecting cubic B-spline tag surfaces from a spatial stack of coupled B-snake grids.

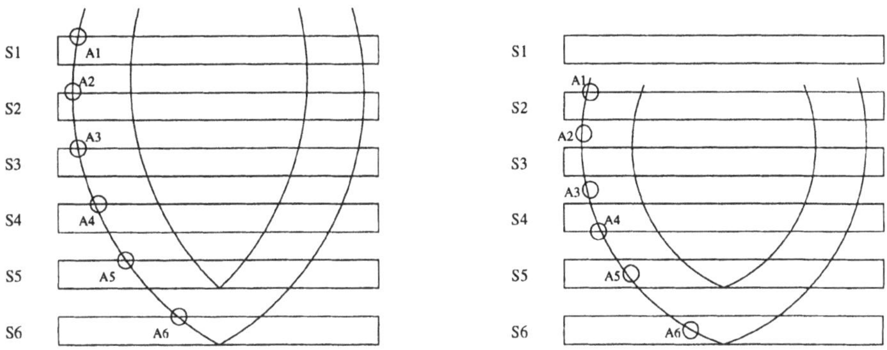

Figure 8.15: Imaging geometry in MRI. The position of slices $(S1, \cdots, S6)$ are fixed relative to the magnet's coordinate system. However, a dynamic organ such as the heart moves in-and-out of the slices. Motion of points $A1, \cdots, A6$ illustrates this.

8.5.3 Computing 3D Coordinates of Myocardial Beads

As in the case of coupled B-snakes of short-axis images, deformations of tag planes in the long-axis orientation are again measured by creating B-spline surfaces from stacks of B-snakes. The difference between short-axis and long-axis image acquisitions however is that there is only one set of parallel tag planes intersecting long-axis images. Figure 8.18 illustrates a tag surface constructed from a spatial sequence of long-axis images.

Coordinates of material points may be obtained by computing intersections of three intersecting B-spline surfaces representing three intersecting tag surfaces. For each triplet of intersecting B-spline surfaces, $(\mathbf{S}_1(u_1, v_1), \mathbf{S}_2(u_2, v_2), \mathbf{S}_3(u_3, v_3))$, the following computation is performed

$$\min_{\mathbf{q}_1, \mathbf{q}_2, \mathbf{q}_3} d^2(\mathbf{S}_1, \mathbf{S}_2) + d^2(\mathbf{S}_1, \mathbf{S}_3) + d^2(\mathbf{S}_2, \mathbf{S}_3) \tag{8.36}$$

where point $\mathbf{q}_i$ belongs to surface $\mathbf{S}_i$ and d is the Euclidean distance metric. The minimization is carried out using the method of Conjugate Gradient Descent which ensures the fast convergence of the method. Note that the overall distance function above can be written as

$$\begin{aligned} &\|\mathbf{S}_1(u_1, v_1) - \mathbf{S}_2(u_2, v_2)\|^2 + \|\mathbf{S}_2(u_2, v_2) - \mathbf{S}_3(u_3, v_3)\|^2 + \\ &\qquad \|\mathbf{S}_1(u_1, v_1) - \mathbf{S}_3(u_3, v_3)\|^2 \end{aligned} \tag{8.37}$$

with the goal of finding the parameters (u_i, v_i) for the triplet of surfaces. The computed parameters will in fact be surface parameters of the intersection point. For the iterative optimization process, a good initial set of parameters has been found to be parameters of the intersection point assuming linear B-spline bases.

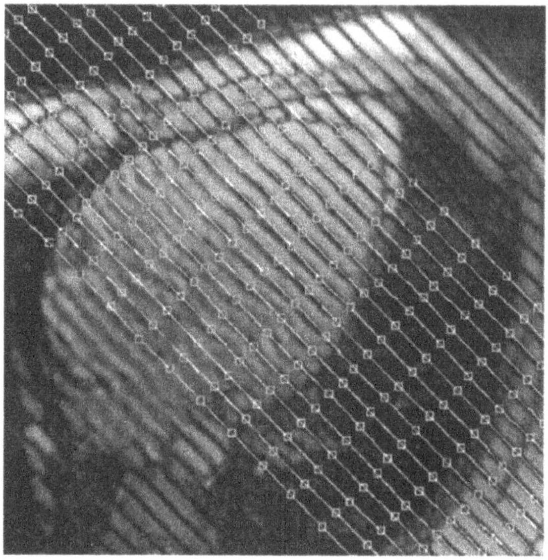

Figure 8.16: Position of short-axis image slices at the time of tag placement is drawn on a long-axis image acquired at the same time point in the cardiac cycle.

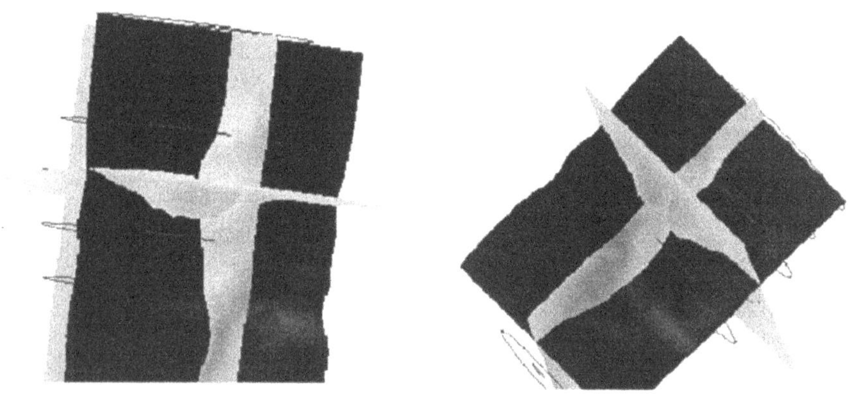

Figure 8.17: This figure illustrates the reconstruction of two orthogonal short-axis tag surfaces from a sequence of coupled B-spline curves in short-axis image slices. Two views of the same tag planes are shown. The bright horizontal surface is a long-axis tag plane.

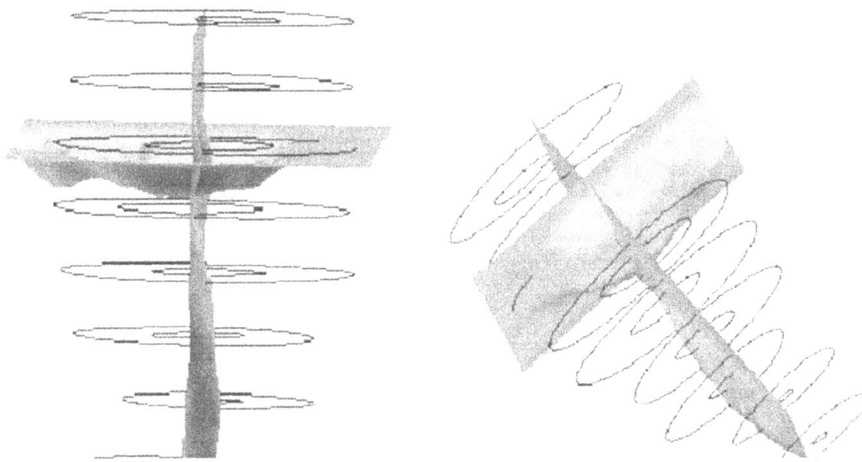

Figure 8.18: B-spline surface representation of a long-axis tag plane reconstructed from a spatial stack of B-snakes. Two views of a reconstructed long-axis tag surface is displayed (horizontal surface on the left). "Out-of-plane" movement of the heart is visualized by the deviation from flatness of the long-axis B-surface. The vertical surface on the left is a short-axis tag surface. The short-axis myocardial contours are also displayed.

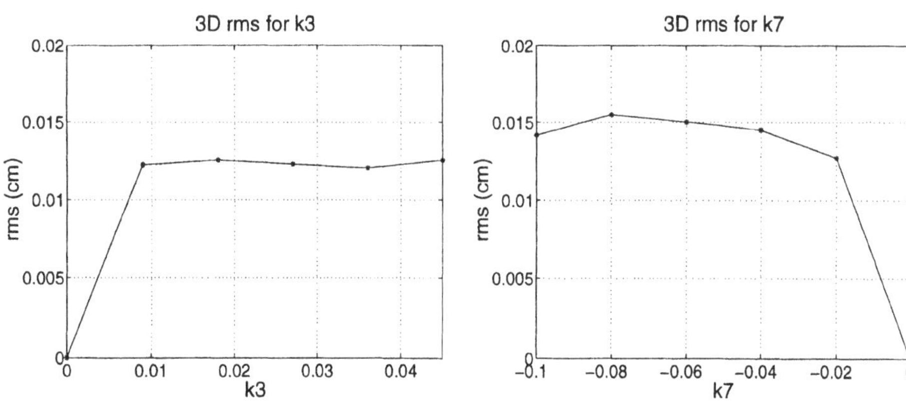

Figure 8.19: RMS error plots (Equation (8.38)) as a function of k_3 and k_7. To generate these error curves, the deformation matrix ([22]) was directly applied to the locations of tag line control points in the undeformed reference state. Intersections of the triplet of tag surfaces were then found and the RMS error between the computed and theoretical intersections were calculated. In both cases, $k_i = 0$ represents the undeformed reference state at time 0. Please note that in the above plots, depending on whether k_i increases or decreases from zero, time increases from left to right, or right to left.

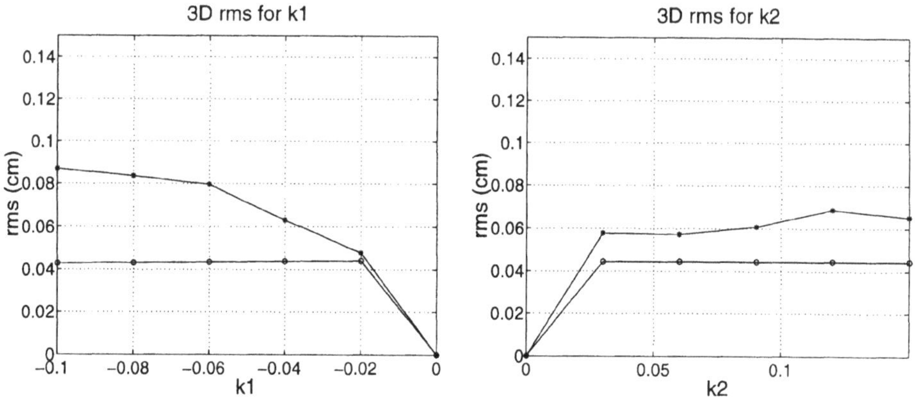

Figure 8.20: RMS error plots for all the simulated myocardial material points as a function of k_1 and k_2 with tag detection and manual correction. In all cases, $k_i = 0$ represents the undeformed reference state at time 0. For the k_1 plot, time increases from right to left and for k_2 plot, time increases from left to right. In each case, the top plot represents the RMS error with tag spacing of 0.785 cm and the bottom plot is the error curve with tag spacing of 0.393 cm.

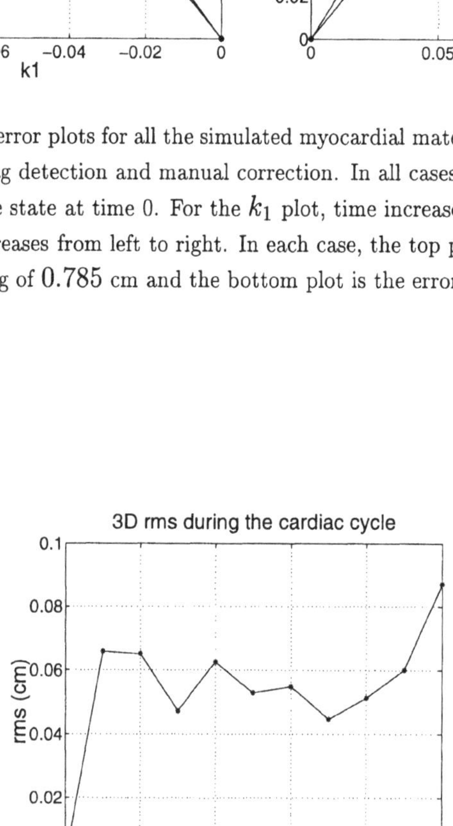

Figure 8.21: RMS error plots for all the simulated myocardial material points during the whole cardiac cycle when all the k parameters are concurrently varied. The k parameters for each time point were found by least-squares fitting to an *in-vivo* canine heart over the entire ECG cycle [6].

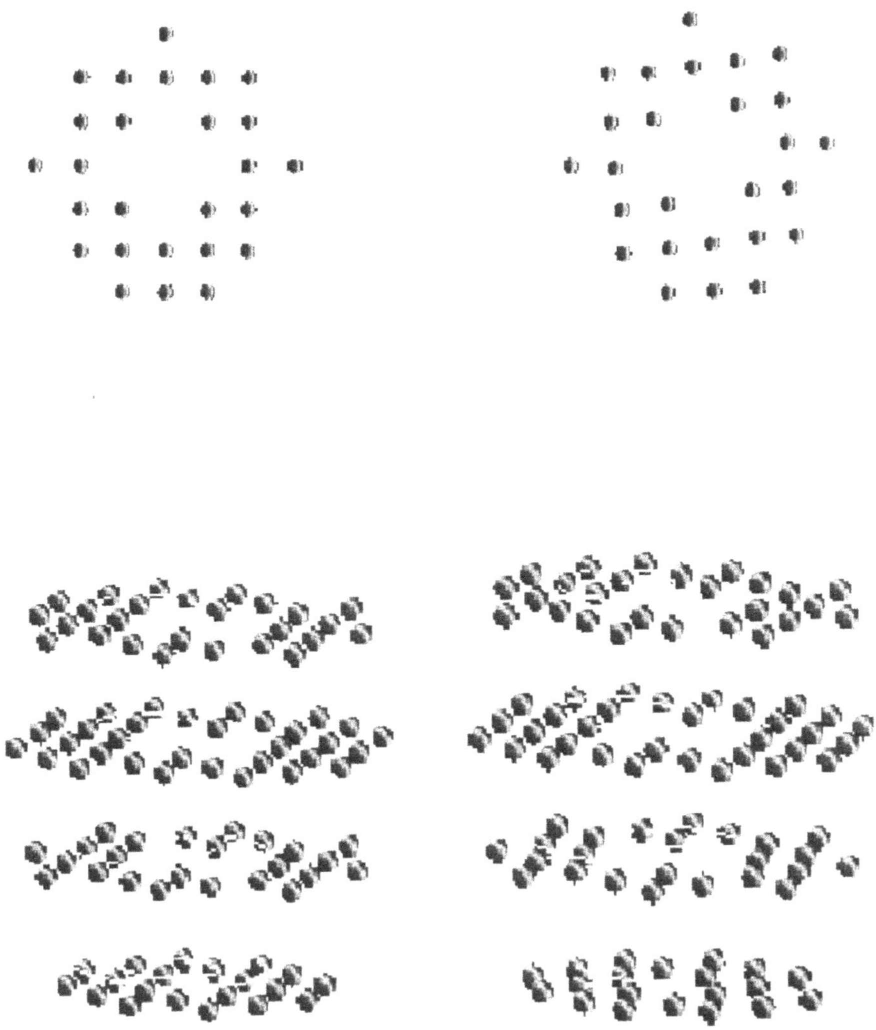

Figure 8.22: Intersections computed for the k_2 simulated sequence: slice 0 of the spatial stack at times 0 ($k_2 = 0$) and 5 ($k_2 = 0.15$) (top). Slices 0, 2, 4, and 6 at times 0 and 5 (bottom).

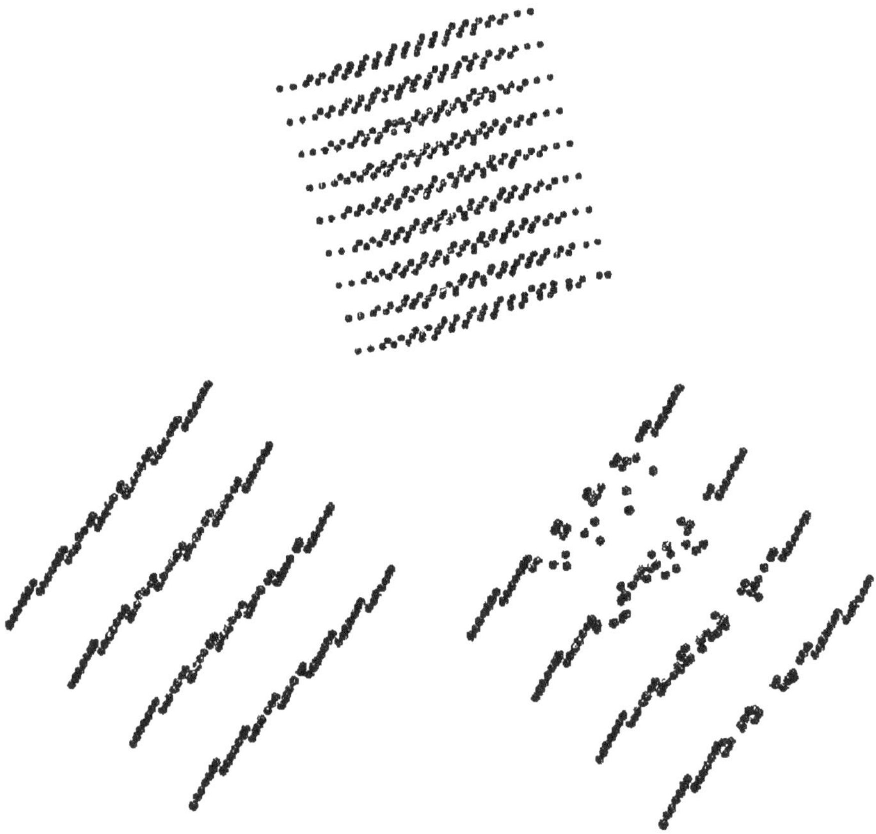

Figure 8.23: Initial 3D location of material points shown on every second slice of the MRI data in a healthy volunteer (top). Location of the material points, for every fourth slice, of the MRI data is displayed on the left. New computed location of material points, one-third through systole, is shown on the right. The non-rigid motion of the material points of the heart can be seen: points further up in slices (around the base) move downwards, whereas points near the heart's apex are relatively stationary.

8.5.4 Validations

In order to validate the accuracy of the method in measuring 3D motion of myocardial material points, the cardiac motion simulator was used to generate SA and LA images as prescribed by the imaging protocol of Section 8.5.1.

The correspondence of LA tag planes and SA image slices as well as one set of SA tag planes and the LA image slices in the undeformed state was ensured by computing the exact location of the tag plane intersecting the 3D model using Equation (11) of [22]. The location of the image slice in each case was chosen to be identical to this position. The SA image planes were located at: $z = -1.57, -0.785, 0, 0.785, 1.57, 2.355, 3.14, 3.925$ (all locations in cm) which coincide with position of LA tag planes in the undeformed state. The LA image planes were located at: $y = -2.355, -1.57, -0.785, 0, 0.785, 1.57, 2.355$ (all locations in cm) which coincided with position of one set of SA tag planes. Therefore, there were eight SA slices and seven LA slices. The slice separation as well as the tag separations in SA and LA images were 0.785cm.

To compute a figure of merit for the algorithm, the RMS error between theoretical intersections, $\mathbf{q}_i^t$ and the computed intersections, $\mathbf{q}_i^c$, were calculated

$$RMS = \sqrt{\frac{1}{N}\sum_{i=1}^{N} |\mathbf{q}_i^t - \mathbf{q}_i^c|^2} \tag{8.38}$$

where the sum is over all myocardial material points across all spatial slices for a given volumetric time frame.

Because the accuracy of the intersection calculations are affected by both the tag line detection/tracing procedure as well as tag spacings, and in order to remove the effect of errors in tag line detection/tracing, we used the theoretical tag line locations (known from the simulator parameters) for validating the computed intersections for each of the six image collection time points for k_3, k_7, and k_9 sequences. The 3D RMS error curves are shown in Figure 8.19. The plots indicate that these errors, which are solely due to numerical optimization and round-off errors in computing the location of myocardial beads, are truly negligible (on the order of 0.01cm). Figure 8.20 displays how the RMS error varies with the tag spacing under tag line detection/manual correction for k_1 and k_2 sequences.[1] The error curves in this case clearly indicate larger errors than those in Figure 8.19. However, note that when tag spacing is reduced by half, the RMS error is reduced by half or by a third for for the parameters k_1 and k_2 respectively. Figure 8.21 shows the RMS error for the entire cardiac cycle when all the 13 k parameters are concurrently varied. The time evolution of the 13 k parameters are as those reported in [6]

1 - For k_3, k_7 and k_9 image sequences, it is possible to obtain the exact location of the B-snake grid control point locations (and consequently 3D coordinates of tag curves) for all time points by directly applying the simulator deformation matrix [22] to the coordinates of the control points in the undeformed state. However, due to the structure of B-spline bases, for k_1 and k_2 (radially-dependent compression and torsion) parameters, this can not be achieved.

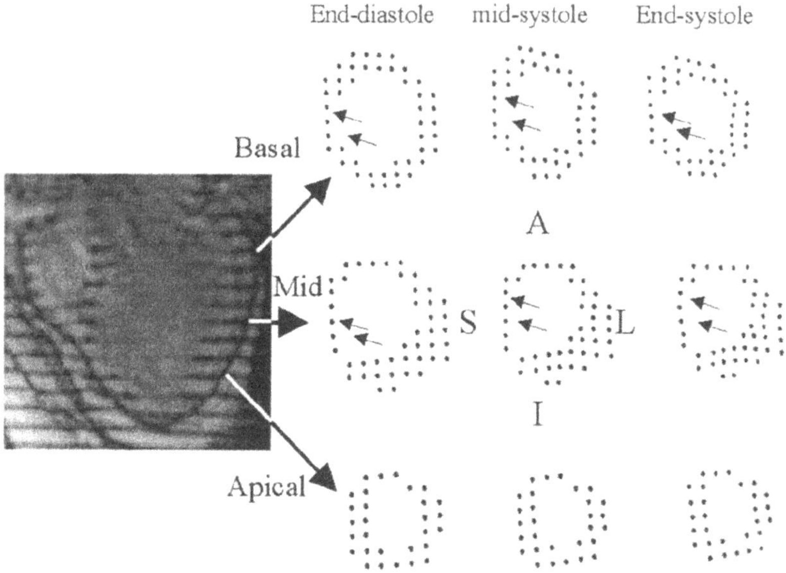

Figure 8.24: MRI of the left-ventricular long-axis view with tissue-tagging (left) in a patient with a history of an antero-septal myocardial infarction. The antero-septal wall (arrows) shows no motion of the beads during the systolic phase of the cardiac cycle (end-diastole to mid-systole to end-systole), reflecting akinesis of these segments, compatible with myocardial infarction (right). Please note that the location of beads at end-diastole correspond to short-axis slice positions as shown on the long-axis image.

and [22], representing canonical deformations of an *in-vivo* canine LV. Figure 8.22 shows intersections computed from k_2 simulated images from frame 0 to from 5.

The algorithm was also tested on a normal human image sequence which included 17 slices and 19 frames (17×19 images) yielding temporal position of around 250 beads over the heart cycle. In a movie of these material points, the 3D motion of individual SPAMM points of the myocardium is clearly apparent. Figure 8.23 displays results of the intersection computation for a few of the material points. Figure 8.24 shows results from the application of the algorithm to images collected from a patient with an old, healed, antero-septal myocardial infarction.

8.6 Conclusions

In this chapter, we have provided an overview of B-spline based image analysis methods for measurement of deformations of the left-ventricle of the heart from tagged images.

The presented 2D analysis method is a fast approach (one minute compute time) to LV deformation reconstruction based on point and line constraints. Once a dense displacement vector field is reconstructed, the strain of deformation at all myocardial points can easily be computed. Methods were also presented for computing the 3D location of beads encoded within the ventricular wall with a tagging pulse sequence.

Acknowledgments

This work was supported by the NIH under grants HL-57628 and HL-64217 and by the NSF under grant IRI-9796207.

References

[1] A. Amini, R. W. Curwen, and John C. Gore. Snakes and splines for tracking non-rigid heart motion. In *European Conf. on Computer Vision*, pages 251–261, U. of Cambridge, UK, April 1996.

[2] A. Amini and et al. Energy-minimizing deformable grids for tracking tagged MR cardiac images. In *Computers in Cardiology*, Durham, North Carolina, pages 651–654, October 1992.

[3] A. Amini, Y. Chen, R. Curwen, V. Mani, J. Sun, Coupled B-snake grids Coupled B-snake grids and constrained thin-plate splines for analysis of 2-D tissue deformations from tagged MRI. *IEEE-TMI*, 7(3):344-356, June 1998.

[4] A. Amini, Y. Chen, D. Abendschein, Comparison of landmark-based and curve-based thin plate warps for analysis of left ventricular motion from tagged MRI. in *MICCAI*, University of Cambridge, UK, Sept. 1999.

[5] A. Amini, Y. Chen, M. Elayyadi, and P. Radeva, Tag surface reconstruction and tracking of myocardial beads from SPAMM-MRI with parametric B-Spline surfaces. *IEEE-TMI*, 20(2):94-103, February 2001.

[6] T. Arts, W. Hunter, A. Douglas, A. Muijtjens, and R. Reneman. Description of the deformation of the left ventricle by a kinematic model. *J. Biomechanics*, 25(10):1119–1127, 1992.

[7] L. Axel and L. Dougherty. MR imaging of motion with spatial modulation of magnetization. *Radiology*, 171(3):841-845, 1989.

[8] F. Bookstein. Principal warps: Thin-plate splines and the decomposition of deformations. *IEEE T-PAMI*, 11:567–585, 1989.

[9] T. Denney and J. Prince. Reconstruction of 3-d left ventricular motion from planar tagged cardiac MR images: An estimation-theoretic approach. *IEEE-TMI*, 14(4):625-635, December 1995.

[10] M. E. Mortenson. *Geometric Modeling*. Wiley, New York, 1985.

[11] G. Golub, C. V. Loan, *Matrix Computations*. Johns Hopkins University Press, Baltimore, MD, third edition, 1996.

[12] J. Huang, D. Abendschein, V. G. Davila-Roman, and A. Amini. Spatio-temporal tracking of myocardial deformations with a 4D B-spline model from tagged MRI. *IEEE-TMI*, 18(10):957-972, October 1999.

[13] W. Kerwin and J. Prince. Generating 3-D Cardiac Material Markers Using Tagged MRI. Information Processing in Medical Imaging, pp. 313-326, June 1997.

[14] A. Klein, F. Lee, and A. Amini. Quantitative coronary angiography with deformable spline models. *IEEE-TMI*, 16(5):468-482, 1997.

[15] S. Menet, P. Saint-Marc, and G. Medioni. B-snakes: Implementation and application to stereo. In *Proceedings of the DARPA Image Understanding Workshop, Pittsburgh, PA*, pages 720-726, Sept. 1990.

[16] W. O'Dell, C. Moore, W. Hunter, E. Zerhouni, and E. McVeigh. Three-dimensional myocardial deformations: Calculation with displacement field fitting to tagged MR images. *Radiology*, 195(3):829-835, 1995.

[17] J. Park, D. Metaxas, and L. Axel. Volumetric deformable models with parameter functions: A new approach to the 3D motion analysis of the LV from MRI-SPAMM. In *Proc. of ICCV*, pages 700-705, 1995.

[18] P. Radeva, A. Amini, and J. Huang. Deformable B-Solids and implicit snakes for 3D localization and tracking of SPAMM MRI data. *CVIU*, 66(2):163–178, May 1997.

[19] N. Reichek. Magnetic resonance imaging for assessment of myocardial function. *Mag. Res. Quarterly*, 7(4):255–274, 1991.

[20] M. Unser, A. Aldroubi, M. Eden. B-spline signal processing: Part 1 and Part 2. *IEEE T-ASSP*, 41(2):821-847, 1993.

[21] G. Wahba, *Spline methods for observational data*, SIAM CBMS-NSF, Philadephia, 1990.

[22] E. Waks, J. Prince, and A. Douglas. Cardiac motion simulator for tagged MRI. In *Proc. IEEE MMBIA*, pages 182-191, 1996.

[23] Y. Wang and S. L. Lee. Scale-space derived from B-splines. *IEEE T-PAMI*, 21(9):277-285, 1998.

[24] Y. Wang, Y. Chen, and A. Amini, Fast LV Motion Estimation Using Subspace Approximation Techniques, *IEEE-TMI*, (20)6:499-513, June 2001.

[25] A. Young, D. Kraitchman, L. Dougherty, and L. Axel. Tracking and finite element analysis of stripe deformation in magnetic resonance tagging. *IEEE-TMI*, 14(3):413-421, September 1995.

Chapter 9

MR Physics and Imaging of Phase Contrast MRI

Michael Markl, Britta Schneider, and Jürgen Hennig
Uniklinik Freiburg,
Abt. Rontgendiagnostik,
Sect. of Medical Physics,
Hugstetter Str. 55,
D 79106 Freiburg,
Germany

9.1 Introduction

In recent years cardiac magnetic resonance (MR) imaging has become an important method for diagnosis of heart disease not only for morphologic evaluation but also for the characterization of myocardial function. Noninvasive measurement of myocardial wall motion with MRI is a promising method for detection of the mechanical performance of the heart in order to identify abnormal motion and potentially infarcted areas of the left ventricle. Several methods for ventricular motion mapping have already been proposed. An extensive discussion of the various approaches is found in Ref.[1].

The most abundantly used approach are tagging techniques, in which the images of the myocardium are labeled with stripe or grid pattern by spatial modulation of the z-magnetization prior to signal readout. The change in shape of the saturation pattern in the image reflects the local motion of the underlying heart muscle. Such techniques can be used to observe the spatial displacement of the tagging labels over the ECG-cycle. In addition to that, tagging allows the study of the mechanical properties of the heart wall, using a stress-strain analysis of myocardial regions. An intrinsic disadvantage of tagging techniques is the fact that the spatial resolution of the functional information compared to the anatomical resolution of the underlying images is reduced by a factor of 3–5 in linear dimensions or 9–25 if the voxel areas are compared. Nevertheless, tagging methods have been used successfully to describe the mechanical properties of the myocardium in healthy volunteers and

A.A. Amini and J.L. Prince (eds.),
Measurement of Cardiac Deformations from MRI: Physical and Mathematical Models, 219–255.

patients [2–37].

A second approach to characterization of heart wall motion is offered by the sensitivity of the phase of the MR signal to motion. This can be used to directly measure the local velocity of the myocardium by MR-interferometric or phase contrast techniques on a pixel-to-pixel basis [38]. It should be noted that phase contrast techniques and MR interferography are generically equivalent, since both approaches use the phase difference between a motion compensated signal and a motion sensitized signal for measuring velocities. Phase contrast methods offer the advantage that they can be implemented in a way that one measurement can be performed within one breath-hold. Artifacts from breathing motion are thus avoided. Phase contrast techniques have already been used for such velocity measurements. However, the commonly applied procedure to localize myocardial areas with compromised function in velocity based approaches is stress-strain analysis as in tagging techniques. For the detection of local variations in the motional performance of the myocardium pixel wise trajectories are calculated from the measured velocity fields and analyzed [39–48].

This chapter explains how to directly use two- or three-dimensional velocity data for the characterization of myocardial motion. It also explores the feasibility of velocity-based data evaluation for the measurement and characterization of functional deficits caused by focal and global pathologies [49–58].

9.2 Basic Principles of Phase Contrast MRI

Most MR sequences demonstrate more or less significant sensitivity to flow and motion, which can lead to artifacts in many applications. The intrinsic motion sensitivity of MRI can however be used to image vessels as in phase contrast MR-angiography to quantify blood flow and also to measure motion of tissue. Using appropriate velocity encoding gradients the flow or motion dependent phase effect can be used to measure two datasets with different velocity dependent phase with otherwise identical acquisition parameters. Subtraction of the two resulting phase images allows the quantitative assessment of the velocities of the underlying flow or motion [59–71].

The phase dependency of the MR signal to moving spins can be derived from the precession frequency of spins in local magnetic fields. The resulting signal phase can be written as a sum of nth order components ($n = 0, 1, \dots, \infty$).

$$\Phi(\mathbf{r}, t_s) = \Phi(\mathbf{r}, t_0) + \sum_{n=0}^{\infty} \Delta\Phi_n(\mathbf{r}^{(n)}, t_s)\,, \tag{9.1}$$

If the motion of the tissue under investigation does not change fast with respect to the temporal resolution of data acquisition the corresponding velocities can be approximated to be constant during the measurement of each time frame. As a result the evolution of the signal phase is given by zeroth and first order components $\Delta\Phi_0(\mathbf{r}_0, t_s)$ and $\Delta\Phi_0(\nu, t_s)$ which describe the influence of magnetic field gradients on phase components of static spins at $\mathbf{r}_0$ and moving spins with velocities ν, respectively. A more detailed description of the corresponding calculations is given in the appendix at the end of this chapter. Specifically, equations (9.9) and (9.10) in the appendix express the zeroth and first order components of the signal phase.

9.2.1 Flow and Motion Compensation

In order to reduce artifacts resulting from flow or motion induced phase shifts, compensation techniques can be applied to the pulse sequences. Here gradient switching schemes are chosen such that velocity induced phase shifts are refocused. These schemes can be calculated for all orders of $\mathbf{r}(t)$ and designed for all three gradient encoding directions from the boundary condition $\sum \Delta\Phi_n(\mathbf{r}^{(n)}, TE) = 0$ for read and slice direction and $\sum \Delta\Phi_n(\mathbf{r}^{(n)}, TE) = \vartheta_{k-\text{space}}$ for the phase direction. Consequently for mth order motion compensation in the read or slice directions, all signal phases $\Delta\Phi_n$ with $n \leq m$ are required to vanish at the echo time TE (Figure 9.1). In the phase direction, the resulting phase at TE must equal the appropriate phase $\vartheta_{k-\text{space}}$ for encoding of the corresponding k-space line.

Usually first order motion compensation is sufficient for acquisition of artifact free images. However, in comparison to standard pulse sequences additional gradients are necessary and lead to increased echo and repetition time. For higher order compensations even more complicated gradient switching schemes are required.

9.2.2 Velocity Encoding

The velocity encoding gradient is usually bipolar, and thus does not lead to any phase encoding of stationary spins. Moving spins, however, will experience a linear velocity dependent phase change, which is proportional to the amplitude and timing of the gradient. According to Equations (9.9) and (9.10), phase shifts introduced by a bipolar gradient in the k-direction ($k = x, y, z$) with ramp time t_{ramp}, plateau time t_P, and gradient strength G_k are given by

$$\begin{aligned} \Delta\Phi_0(\mathbf{r}_0) &= 0, \\ \Delta\Phi_1(\nu) &= -\gamma G_k(2t_{\text{ramp}}^2 + 3t_{\text{ramp}}t_P + t_P^2)\nu_k(\mathbf{r}_0)\,. \end{aligned} \tag{9.2}$$

Depending on the spatial orientation k of the bipolar encoding gradient, only velocities in the corresponding direction $\nu_k(\mathbf{r}_0)$ contribute to the phase of the MR signal and are thus directly related to the induced first-order phase shift ($\Delta\Phi_1 \sim \nu_k(\mathbf{r}_0)$) (see Figure 9.2).

In order to filter out phase effects from sources other than motion, a non-velocity encoded scan has to be acquired as a reference image. Since velocity sensitization can only be achieved in one direction per experiment, four independent measurements (reference scan and three motion sensitive measurements in x-, y- and z-directions) must be performed to acquire a 3D velocity data set with isotropic

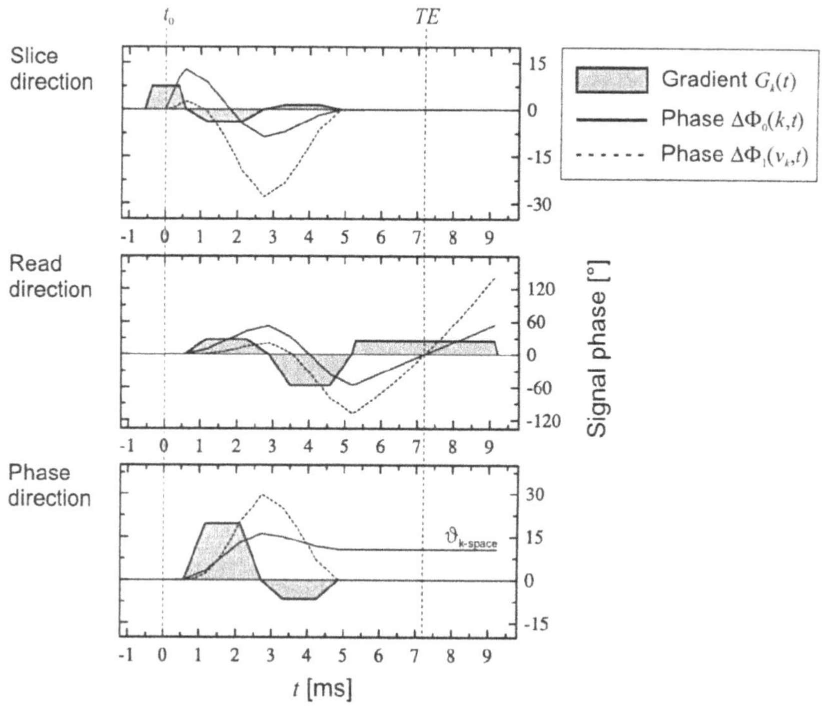

Figure 9.1: Gradient switching schemes for first order motion compensation of a gradient echo pulse sequence. Calculations were performed for a velocity of $\nu_k = 20\text{cm/s}$. In the read and slice direction, three instead of the usual two gradients are required, whereas in the phase encoding direction, two gradients are sufficient to provide the desired signal phases at $t = TE$.

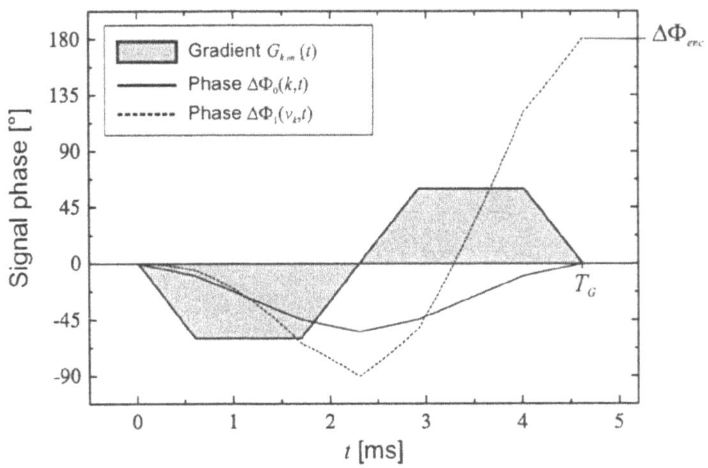

Figure 9.2: Evolution of zero and first order signal phase for a bipolar velocity encoding gradient. Calculations were performed for a velocity of $\nu_k = 20\text{cm/s}$.

flow or motion sensitivity. In order to assess the velocity encoded phase shifts $\Delta\Phi_{\text{enc}}(\mathbf{r}_0)$, phase difference images of a reference scan without a bipolar encoding gradient and a velocity sensitive scan have to be calculated:

$$\Delta\Phi_{\text{enc}}(\mathbf{r}_0) = \Phi_{\text{reference}} - \Phi_{\text{sensitive}} = \Delta\Phi_{1,\text{sensitive}}(\nu_k(\mathbf{r}_0))\,. \tag{9.3}$$

Since the image reconstruction with Fourier transformation resolves signal amplitudes and phases as a function of spatial locations, the encoded velocities are directly assessable as pixel intensities in the calculated phases difference images. Phase contrast MRI also requires knowledge of the magnitude of the velocities that are to be imaged. For velocities that are too large, the velocity-dependent phase shift can exceed $\pm 180^o$, and aliasing occurs. Consequently, the highest velocity that is expected must be used to define the velocity encoding (Venc-factor) in order to avoid unintentional signal cancelation.

9.3 Implementation issues

This section is intended to give an overview of implementation issues concerning respiratory motion, ECG gating, and artifacts from blood flow. In addition to basic gradient echo implementations, measurement timing in the case of phase contrast acquisition and faster imaging modules like segmented EPI as well as view sharing approaches are discussed.

9.3.1 Gradient Echo imaging

The most common and widely used pulse sequences for ECG-gated phase contrast data acquisition are gradient echo (GE) based sequences. Those methods offer

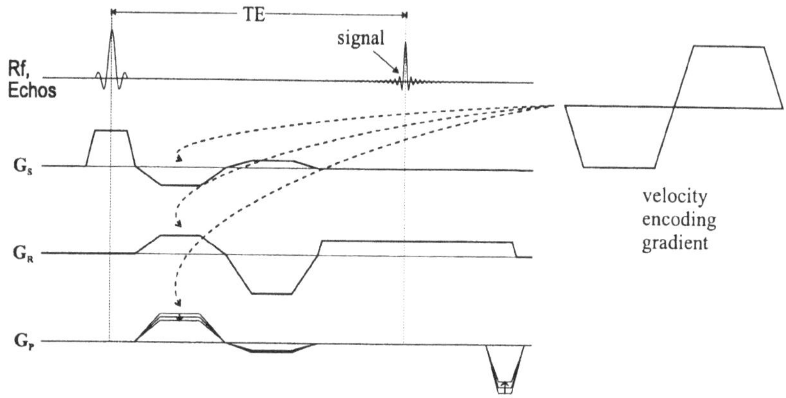

Figure 9.3: Pulse sequence diagram for a gradient-echo sequence with first order motion compensation in all three dimensions. A bipolar velocity encoding gradient is added on top of the sequence gradients in one of the three dimensions for respective motion sensitization.

reliable image quality and can successfully be implemented as breath-hold examinations due to short echo and repetition times as well as low sensitivity to flow, motion and susceptibility artifacts [80,82,91]. For further reduction of flow artifacts, first-order motion compensation along the read, phase, and slice direction is necessary in order to produce reliable reference images. Measurement of velocities are performed by adding a bipolar gradient to the otherwise identical sequence in any of the three dimensions (9.3). The number of k-space lines per cardiac cycle must be chosen in a way that the spatial and temporal resolution of the CINE images is sufficient and that the breath-hold period for each scan is tolerable for patients. If reference and motion sensitive scans are to be acquired successively within a single breath-hold, the duration of the examination of one set of CINE images should not exceed 4–6 heartbeats. Motion sensitization must be performed using a strong bipolar gradient of the order of $\nu_{\text{enc}} = 20$cm/s in order to achieve a sensitivity sufficient for myocardial velocities.

9.3.2 Respiratory Motion

In order to reduce effects from respiratory motion, appropriate measures must be taken to avoid artifacts from bulk motion during breathing. Several approaches to address this problem have been proposed. These include respiratory ordering of phase encoding (ROPE), navigator techniques, and simply collecting all data during a breath-hold [72–79]. We have chosen breath-hold acquisitions for our approach to velocity mapping of myocardial motion because it is a robust and simple method to ensure a constant heart position during examination. The heart position can be reproduced within the range of a few millimeters during successive breath-holds if the measurement is carried out during end expiration. However, fast pulse sequences with high switching rates are necessary to acquire all needed data within a period of maximal 15–20 seconds.

9.3.3 Segmented Scans

A second issue is the motion of the heart itself, which requires image acquisition at an appropriate speed on a frame-to-frame basis. In order to accomplish this task the measurement has to be repeated over a number of ECG cycles to gain a sequence of images representing different phases of cardiac motion. Those ECG-gated CINE images are acquired using k-space segmented scan procedures usually based on gradient echo or segmented EPI pulse sequences. A gating signal derived from the ECG of the patient is used to start acquisition of multiple projections on the same slice with one or more identical phase encoding gradients. The phase encoding gradient is then incremented for the next acquisition cycle following the next gating pulse. After acquiring all phase encoding steps, images can then be reconstructed for each time increment over the ECG-cycle [80–85].

Such CINE images can already be used for visual inspection of myocardial and valvular motion if the resulting images are played phase-by-phase in a movie loop. For phase contrast velocity mapping, however, bipolar gradients have to be introduced at appropriate positions and multiple sets of CINE images have to be acquired for the same slice position since reference and sensitive scans are needed to calculate myocardial velocities. Thus for each slice under investigation either successive breath-hold examinations have to be performed for reference scan and two or three motion sensitized acquisitions (for 2D or 3D velocity fields respectively) or high speed pulse sequences have to be implemented which allow the acquisition of sensitive and reference scans within a single breath-hold measurement.

In order to define reproducible image orientations, the short axis plane of the heart is usually chosen as slice orientation for functional cardiac MRI. This view direction also allows saturation of inflowing blood inside the heart chambers and permits the transformation of the measured velocity into coordinates, which are adapted to the geometry, and function of the myocardium as will be described further down in this chapter.

9.3.4 Black Blood Preparation

Non-periodical blood flow over the several ECG-cycles has proven to be a main problem in the acquisition of motion sensitized images. The high motion sensitivity leads to image artifacts resulting from signals of flowing blood inside of the ventricles as a consequence of phase jitters caused by poorly reproducible blood flow [86]. Several techniques have been proposed to address this problem [87–90].

Conventional black-blood preparation is based on the T1 of blood and uses two by 180° phase cycled inversion recovery pre-pulses with an inversion delay of about 500 ms. This approach leads either to a lengthening of the overall examination time by acquiring image data only every other ECG-cycle or to insufficient

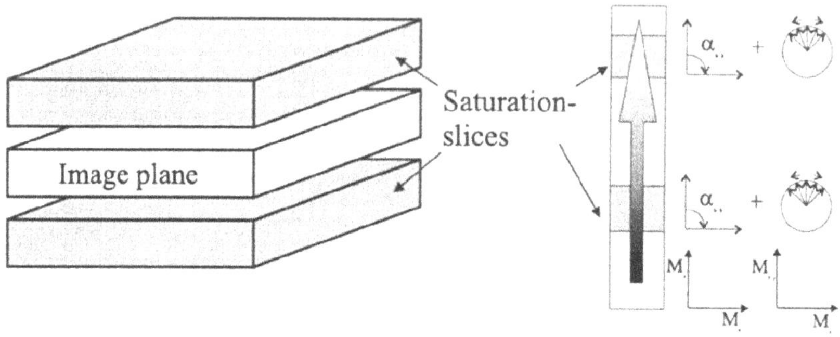

Figure 9.4: Schematic slice profile produced by a Black Blood preparation pulse. Magnetization of spins above and below the investigated slice is flipped into the transverse plane and dephased by spoiler gradients.

blood saturation during systole if the inversion pulses are applied at the beginning of the ECG cycle. Both alternatives were found to be inappropriate for the purpose of assessing myocardial motion with breath-hold examinations. Strategies for suppressing blood signal by applying broad spatial saturation pulses across the left atrium and the pulmonary veins have not turned out to give consistently good suppression for fast gradient echo and segmented echo planar imaging (EPI) sequences.

Thus a slightly different approach can be chosen using a spatially selective preparation pulse, which nulls all signal from blood directly outside of the observed slice. This was achieved by using a "sandwich-pulse", in which the profiles of a 90°-pulse acting on the slice under observation was added to that of a −90°-pulse acting on a concentric thicker slice (see Figure 9.4). As a result, spins inside of the examined slice are not affected and the z-magnetization immediately adjacent to the observed slice is nulled. The transverse magnetization generated by the pulse is destroyed with an appropriate spoiler gradient. The width of the saturation slice was experimentally optimized to 3.2 mm for an observation slice thickness of 8 mm [51].

9.3.5 Measurement Timing and Pulse Sequence Design

For assessment of phase contrast data, a set of pulse sequences is necessary for each slice under examination. A motion compensated reference scan without velocity encoding and sequences with added bipolar encoding gradients along x-, y-, and z-directions are necessary to gain the desired functional information. Figure 9.6 displays velocity-encoded short-axis images obtained with a black blood prepared segmented gradient echo sequence and phase-contrast images for the given slice location along three spatial orientations.

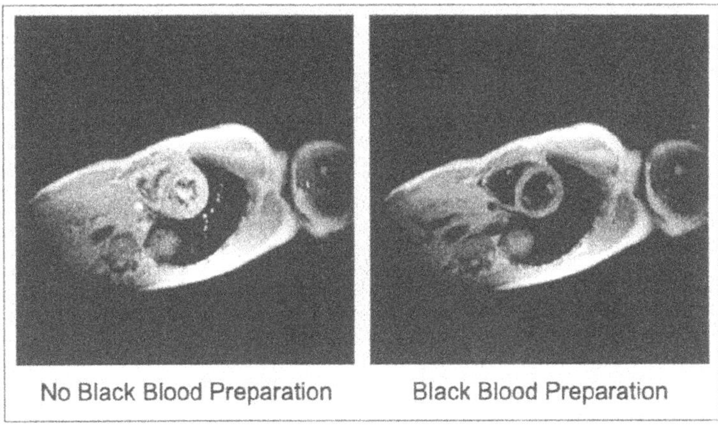

Figure 9.5: Diastolic frame of a set of phase contrast gradient echo CINE images of a healthy volunteer's heart without (left) and with (right) black blood preparation. The images demonstrate adequate suppression of the blood signal using the spatially selective sandwich-pulse. In general the suppression works better in the slices close to the heart base where stronger exchange of blood across the slice occurs compared to slices closer to the apex.

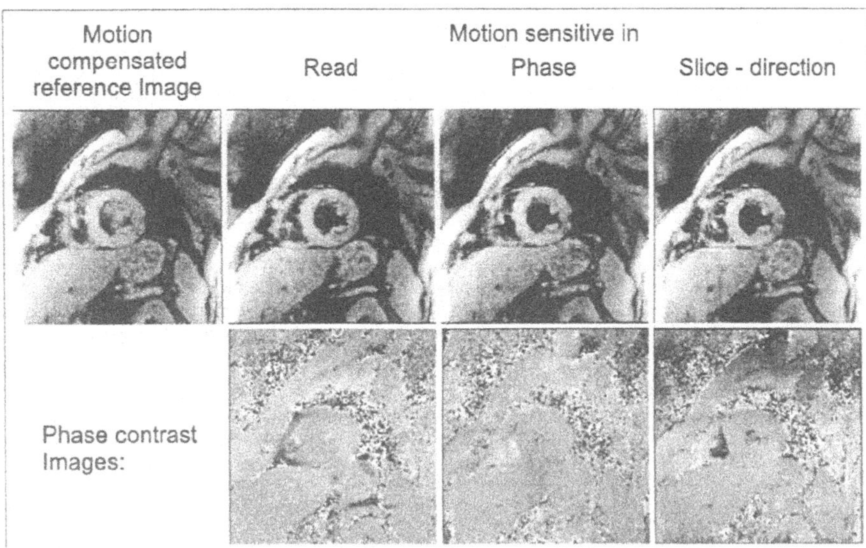

Figure 9.6: Short axis images of the left ventricle of a normal volunteer during systole ($t_{ecg} = 90$ ms) acquired with a black blood prepared segmented gradient echo sequence. The motion-compensated reference scan and images with velocity encoding in x-,y- and z-direction respectively are shown in the top row. The bottom row represents the phase difference images of motion sensitive and reference images in three spatial orientations.

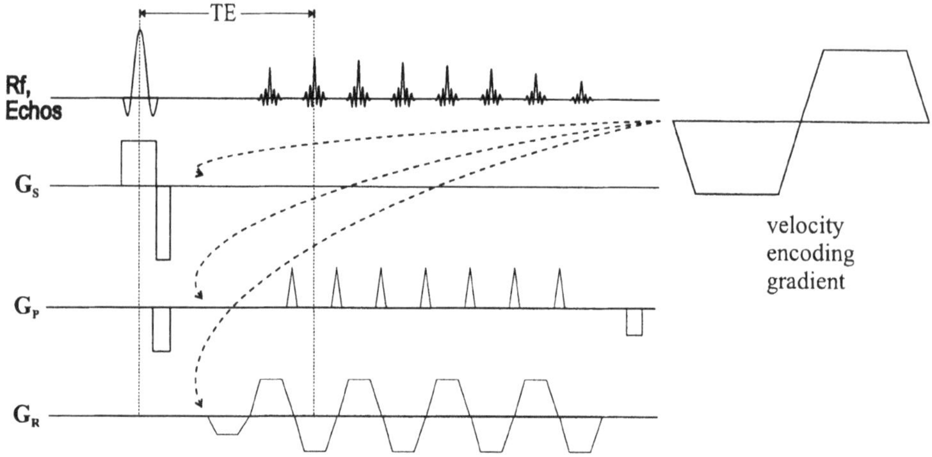

Figure 9.7: Pulse sequence diagram for a segmented EPI sequence with an echo train length of eight echoes per RF excitation. The phase encoding gradient is rewinded for every excitation. Flow encoding is implemented similar to the gradient echo sequence in Figure 9.3.

In the following section different imaging techniques are described and examples of corresponding pulse sequences are given.

9.3.6 Multi Echo Approaches

One possible solution to improve temporal and/or spatial resolution or to reduce the duration of the breath-hold period is the use of echo planar imaging (EPI) sequences for image acquisition. Despite problems concerning image quality arising from properties of the EPI acquisition technique (artifacts due to flow, off-resonance and susceptibility effects) several improvements and applications have already been proposed [92–101]. For cardiac phase contrast applications k-space segmented EPI sequence with Black Blood preparation for multi-phase imaging are a suitable alternative to gradient echo approaches.

As shown in Figure 9.7, velocity encoding is done similar to the gradient echo sequences (Figure 9.3) by adding a bipolar gradient after the RF excitation pulse.

Examples for both imaging modalities (Figure 9.8) include a RF-spoiled k-space segmented gradient echo sequence with first order motion compensation along read and phase direction. Fourteen phase encoding steps per cardiac phase were acquired within each ECG cycle, such that over five ECG cycles a 70×256 matrix could be collected. Images were reconstructed to a matrix of 192×256 for a field of view of 300×400 mm using zero padding. The black blood preparation pulse was introduced at the beginning of each cardiac phase.

The segmented EPI pulse sequence consisted of a blipped multi-shot scan with an echo train length of 8 echoes per excitation (flip angle $= 25°$, bandwidth $=$

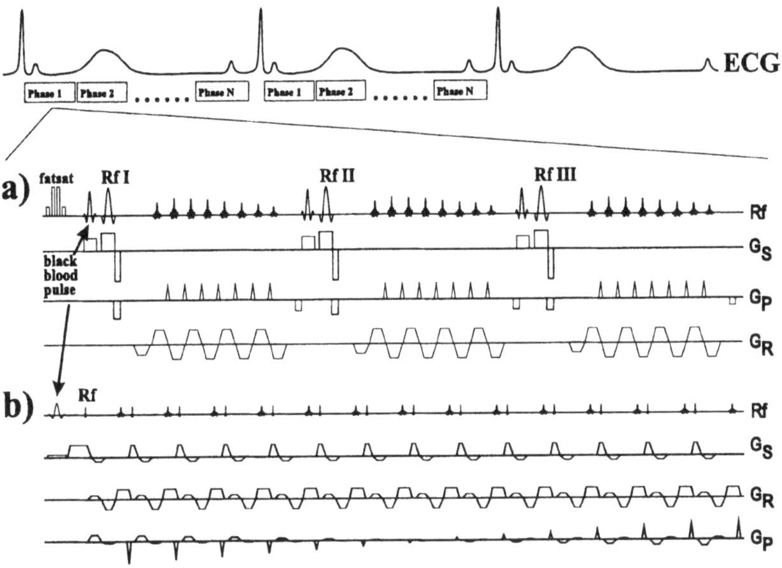

Figure 9.8: Sequence design and measurement timing. ECG gated multi-phase data acquisition and pulse sequence for **a)** EPI and **b)** gradient echo acquisition.

780 Hz/pixel). Phase encoding gradients were rewinded for each excitation. In order to achieve short overall scan times data was read out with three shots per phase, which results in an acquisition of 24 k-space lines per cardiac phase.

Five ECG cycles were thus required to collect a 120×256 matrix in an interleaved manner which was then reconstructed to 192×256 using zero padding. In order to achieve short echo times the second echo was positioned in the center of k-space resulting in asymmetric sampling in the phase encoding direction. An even-odd phase correction was performed using a calibration scan acquired under reversed switching gradients. Fat saturation using four rectangular pulses was applied for every cardiac phase. These parameters allow multi-phase images to be acquired in six heartbeats during a breath-hold. The measurement during the first ECG cycle serves as a dummy scan including acquisition of 2 lines of data per time frame for even-odd phase correction [53,102].

The most limiting part concerning echo and repetition time is the switching time needed for the strong bipolar velocity encoding gradient. If both gradient echo and segmented EPI have similar temporal resolutions, echo planar imaging techniques provide a much higher spatial resolution. More k-space lines can be received since acquisition times are shorter mainly because only one bipolar gradient is needed for the velocity encoding of several echoes.

Figure 9.9 demonstrates the result of a multi-phase measurement of a healthy volunteer's heart in short axis view. The temporal resolution of the ventricular motion was 92 ms for the EPI and 99 ms for the gradient echo sequence.

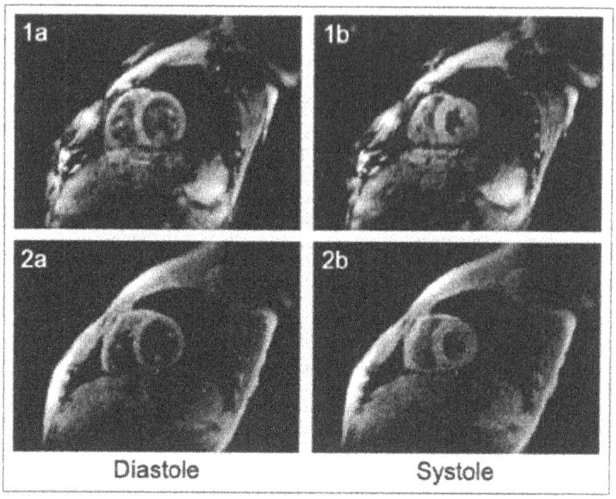

Figure 9.9: Black blood images for a diastolic **(a)** and systolic phase **(b)**. The top row **(1)** displays EPI, the bottom row **(2)** displays gradient echo images.

The gradient echo approach has proven to be more robust than EPI to the effects of blood flow, off-resonance, and susceptibility. EPI provides a higher SNR and spatial resolution but is more sensitive to artifacts and quality of the shim. Segmentation of the left ventricle, which is necessary for data processing, is thus more demanding and artifacts are more likely to interfere with the velocity encoded phases. In order to receive reliable image quality, it has been shown that length of the echo train for segmented EPI should not exceed 10–15 ms. If in addition the central k-space lines are acquired in an early echo (asymmetric sampling resulting in short TE artifacts from blood flow and susceptibility effects can be reduced significantly. Since signal to noise ratio (SNR) is directly proportional to the total acquisition time, further reduction of temporal resolution with fast segmented EPI sequences can be accompanied with losses in SNR.

9.3.7 Measurement Timing

Using state-of-the art gradient systems high speed GE and EPI pulse sequences with optimized strong gradients and high switching rates permit the acquisition of one data set within a few cardiac cycles. Thus black blood prepared gradient echo or echo planar phase contrast sequences can be implemented which allow the acquisition of one reference scan plus scans with velocity encoding in multiple directions within a single breath hold. The pulse sequences introduced above permit the assessment of the full in plane 2D velocity information over 16–19 heartbeats (depending on the spatial or temporal resolution of the resulting images).

The protocol for velocity mapping measurements for both EPI and gradient echo imaging is shown in Figure 9.10. It consists of four blocks, in which the first one

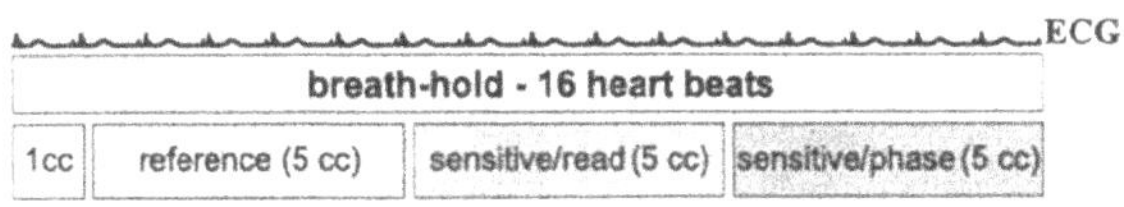

Figure 9.10: Measurement timing for 2D phase contrast velocity mapping within a breath-hold period of 16 heartbeats (1cc: steady state preparation, cc: Cardiac Cycle).

is just one cardiac cycle. This part serves as steady state preparation and in case of EPI phase correction data is acquired within this heartbeat. In the following three blocks the reference and motion sensitive scans are executed consecutively over five cardiac cycles each. This leads to a total acquisition time of 16 ECG cycles. Thus CINE images and full in-plane velocity information of the moving heart are obtained with a single breath-hold measurement. As a result, three identical CINE series of magnitude images are obtained. These can be averaged and lead to a gain in SNR of $\sqrt{3}$. The functional information is contained in the phase difference images of sensitive and reference scans.

Breath-hold examinations which are performed for each of the reference scan and the two motion sensitized acquisitions may result in a slight variability of heart position between successive breath-holds. The measurements during one breath-hold resolves drawbacks of such implementations and provides a constant heart position for reference and sensitive scans [51,52].

9.3.8 View Sharing Approaches

The temporal and spatial resolution of the phase contrast CINE images can be further increased by the use of view sharing techniques for data acquisitions. Here, central parts of k-space are updated more frequently if compared to outer regions of the raw data matrix. Several applications of this technique have already been proposed and are generally used for reduction of total imaging time [63,103–105]. For cardiac CINE MRI these methods exploit the high degree of inter-frame correlation that exists between time-resolved cardiac images. In addition it can be shown, that the velocity induced phase shift in phase contrast techniques is mainly encoded in the central section of k-space which makes view sharing also suitable for velocity mapping.

To reconstruct each phase of the cardiac cycle a full k-space data set is required. In the case of view sharing, however, certain outer regions of k-space are not directly sampled with the corresponding time frame. Thus, for image reconstruction, the full data matrices have to be generated by filling in signals from earlier and later cardiac phases. In case of two fold sampling of the center of k-space if compared to outer sections data from these areas are shared by neighboring frames. Even with this simple sampling scheme the time corresponding to one frame of a given k-space segmented pulse sequence can be significantly reduced. The improvement

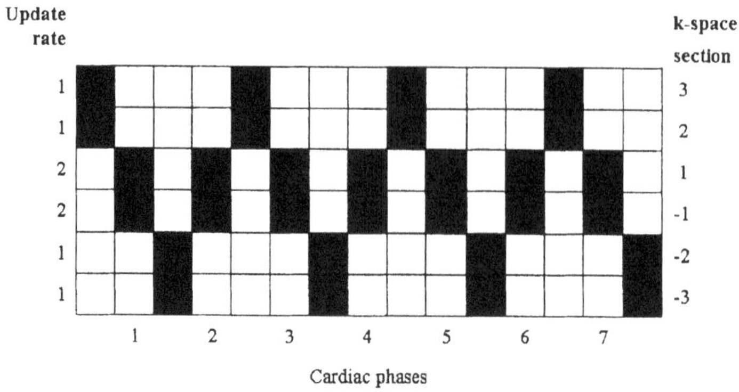

Figure 9.11: k-space sampling scheme for seven cardiac phases for a sampling rate of two for the central region of k-space. Images for each cardiac phase are reconstructed using data of the central part and from the two neighboring outer sections.

in temporal resolution depends on the size of the sections in k-space with higher sampling frequencies. Figure 9.11 shows an example of the distribution of data in k-space as a function of cardiac phases within the ECG cycle. Here, one third of the raw data is updated twice as much within a certain time frame in comparison to the rest of k-space, which leads to a time reduction of approximately 30%.

Based on a similar approach for a k-space segmented phase contrast gradient echo sequence with 16 phase encoding steps for each frame of the cardiac cycle a temporal resolution of 64 ms could be achieved. For this implementation a doubled update rate of the central part of k-space corresponding to 1/4 of the whole data set was used. Figure 9.12 demonstrates black blood CINE images acquired with the view sharing technique.

In comparison to the previously described gradient echo sequence this results in a clear increase of temporal resolution with an even higher spatial resolution. If the view sharing method is directly compared to a pulse sequence with identical parameters using standard reconstruction the gain in acquisition speed is 40%. Table 9.1 summarizes parameters for different implementations of pulse sequences used for data acquisition according to the above described measurement timing.

For all implemented pulse sequences, the sensitivity to motion velocities can be verified by measurements on a rotating phantom. The results demonstrate a high consistency of the measured and theoretical velocities, which are known from the rotational frequency and diameter of the phantom.

9.4 Data Processing

In order to evaluate the functional information of the phase contrast images post-processing of the acquired images is necessary. The ultimate goal in designing an

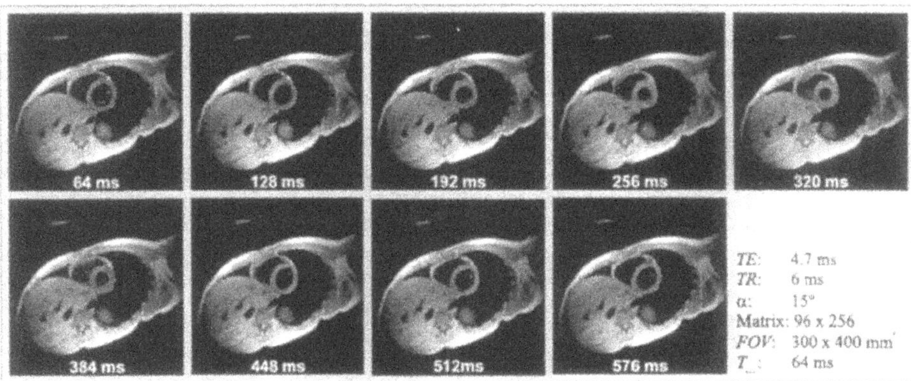

Figure 9.12: CINE series of magnitude images measured with a view shared gradient echo sequence. The examination was performed within a breath-hold period of 19 cardiac cycles. The time after the R wave corresponding to the reception of the central regions of k-space is indicated in the bottom part of each time frame.

Table 9.1: Pulse sequence parameters for different implementations of phase contrast pulse sequences with k-space segmentation and black blood preparation. All parameters correspond to a breath hold period of 16 cardiac cycles for successive reference and two motion sensitive scans (# 3 excitations, 24 k-space lines for each cardiac phase).

	GE	Segmented EPI	GE View Sharing
TE	5.5 ms	9.1 ms	4.7 ms
TR	6.7 ms	22.9 ms	6 ms
k-space segments	14	8#	16
Matrix (data acquisition)	70 × 256	120 × 256	80 × 256
Matrix (reconstructed image)	192 × 256	192 × 256	192 × 256
FOV	300 X 400mm^2	300 X 400mm^2	300 X 400mm^2
Bandwidth	780 Hz/pixel	780 Hz/pixel	560 Hz/pixel
Flip angle α	15°	25°	15°
Fat saturation	-	+	
Temporal resolution	99 ms	92 ms	64ms

appropriate software package is to calculate a set of parameters, which can be used to characterize the mechanical performance of the heart and to aid diagnosis in patients with functional deficits. The working hypothesis in the development of our program was that in order to obtain meaningful velocity data for the description of the internal dynamics of myocardial motion, the measured velocities in the laboratory frame must be translated into an internal coordinate system positioned at the center of mass of the moving myocardium in order to remove bulk motion components, which reflect the overall movement of the heart and its attachment to the surrounding tissue more than the actual internal performance of the heart muscle.

A standard evaluation procedure consists of three basic steps and offers a variety of different ways of presenting the velocity data and/or further data processing. The first step in data analysis is the semi-automatic segmentation of the myocardium. Usually some user interaction is required to set initial parameters points inside and at the inside and outside of the left ventricular wall. The inner and outer contours of the myocardial wall are then found automatically using a contour-tracing algorithm. The resulting segmentation mask can be displayed as semitransparent overlay onto the left ventricle and further interactively edited and optimized with various tools.

In the second step, the phase difference images of the reference scan and the motion sensitive scans are calculated which already contain the velocity information ν_x, ν_y, and ν_z in cartesian coordinates (x, y, z). In order to remove bulk motion from the velocity fields a correction based on subtraction of global translation velocities from the local velocity components is performed.

The third step includes the transformation of the velocities measured in the laboratory frame into an internal polar coordinate system positioned at the center of mass of the inner hull of the myocardium. Thus myocardial motion can now be described by radial and angular velocities $\nu(r, \phi, z)$, which are more adapted to the motion of the left ventricle than velocities $\nu(x, y, z)$ in a cartesian system. Here, radial velocities are defined as positive for contraction, and tangential velocities as positive for clockwise rotation.

After the steps of segmentation and conversion, the results can be viewed in various presentation modes. Examples of available visualization tools for the display of parametric images and further processing options for the interpretation of the results can be summarized as follows.

- The overall performance of the myocardium is characterized by plots of averaged radial and tangential velocities of the whole left ventricle as a function of time after the R-wave.
- Pixel-wise diagrams of ν_ϕ and ν_r as a function of ϕ and r can be used to visualize the uniformity of motion.
- All calculated velocity components can be displayed as color coded velocity maps for each phase of the cardiac cycle in order to visually inspect any

regional variations.

- The cartesian velocity components are used to create pixel-by-pixel velocity vector field plots, which display the in-plane velocity data along the segmented left ventricle. Length of the arrows corresponds to the magnitude and the orientation to the direction of the velocity for each pixel.
- Mean values of radial and rotational velocities in selected regions of interest (ROIs) are averaged for every cardiac phase in order to visualize motion patterns of selected areas over the ECG cycle.
- Transmural velocity gradients $d\nu_r/dr$ are calculated and can be visualized as mean values in certain ROIs over the ECG cycle or as color-coded parametric image for each cardiac phase. The velocity gradients are calculated for 24 predefined angular areas by application of linear regression to the radial velocity components as a function of the radius.

Since myocardial contours are detected for the processing of the phase contrast data the resulting segmentation masks can also be used for the assessment of parameters, which are accessible from the magnitude images and characterize the heart function. The end systolic and diastolic volumes of the left ventricle permit the evaluation of global parameters like stroke volume and ejection fraction (EF). In addition regional left ventricular wall parameters like wall thickness and wall thickening can be calculated from the segmentation masks. In our software package, automatic evaluation of systolic wall thickness and wall thickening for predefined regions of the left ventricle was implemented.

The different possibilities for visualization of the results will be demonstrated for an examination of a healthy volunteer's heart. Pixel by pixel arrow plots display the total in-plane velocity information in one plot for each phase of the ECG cycle. Figure 9.13 shows an example for a normal volunteer with two selected arrow plots for cardiac phases with nearly pure clockwise rotation (top) and expansion (bottom) of the left ventricle. Combined with global motion parameters like average radial ($\bar{\nu}_r$) and rotational ($\bar{\nu}_\phi$) velocities the exact motion patterns for compression and rotation of the left ventricle can be examined.

Color-coded velocity maps contain the same information as an arrow plot, but two images per ECG phase are necessary to display the in-plane velocities. The advantages of this visualization technique are the better recognizable deviations or variations of motion patterns along the myocardium. The ventricular contraction and clockwise rotation during systole as well as expansion and anti-clockwise rotation during diastole are displayed in Figure 9.14.

To investigate regional motion evolution, ROIs of any size and position can be selected by the user. The average radial and rotational velocities in the selected ROIs are displayed and reflect the compression and rotation of these regions over the ECG cycle. Note the high consistency between the motion patterns of different regions of the left ventricle in a healthy volunteer (see Figure 9.15).

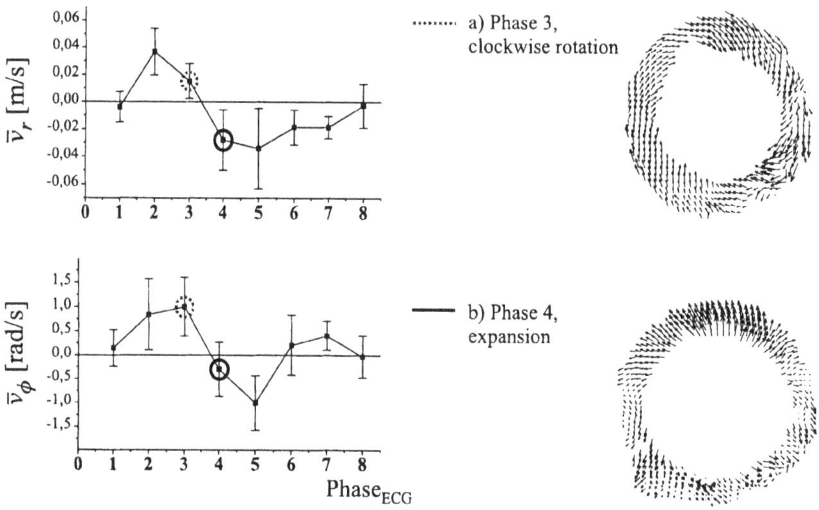

Figure 9.13: Average radial ($\bar{\nu}_r$) and rotational ($\bar{\nu}_\phi$) velocities in a healthy volunteer (left) with positive values for inward motion and clockwise rotation and negative values for outward motion and anti-clockwise rotation. For two selected phases, corresponding pixel-by-pixel arrow plots are displayed. They demonstrate nearly pure clockwise rotation (a) and expansion (b) of the left ventricle.

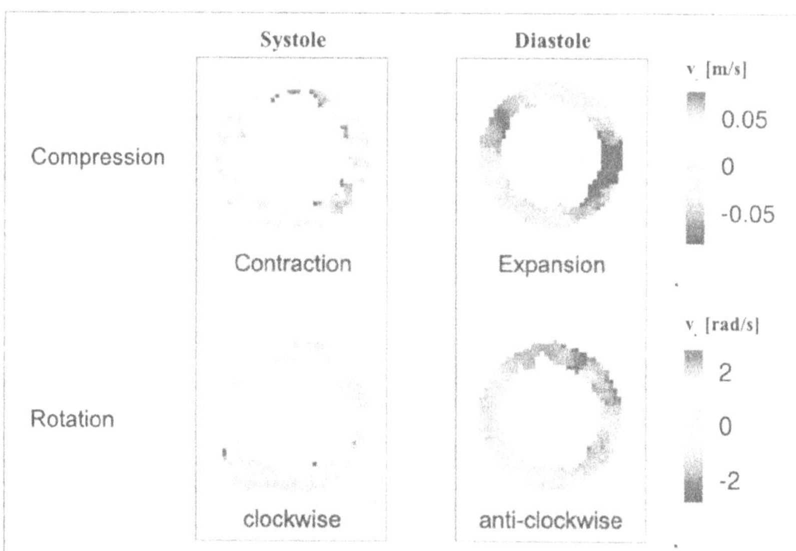

Figure 9.14: Color coded velocities for a healthy volunteer. Positive values correspond to inward and clockwise, and negative values to outward and anti-clockwise motion respectively. The range of the velocities is indicated by the color bars. See color Plate 4.

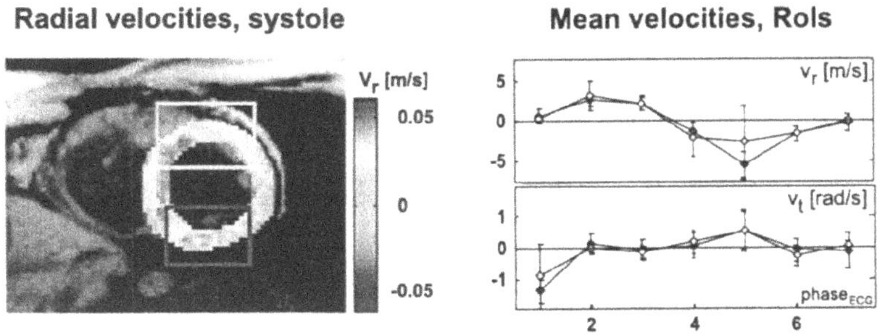

Figure 9.15: Averaged compression ($\bar{\nu}_r$) and tangential ($\bar{\nu}_\phi$) velocities in two selected ROIs in a normal volunteer. Radial velocities of a systolic phase are displayed as color coded image, which is superimposed on the corresponding magnitude image. Time evolution of the average velocity components over the cardiac cycle inside the ROIs is displayed in the plots (red = posterior wall, yellow = anterior wall) on the right. The motion parameters exhibit coincident temporal evolution for both velocity components. See color Plate 5.

9.5 Results

In this section a brief summary of results in a study with healthy volunteers and patients suffering from myocardial infarction is given. The overall left ventricular motion can be characterized by appropriate parameters describing the rotation and contraction or expansion respectively. Regional motion disturbances are visualized using parametric images. In contrast to the highly consistent interindividual data in normal volunteers, patients showed significant localized motion deficits [50–52,58].

9.5.1 Volunteers

The measurement technique and the postprocessing options have been evaluated in a study with 11 normal volunteers. For these examinations a gradient echo based pulse sequence with a temporal resolution of 90 ms per cardiac phase was used. The cumulative result of the average rotational and radial velocities ν_t and ν_r over 11 normal volunteers is demonstrated in Figure 9.16.

Note the small error bars, which show the very high consistency of interindividual motion. This is in marked contrast to the measured velocities in the laboratory frame, which varied considerably between volunteers and did not reveal any significant interindividual reproducibility. The diagrams show that normal heart action begins with anti-clockwise rotation even before the onset of contraction (time frame 1). Immediately after the onset of systole, the rotational velocity is reduced and even slightly inverted in the more basal slices.

The interindividual transmural gradients of the radial velocity are found to be less consistent between individuals (see Figure 9.17), which results in larger error

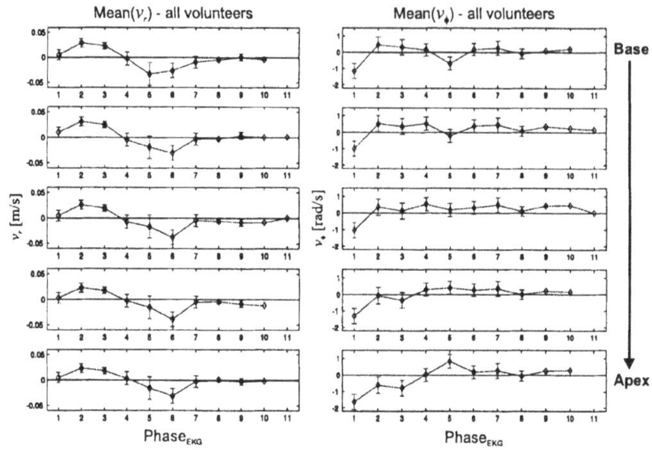

Figure 9.16: Average values for the mean radial and rotational velocities ν_r and ν_t for 11 volunteers. The error bars represent the standard deviation. The diagram at the top represents a slice two cm from the base of the heart, the position moves downward in 1cm intervals towards the apex.

bars if compared to mean radial and rotational velocities.

The variations of the transmural velocity gradients do not necessarily reflect a greater interindividual variability of motion, but might be an artifact of the simple calculation method. A reliable calculation of the transmural gradient for the basal slices therefore requires more sophisticated analysis, which takes the anatomical eccentricity into account. For all slices Figure 9.17 nevertheless demonstrates higher compression velocities of the inner myocardium in systole and a reversal in diastole as expected for compression and expansion accompanied by wall thickening (systole) and thinning (diastole).

Finally the "velocity twist" $d\nu_\phi/dz$ in the apical-to-basal rotation velocities can be calculated by linear regression of the mean rotational velocities at each time point ν_ϕ as a function of the long-axes z-coordinate (see Figure 9.18).

Again a very high interindividual consistency of the data is observed and a counter rotation of the basal versus the apical slices could be demonstrated. The twisting motion is mostly dominant at $t_{ecg} = 90$ and 180 ms and again at $t_{ecg} =$ 450 ms.

9.5.2 Patients

In this section exemplary results of examinations in patients with global and focal pathologies are given in order to demonstrate the potential of phase contrast measurements to detect disturbances in regional as well as the global motion patterns. Pronounced regional variations in the motional components as well as significant deviations of the global motion parameters compared to the volunteers could be

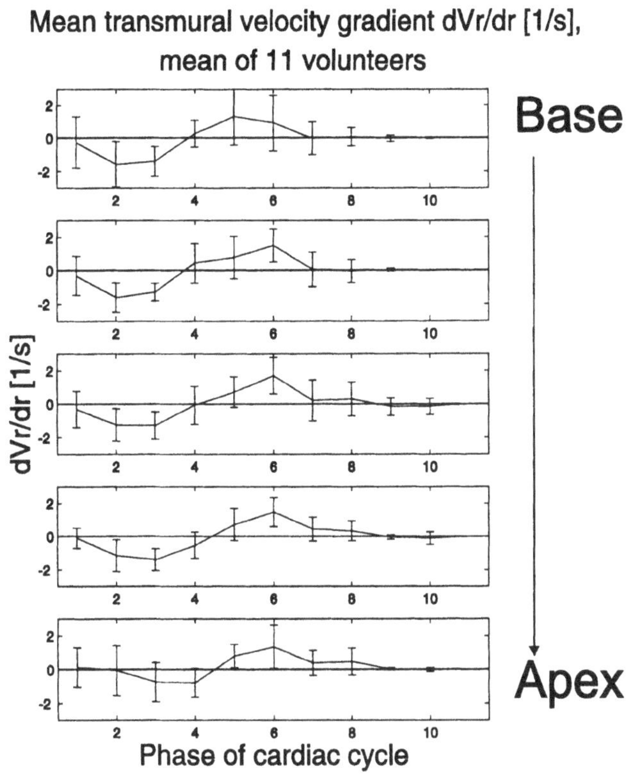

Figure 9.17: Average values for the transmural velocity gradient dv_r/dr over 12 volunteers. Slice positions are identical to those in Figure 9.14.

demonstrated in several studies.

Figure 9.19 shows the average radial velocities ($\bar{v}_r$) in a 60-year old patient who suffers from posterior myocardial infarction and has an echocardiographic diagnosis of a globally reduced left ventricular function with an ejection fraction (EF) of 45 % (thin line). In comparison to the much younger normal volunteers (thick line) the radial velocities are significantly reduced. The larger error bars reflect the increasing variation of velocities along the myocardium in such patients. This can be considered as an example for global pathological motion in patients with heart disease. Qualitatively similar results were received from other patients.

The same patient as in Figure 9.19 provides a good example for the detection of infarcted regions due to localized akinetic or even dyskinetic motion (see Figure 9.20). In the infarcted region both color-coded compression velocities and arrow plot clearly demonstrate areas of opposite motion if compared to the remaining part of the myocardium. Out of eight measured phases of the ECG cycle a diastolic time frame was chosen which exhibited the highest local motional disturbances.

Figure 9.21 shows a color coded velocity image (top) of a 68-year old patient with a posterior myocardial infarction in comparison with a Tl-201 SPECT ex-

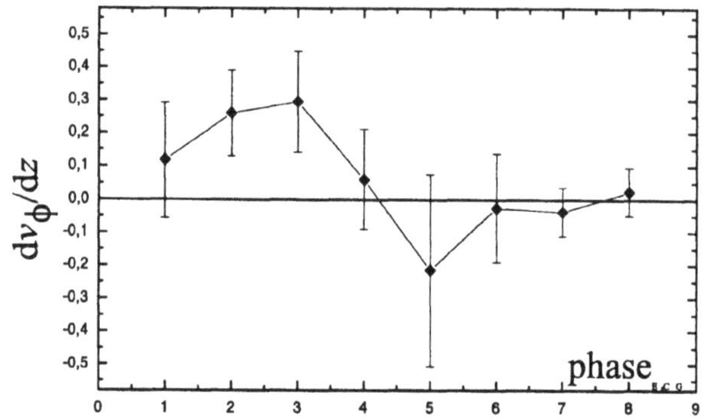

Figure 9.18: Average values of the rotational velocity twist $\frac{d\nu_\phi}{dz}$ defined as the linear gradient of the mean rotational velocity as a function of the long axis z-position over 11 volunteers along the ECG-cycle. Positive values of $\frac{d\nu_\phi}{dz}$ represent higher (anti-clockwise) rotation velocities of the apical slices.

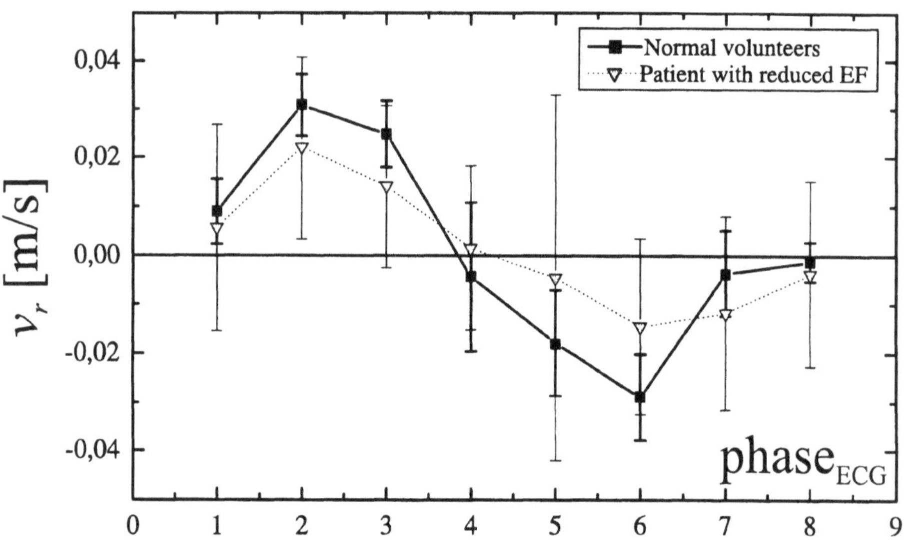

Figure 9.19: Globally reduced compression velocities in a patient (red line) in comparison to the interindividual average radial motion of 12 healthy volunteers (black line) over the ECG cycle.

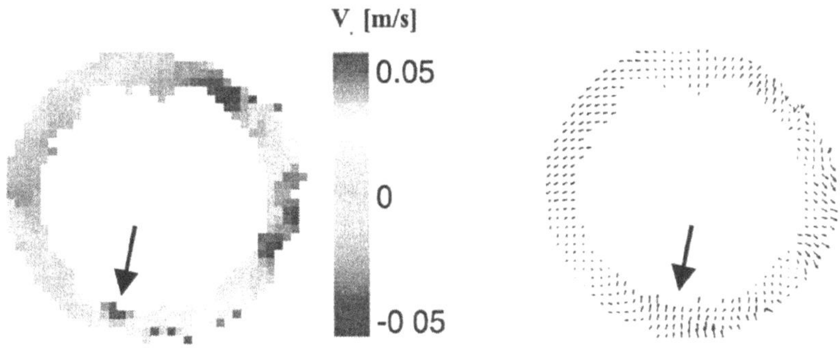

Figure 9.20: Color coded image (left) and arrow plot (right) in a diastolic phase of a patient with posterior infarction. The arrows point towards the regions, which demonstrate dyskinetic motion in the infarcted region. See color Plate 6.

amination (bottom) displaying a local perfusion deficit. The patient had a mildly reduced ejection fraction (EF) of 40% and no pathological findings in FDG-PET. The MR-images show reduced velocities in the hypoperfused area. No major deviations of the global motional parameters from the values measured in volunteers were observed.

If the temporal evolution is viewed as a function of time after the R-wave also abnormal motion patterns over the whole cardiac cycle can be found in ischemic regions as shown in Figure 9.22. For a patient with posterior infarction as demonstrated by NH_3-PET, radial velocities of a diastolic phase are shown as color coded overlay on the corresponding magnitude image. The infarcted area can already be identified by the thinned postero-lateral wall. The infarcted region (red ROI) demonstrates an inward motion that lags behind the already expanding rest of the ventricle. The averaged radial motion in the infarcted posterior region (red ROI) evolves contrary to the non-pathological area in the lateral wall (yellow ROI). It deviates clearly from the regional motion patterns in a normal volunteer (see Figure 9.15). Here, different left ventricular areas move nearly coincidentally over the cardiac cycle. For the patient, the rotational velocities are similar for both areas whereas the radial velocities show a dyskinetic motion of the infarcted region, shown in red, if compared to the anterior wall, shown in yellow. The area corresponds well to the localization and extent of the infarcted area in PET images.

Van der Geest and colleagues [54] examined impaired myocardial function in six pigs with surgically induced myocardial infarction using a similar technical approach and compared the velocity data with the results of a post mortem pathological examination of the left ventricular myocardium. In this animal model high sensitivities and specificities for the detection of impaired myocardial function due to infarction were demonstrated. The analysis of mean regional radial velocities

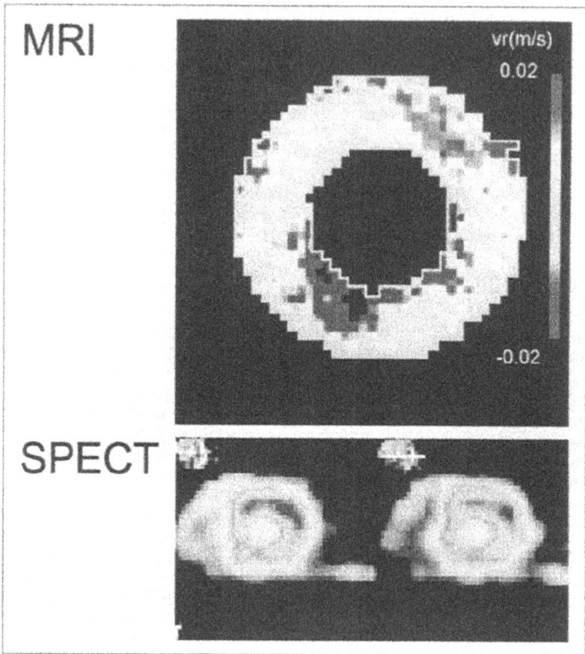

Figure 9.21: Color-coded image of v_r in a slice 3 cm from the base of the left ventricle in a patient with a posterior infarction acquired at $t_{ecg} = 90$ ms (top) compared to a TI-201-SPECT examination (bottom). The scintigrams represent two parallel sections during a time frame in systole. A comparison of the velocity scale with Figure 9.14 shows the much higher variation of v_r over the myocardium. The infarcted region is akinetic or even dyskinetic (outward motion = blue). See color Plate 7.

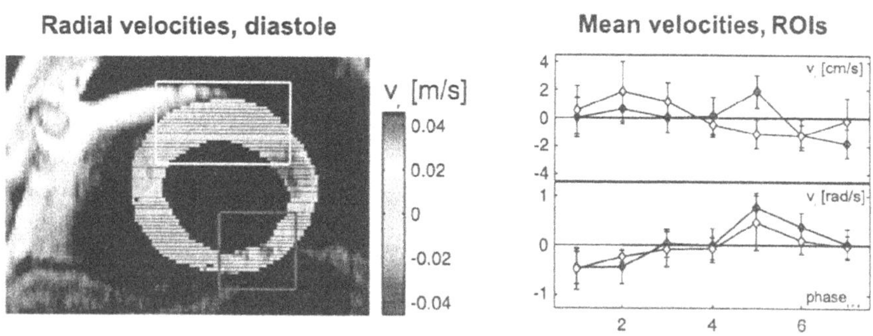

Figure 9.22: Averaged compression ν_r and tangential ν_t velocities in two selected ROIs in a patient with posterior infarction. Temporal evolution of the average velocity components over the cardiac cycle inside the ROIs is displayed in the plots (red = postero-lateral wall, yellow = anterior wall). The radial velocities of the infarcted region show an opposite motion pattern compared to the lateral wall. See color Plate 8.

could even be shown to be more accurate than the analysis of systolic wall thickening.

9.6 Discussion

Segmented breath-hold phase contrast measurements have been shown to produce reliable data and a consistent image quality in both healthy volunteers and patients. Although rotation and contraction/expansion are a quite crude approximation to the actual biophysical mechanism of the contractile motion of the myocardial muscles, they seem to give an adequate and sensitive parameter for the parameterization of myocardial motion.

The absolute values of the measured velocities (2–4 cm/s) seem to be quite low at first glance. This is in part due to the fact that the velocity vectors nearly never point directly to the center of the myocardium. Typical systolic absolute velocity values were observed to be in the order of 4–6 cm/s. In addition, it should be kept in mind that the segmented acquisition mode necessary for doing breath-hold scans leads to a temporal resolution, which is limited by the performance of the scanner hardware and desired spatial resolution. Depending on the duration of the time frames corresponding to a single measured cardiac phase, peak velocities therefore can suffer quite significantly from low-pass filtering.

In patients suffering from myocardial infarction a high sensitivity for the detection of localized disturbance of heart wall motion could be demonstrated. In several studies radial velocities proved to be a good indicator for regional disturbances of motion whereas rotational velocities did not show significant regional deviations. Passive movement of the post-myocardial infarction scar tissue that is being pulled along by the neighboring healthy myocardium can explain the homogeneity of rotational velocities over the circumference of the left ventricle. The most significant deviation of left ventricular wall motion was almost exclusively demonstrated in early diastole. Systolic deviations of left ventricular wall motion were either less pronounced compared to the diastolic deviations or were completely absent. This is most likely to be due to the limited temporal resolution of the phase contrast technique (60–100 ms). Due to the limited temporal resolution subtle differences in myocardial velocities, especially in systole, can be missed. However, comparison of motion patterns of mean radial velocities for different myocardial areas permit the assessment of hypokinetic, akinetic and even dyskinetic left ventricular contractility for interactively selected regions.

Despite the high consistency of data there are some technical limitations to the phase contrast approaches described here. For some patients standard acquisition time may prove to be too long. In patients unable to tolerate the required breath-hold period the duration of the breath-hold interval can be reduced by acquiring fewer lines of k-space using zero filling. This, however, goes along with a loss of spatial resolution resulting in less velocity information along the left ventricle.

The use of faster imaging modules using more sophisticated view sharing techniques including segmented EPI based approaches will also yield improved temporal resolution within the ECG cycle. This might allow the assessment of regional motion defects during systole, which could not be reliably detected with currently available implementations. In addition, respiratory compensated or gated sequences for patients who cannot hold their breath for a longer time could be developed and implemented. In order to further decrease acquisition times, high speed imaging techniques like spiral MRI with short readout period for cardiac applications and reconstruction based acceleration techniques like SMASH or SENSE could be used to increase spatial and/or temporal resolution of the functional examination techniques.

For all described techniques fast imaging sequences are an essential condition. Imaging conditions set high standards concerning scanner hardware and require especially strong magnetic field gradients and high slew rates.

Phase contrast measurements permit the measurement of tissue velocities in all three spatial dimensions. Information on through-plane motion (along the long axis of the heart), however, did not show to be helpful in earlier studies [51,52]. Postprocessing is therefore set out to characterize in-plane motion (short axis view), automatically providing radial and angular (rotational) velocities, respectively. Data processing can be implemented with a high degree of automation. Manifold modes for visualization and processing of motion parameters provide a good platform for investigation of heart wall motion. However, postprocessing is still time consuming with the segmentation process being the main reason. To improve the performance of data analysis future software packages are required to include more sophisticated segmentation algorithms in order to reduce time needed for data evaluation.

Compared to tagging techniques phase contrast MRI offers the advantage of significantly higher functional resolution and the opportunity for a much more direct, automatic and robust assessment of myocardial function. On the experimental side, tagging techniques provide higher temporal resolutions and less sensitivity to artifacts whereas phase contrast imaging is more demanding and requires improved scanner performance.

In summary, phase contrast techniques provide a robust and reliable platform to study cardiac wall motion in healthy subjects and allow the definition and assessment of motion related parameters in order to identify global and local myocardial pathologies in patients with ischemic heart disease.

Appendix: Signal Phase

The phase dependency of the MR signal to moving spins can be derived from the precession frequency of spins in local magnetic fields. The Larmor frequency ω_L of spins at the spatial location $\mathbf{r}$ in a static magnetic field B_0 with an added magnetic field gradient $\mathbf{G}$ is given by

$$\omega_L(\mathbf{r},t) = \gamma B_z(\mathbf{r},t) = \gamma B_0 + \gamma \mathbf{r}(t)\mathbf{G}(t)\,, \quad \text{with} \quad \gamma B_0 = \omega_{L,0}\,. \tag{9.4}$$

Since flow or motion is taken into account the spin positions are described by the time dependent vector $\mathbf{r(t)}$. The received signal in a MR experiment corresponds to voltage induced by precessing magnetization vector in a receiver coil. Therefore, integration of this equation results in the phase of the precessing magnetization and thus the phase of the measured MR signal after an excitation pulse (at t_0) at a given time t_S:

$$\Phi(\mathbf{r},t_s) - \Phi(\mathbf{r},t_0) = \int_{t_0}^{t_s} \omega_L(\mathbf{r},t)dt = \gamma B_0(t_s - t_0) + \gamma \int_{t_0}^{t_s} \mathbf{G}(t)\mathbf{r}(t)dt\,. \tag{9.5}$$

After signal reception, the acquired FID is demodulated with respect to the Larmor frequency $\omega_{L,0}$ associated with the static magnetic field B_0. This corresponds to a transformation of the MR signal into a rotating reference frame. In terms of signal phase, this transformation results

in $\gamma B_0(t_S - t_0) = 0$ in Equation (9.5), which can now be expanded in the following Taylor series:

$$\begin{aligned} \Phi(\mathbf{r},t_s) &= \Phi(\mathbf{r},t_0) + \sum_{n=0}^{\infty} \Delta\Phi_n(\mathbf{r}^{(n)},t)\,, \\ &= \Phi(\mathbf{r},t_0) + \sum_{n=0}^{\infty} \gamma \frac{\mathbf{r}^{(n)}}{n!} \int_{t_0}^{t_s} \mathbf{G}(t)(t-t_0)^n dt\,, \end{aligned} \tag{9.6}$$

with $\mathbf{r}^{(n)}$ being the n-th derivative of the time dependent spin position and $\Delta\Phi_n$ the corresponding n-th order phase.

If the motion of the tissue under investigation does not change fast with respect to the temporal resolution of data acquisition, the corresponding velocities can be approximated to be constant during the measurement of each time frame. Thus $\mathbf{r}(t)$ can be introduced as first-order displacement $\mathbf{r}$ with a constant velocity $\mathbf{v}$. Equation (9.6) then simplifies to

$$\Phi(\mathbf{r},t_s) = \Phi_0 + \Delta\Phi_0(\mathbf{r}_0,t_s) + \Delta\Phi_1(\nu,t_s)\,, \tag{9.7}$$

with zero and first-order phase components

$$\Phi_0 = \Phi(\mathbf{r}, t_0), \tag{9.8}$$

$$\Delta\Phi_0(\mathbf{r}_0, t_s) = \gamma \mathbf{r}_0 \int_{t_0}^{t_s} \mathbf{G}(t)dt, \tag{9.9}$$

$$\Delta\Phi_1(\nu, t_s) = \gamma \cdot \nu \int_{t_0}^{t_s} \mathbf{G}(t)(t - t_0)dt. \tag{9.10}$$

This approximation has a signal phase related to the Larmor frequency of stationary spins (Equation 9.9), an initial phase offset Φ_0, and another phase $\Delta\Phi_1(\mathbf{v})$, which is directly proportional to the velocity of moving spins. This first-order approximation of $r(t)$ is only valid if the involved velocities do not change significantly with respect to the temporal resolution of the pulse sequence. Thus, image acquisition has to be fast enough to ensure that the velocities of moving spins can be assumed to be constant while data corresponding to a certain time frame of flow or motion patterns is received.

References

[1] E. R. McVeigh. MRI of myocardial function: motion tracking techniques. Magn Reson Imaging, vol. 14, pp. 137-50, 1996.

[2] A. A. Amini, Y. Chen, R. W. Curwen, V. Mani, and J. Sun. Coupled B-snake grids and constrained thin-plate splines for analysis of 2-D tissue deformations from tagged MRI. IEEE Trans Med Imaging, vol. 17, pp. 344-56, 1998.

[3] L. Axel, R. C. Goncalves, and D. Bloomgarden. Regional heart wall motion: two-dimensional analysis and functional imaging with MR imaging. Radiology, vol. 183, pp. 745-50, 1992.

[4] H. Azhari, J. L. Weiss, and E. P. Shapiro. Distribution of myocardial strains: an MRI study. Adv Exp Med Biol, vol. 382, pp. 319-28, 1995.

[5] A. Bazille, M. A. Guttman, E. R. McVeigh, and E. A. Zerhouni. Impact of semiautomated versus manual image segmentation errors on myocardial strain calculation by magnetic resonance tagging. Invest Radiol, vol. 29, pp. 427-33, 1994.

[6] P. Croisille, M. A. Guttman, E. Atalar, E. R. McVeigh, and E. A. Zerhouni. Precision of myocardial contour estimation from tagged MR images with a black-blood technique. *Acad Radiol*, vol. 5, pp. 93-100, 1998. Acad Radiol, vol. 5, pp. 93-100, 1998.

[7] Z. A. Fayad, V. A. Ferrari, D. L. Kraitchman, A. A. Young, H. I. Palevsky, D. C. Bloomgarden, and L. Axel. Right ventricular regional function using MR tagging: normals versus chronic pulmonary hypertension. Magn Reson Med, vol. 39, pp. 116-23, 1998.

[8] S. E. Fischer, G. C. McKinnon, M. B. Scheidegger, W. Prins, D. Meier, and P. Boesiger. True myocardial motion tracking. *Magn Reson Med*, vol. 31, pp. 401-13, 1994. Magn Reson Med, vol. 31, pp. 401-13, 1994.

[9] M. A. Fogel, K. B. Gupta, P. M. Weinberg, and E. A. Hoffman. Regional wall motion and strain analysis across stages of Fontan reconstruction by magnetic resonance tagging. *Am J Physiol*,vol. 269, pp. H1132-52, 1995. Am J Physiol,vol. 269, pp. H1132-52, 1995.

[10] F. D. Knollmann, J. Maurer, W. Wlodarczyk, J. C. Bock, and R. Felix. Fourier phase mapping of the human heart. The use of spatial modulation of magnetization cine magnetic resonance imaging. Invest Radiol, vol. 31, pp. 743-8, 1996.

[11] C. M. Kramer, W. J. Rogers, T. M. Theobald, T. P. Power, S. Petruolo, and N. Reichek. Remote noninfarcted region dysfunction soon after first anterior myocardial infarction. A magnetic resonance tagging study. Circulation, vol. 94, pp. 660-6, 1996.

[12] C. M. Kramer, W. J. Rogers, G. Geskin, T. P. Power, T. M. Theobald, Y. L. Hu, and N. Reichek. Usefulness of magnetic resonance imaging early after acute myocardial infarction. Am J Cardiol, vol. 80, pp. 690-5, 1997.

[13] J. P. Kuijer, J. T. Marcus, M. J. Gotte, A. C. van Rossum, and R. M. Heethaar. Simultaneous MRI tagging and through-plane velocity quantification: a three-dimensional myocardial motion tracking algorithm. J Magn Reson Imaging, vol. 9, pp. 409-19, 1999.

[14] J. A. Lima, V. A. Ferrari, N. Reichek, C. M. Kramer, L. Palmon, M. R. Llaneras, B. Tallant, A. A. Young, and L. Axel. Segmental motion and deformation of transmurally infarcted myocardium in acute postinfarct period. Am J Physiol, vol. 268, pp. H1304-12, 1995.

[15] G. A. MacGowan, D. Burkhoff, W. J. Rogers, D. Salvador, H. Azhari, P. S. Hees, J. L. Zweier, H. R. Halperin, C. O. Siu, J. A. Lima, J. L. Weiss, and E. P. Shapiro. Effects of afterload on regional left ventricular torsion. Cardiovasc Res, vol. 31, pp. 917-25, 1996.

[16] S. E. Maier, S. E. Fischer, G. C. McKinnon, O. M. Hess, H. P. Krayenbuehl, and P. Boesiger. Acquisition and evaluation of tagged magnetic resonance images of the human left ventricle. Comput Med Imaging Graph, vol. 16, pp. 73-80, 1992.

[17] S. E. Maier, S. E. Fischer, G. C. McKinnon, O. M. Hess, H. P. Krayenbuehl, and P. Boesiger. Evaluation of left ventricular segmental wall motion in hypertrophic cardiomyopathy with myocardial tagging. Circulation, vol. 86, pp. 1919-28, 1992.

[18] J. T. Marcus, M. J. Gotte, A. C. Van Rossum, J. P. Kuijer, R. M. Heethaar, L. Axel, and C. A. Visser. Myocardial function in infarcted and remote regions early after infarction in man: assessment by magnetic resonance tagging and strain analysis. Magn Reson Med, vol. 38, pp. 803-10, 1997.

[19] C. Matter, E. Nagel, M. Stuber, P. Boesiger, and O. M. Hess. Assessment of systolic and diastolic LV function by MR myocardial tagging. Basic Res Cardiol, vol. 91, pp. 23-8, 1996.

[20] G. C. McKinnon, S. E. Fischer, and S. E. Maier. Non invasive measurement of myocardial motion using magnetic resonance tagging. Australas Phys Eng Sci Med, vol. 14, pp. 189-96, 1991.

[21] E. R. McVeigh and E. A. Zerhouni. Noninvasive measurement of transmural gradients in myocardial strain with MR imaging. Radiology, vol. 180, pp. 677-83, 1991.

[22] E. R. McVeigh and E. Atalar. Cardiac tagging with breath-hold cine MRI. Magn Reson Med, vol. 28, pp. 318-27, 1992.

[23] T. J. Mosher and M. B. Smith. A DANTE tagging sequence for the evaluation of translational sample motion. Magn Reson Med, vol. 15, pp. 334-9, 1990.

[24] J. Park, D. Metaxas, and L. Axel. Analysis of left ventricular wall motion based on volumetric deformable models and MRI-SPAMM. Med Image Anal, vol. 1, pp. 53-71, 1996.

[25] T. P. Power, C. M. Kramer, A. L. Shaffer, T. M. Theobald, S. Petruolo, N. Reichek, and W. J. Rogers, Jr. Breath-hold dobutamine magnetic resonance myocardial tagging: normal left ventricular response. Am J Cardiol, vol. 80, pp. 1203-7, 1997.

[26] F. E. Rademakers, W. J. Rogers, W. H. Guier, G. M. Hutchins, C. O. Siu, M. L. Weisfeldt, J. L. Weiss, and E. P. Shapiro. Relation of regional cross-fiber shortening to wall thickening in the intact heart. Three-dimensional strain analysis by NMR tagging. Circulation, vol. 89, pp. 1174-82, 1994.

[27] F. E. Rademakers and J. Bogaert. Left ventricular myocardial tagging. Int J Card Imaging, vol. 13, pp. 233-45, 1997.

[28] N. Reichek. MRI myocardial tagging. J Magn Reson Imaging, vol. 10, pp. 609-16, 1999.

[29] M. Stuber, S. E. Fischer, M. B. Scheidegger, and P. Boesiger. Toward high-resolution myocardial tagging. Magn Reson Med, vol. 41, pp. 639-43, 1999.

[30] M. Stuber, M. A. Spiegel, S. E. Fischer, M. B. Scheidegger, P. G. Danias, E. M. Pedersen, and P. Boesiger. Single breath-hold slice-following CSPAMM myocardial tagging. Magma, vol. 9, pp. 85-91, 1999.

[31] A. A. Young, L. Axel, L. Dougherty, D. K. Bogen, and C. S. Parenteau. Validation of tagging with MR imaging to estimate material deformation. Radiology, vol. 188, pp. 101-8, 1993.

[32] A. A. Young, C. M. Kramer, V. A. Ferrari, L. Axel, and N. Reichek. Three-dimensional left ventricular deformation in hypertrophic cardiomyopathy. Circulation, vol. 90, pp. 854-67, 1994.

[33] A. A. Young, H. Imai, C. N. Chang, and L. Axel. Two-dimensional left ventricular deformation during systole using magnetic resonance imaging with spatial modulation of magnetization [published erratum appears in Circulation 1994 Sep;90(3):1584]. Circulation, vol. 89, pp. 740-52, 1994.

[34] A. A. Young, Z. A. Fayad, and L. Axel. Right ventricular midwall surface motion and deformation using magnetic resonance tagging. Am J Physiol, vol. 271, pp. H2677-88, 1996.

[35] E. A. Zerhouni, D. M. Parish, W. J. Rogers, A. Yang, and E. P. Shapiro. Human heart: tagging with MR imaging–a method for noninvasive assessment of myocardial motion. Radiology, vol. 169, pp. 59-63, 1988.

[36] L. Axel and L. Dougherty. MR imaging of motion with spatial modulation of magnetization. Radiology, vol. 171, pp. 841-5, 1989.

[37] L. Axel and L. Dougherty. Heart wall motion: improved method of spatial modulation of magnetization for MR imaging. Radiology, vol. 172, pp. 349-50, 1989.

[38] J. Hennig. Generalized MR interferography. Magn Reson Med, vol. 16, pp. 390-402, 1990.

[39] R. T. Constable, K. M. Rath, A. J. Sinusas, and J. C. Gore. Development and evaluation of tracking algorithms for cardiac wall motion analysis using phase velocity MR imaging. Magn Reson Med, vol. 32, pp. 33-42, 1994.

[40] N. J. Pelc, R. J. Herfkens, A. Shimakawa, and D. R. Enzmann. Phase contrast cine magnetic resonance imaging. Magn Reson Q, vol. 7, pp. 229-54, 1991.

[41] L. R. Pelc, J. Sayre, K. Yun, L. J. Castro, R. J. Herfkens, D. C. Miller, and N. J. Pelc. Evaluation of myocardial motion tracking with cine-phase contrast magnetic resonance imaging. Invest Radiol, vol. 29, pp. 1038-42, 1994.

[42] Y. Zhu and N. J. Pelc. Three-dimensional motion tracking with volumetric phase contrast MR velocity imaging. J Magn Reson Imaging, vol. 9, pp. 111-8, 1999.

[43] Y. Zhu, M. Drangova, and N. J. Pelc. Estimation of deformation gradient and strain from cine-PC velocity data. IEEE Trans Med Imaging, vol. 16, pp. 840-51, 1997.

[44] Y. Zhu, M. Drangova, and N. J. Pelc. Fourier tracking of myocardial motion using cine-PC data. Magn Reson Med, vol. 35, pp. 471-80, 1996.

[45] L. Wigstrom, T. Ebbers, A. Fyrenius, M. Karlsson, J. Engvall, B. Wranne, and A. F. Bolger. Particle trace visualization of intracardiac flow using time-resolved 3D phase contrast MRI. Magn Reson Med, vol. 41, pp. 793-9, 1999.

[46] M. Drangova, Y. Zhu, B. Bowman, and N. J. Pelc. In vitro verification of myocardial motion tracking from phase-contrast velocity data. Magn Reson Imaging, vol. 16, pp. 863-70, 1998.

[47] M. Drangova, Y. Zhu, and N. J. Pelc. Effect of artifacts due to flowing blood on the reproducibility of phase-contrast measurements of myocardial motion. J Magn Reson Imaging, vol. 7, pp. 664-8, 1997.

[48] N. J. Pelc, M. Drangova, L. R. Pelc, Y. Zhu, D. C. Noll, B. S. Bowman, and R. J. Herfkens. Tracking of cyclic motion with phase-contrast cine MR velocity data. J Magn Reson Imaging, vol. 5, pp. 339-45, 1995.

[49] A. E. Arai, C. C. Gaither, 3rd, F. H. Epstein, R. S. Balaban, and S. D. Wolff. Myocardial velocity gradient imaging by phase contrast MRI with application to regional function in myocardial ischemia. Magn Reson Med, vol. 42, pp. 98-109, 1999.

[50] J. Hennig, M. Markl, B. Schneider, and S. Peschl. Regional myocardial function with tissue phase mapping. Magma, vol. 6, pp. 145-6, 1998.

[51] J. Hennig, B. Schneider, S. Peschl, M. Markl, T. Krause, and J. Laubenberger. Analysis of myocardial motion based on velocity measurements with a black blood prepared segmented gradient-echo sequence: methodology and applications to normal volunteers and patients. J Magn Reson Imaging, vol. 8, pp. 868-77, 1998.

[52] M. Markl, B. Schneider, J. Hennig, S. Peschl, J. Winterer, T. Krause, and J. Laubenberger. Cardiac phase contrast gradient echo MRI: measurement of myocardial wall motion in healthy volunteers and patients. Int J Card Imaging, vol. 15, pp. 441-52, 1999.

[53] M. Markl and J. Hennig. Fast Velocity Mapping of Myocardial Motion with k-Space Segmented Black Blood Echo Planar and Gradient Echo Imaging.

presented at 7th Scientific Meeting International Society of Magnetic Resonance in Medicine, Philadelphia, USA, 1999.

[54] R. Van der Geest, L. Kroft, H. Kayser, E. van der Wall, A. de Roos, and J. Reiber. Detection of regions of myocardial infarction in pigs. Higher sensitivity and specificity using 3D velocity-encoded cine MR imaging compared to wall thickening. presented at 7th Ann.Meeting ISMRM, Philadelphia, 1999.

[55] R. Van der Geest, H. Kayser, E. van der Wall, J. Reiber, and A. de Roos. Measurement of regional and transmural variation in left ventricular myocardial motion in normal volunteers using 3D velocity encoded cine MRI. presented at 6th Ann.Meeting ISMRM, Sidney, 1998.

[56] H. Kayser, R. van der Geest, E. van der Wall, J. Reiber, and A. de Roos. Assessment of right ventricular wall motion using 3D phase contrast MR velocity mapping. presented at 6th Ann.Meeting ISMRM, Sidney, 1998.

[57] H. Kawamitsu, K. Sugimura, and K. Ochiai. Myocardial wall motion analysis with phase shift imaging: cine phase contrast technique. Nippon Rinsho, vol. 55, pp. 1794-9, 1997.

[58] B. Schneider, M. Markl, C. Geiges, J. Winterer, J. Hennig, and M. Langer. Left Ventricular Phase Contrast Velocity Mapping in 34 Patients with Ischaemic Heart Disease. presented at 8th Scientific Meeting International Society of Magnetic Resonance in Medicine, Denver, USA, 2000.

[59] C. L. Dumoulin. Phase contrast MR angiography techniques. Magn Reson Imaging Clin N Am, vol. 3, pp. 399-411, 1995.

[60] M. F. Walker, S. P. Souza, and C. L. Dumoulin. Quantitative flow measurement in phase contrast MR angiography. J Comput Assist Tomogr, vol. 12, pp. 304-13, 1988.

[61] D. N. Firmin, G. L. Nayler, R. H. Klipstein, S. R. Underwood, R. S. Rees, and D. B. Longmore. In vivo validation of MR velocity imaging. J Comput Assist Tomogr, vol. 11, pp. 751-6, 1987.

[62] D. N. Firmin, G. L. Nayler, P. J. Kilner, and D. B. Longmore, The application of phase shifts in NMR for flow measurement. Magn Reson Med, vol. 14, pp. 230-41, 1990.

[63] V. S. Lee, C. E. Spritzer, B. A. Carroll, L. G. Pool, M. A. Bernstein, S. K. Heinle, and J. R. MacFall. Flow quantification using fast cine phase-contrast MR imaging, conventional cine phase-contrast MR imaging, and Doppler sonography: in vitro and in vivo validation. AJR Am J Roentgenol, vol. 169, pp. 1125-31, 1997.

[64] A. Lingamneni, P. A. Hardy, K. A. Powell, N. J. Pelc, and R. D. White. Validation of cine phase-contrast MR imaging for motion analysis. J Magn Reson Imaging, vol. 5, pp. 331-8, 1995.

[65] R. H. Mohiaddin and D. J. Pennell. MR blood flow measurement. Clinical application in the heart and circulation Cardiol Clin, vol. 16, pp. 161-87, 1998.

[66] G. L. Nayler, D. N. Firmin, and D. B. Longmore. Blood flow imaging by cine magnetic resonance. J Comput Assist Tomogr, vol. 10, pp. 715-22, 1986.

[67] S. R. Underwood, D. N. Firmin, R. S. Rees, and D. B. Longmore. Magnetic resonance velocity mapping. Clin Phys Physiol Meas, vol. 11, pp. 37-43, 1990.

[68] C. Thomsen, M. Cortsen, L. Sondergaard, O. Henriksen, and F. Stahlberg. A segmented K-space velocity mapping protocol for quantification of renal artery blood flow during breath-holding. J Magn Reson Imaging, vol. 5, pp. 393-401, 1995.

[69] G. B. Pike, C. H. Meyer, T. J. Brosnan, and N. J. Pelc. Magnetic resonance velocity imaging using a fast spiral phase contrast sequence. Magn Reson Med, vol. 32, pp. 476-83, 1994.

[70] S. Kozerke, M. B. Scheidegger, E. M. Pedersen, and P. Boesiger. Heart motion adapted cine phase-contrast flow measurements through the aortic valve. Magn Reson Med, vol. 42, pp. 970-8, 1999.

[71] K. S. Nayak, J. M. Pauly, A. B. Kerr, B. S. Hu, and D. G. Nishimura. Real-time color flow MRI. Magn Reson Med, vol. 43, pp. 251-8, 2000.

[72] A. Huber, K. Nikolaou, P. Gonschior, A. Knez, M. Stehling, and M. Reiser. Navigator echo-based respiratory gating for three-dimensional MR coronary angiography: results from healthy volunteers and patients with proximal coronary artery stenosis. AJR Am J Roentgenol, vol. 173, pp. 95-101, 1999.

[73] E. M. Haacke and J. L. Patrick. Reducing motion artifacts in two-dimensional Fourier transform imaging. Magn Reson Imaging, vol. 4, pp. 359-76, 1986.

[74] M. H. Cho, W. S. Kim, and Z. H. Cho. CSF flow artifact reduction using cardiac cycle ordered phase-encoding method. Magn Reson Imaging, vol. 8, pp. 395-405, 1990.

[75] R. L. Ehman and J. P. Felmlee. Adaptive technique for high-definition MR imaging of moving structures. Radiology, vol. 173, pp. 255-63, 1989.

[76] H. W. Korin, J. P. Felmlee, R. L. Ehman, and S. J. Riederer. Adaptive technique for three-dimensional MR imaging of moving structures. Radiology, vol. 177, pp. 217-21, 1990.

[77] J. P. Felmlee, R. L. Ehman, S. J. Riederer, and H. W. Korin. Adaptive motion compensation in MRI: accuracy of motion measurement. Magn Reson Med, vol. 18, pp. 207-13, 1991.

[78] Y. Wang, P. J. Rossman, R. C. Grimm, S. J. Riederer, and R. L. Ehman. Navigator-echo-based real-time respiratory gating and triggering for reduction of respiration effects in three-dimensional coronary MR angiography. Radiology, vol. 198, pp. 55-60, 1996.

[79] A. M. Taylor, P. Jhooti, F. Wiesmann, J. Keegan, D. N. Firmin, and D. J. Pennell. MR navigator-echo monitoring of temporal changes in diaphragm position: implications for MR coronary angiography. J Magn Reson Imaging, vol. 7, pp. 629-36, 1997.

[80] V. Schulen, F. Schick, J. Loichat, U. Helber, P. E. Huppert, G. Laub, and C. D. Claussen. Evaluation of K-space segmented cine sequences for fast functional cardiac imaging. Invest Radiol, vol. 31, pp. 512-22, 1996.

[81] J. Hennig. K-space sampling strategies. Eur Radiol, vol. 9, pp. 1020-31, 1999.

[82] D. J. Atkinson and R. R. Edelman. Cineangiography of the heart in a single breath hold with a segmented turboFLASH sequence. Radiology, vol. 178, pp. 357-60, 1991.

[83] D. A. Bluemke, J. L. Boxerman, T. Mosher, and J. A. Lima. Segmented K-space cine breath-hold cardiovascular MR imaging: Part 2. Evaluation of aortic vasculopathy. AJR Am J Roentgenol, vol. 169, pp. 401-7, 1997.

[84] D. A. Bluemke, J. L. Boxerman, E. Atalar, and E. R. McVeigh. Segmented K-space cine breath-hold cardiovascular MR imaging: Part 1. Principles and technique. AJR Am J Roentgenol, vol. 169, pp. 395-400, 1997.

[85] D. Chien, D. J. Atkinson, and R. R. Edelman. Strategies to improve contrast in turboFLASH imaging: reordered phase encoding and k-space segmentation. J Magn Reson Imaging, vol. 1, pp. 63-70, 1991.

[86] T. A. Tasciyan and D. G. Mitchell. Pulsatile flow artifacts in fast magnetization-prepared sequences. J Magn Reson Imaging, vol. 4, pp. 217-22, 1994.

[87] S. Sinha and U. Sinha. Black blood dual phase turbo FLASH MR imaging of the heart. J Magn Reson Imaging, vol. 6, pp. 484-94, 1996.

[88] J. P. Finn and R. R. Edelman. Black-blood and segmented k-space magnetic resonance angiography. Magn Reson Imaging Clin N Am, vol. 1, pp. 349-57, 1993.

[89] R. R. Edelman, D. Chien, and D. Kim. Fast selective black blood MR imaging. Radiology, vol. 181, pp. 655-60, 1991.

[90] D. Chien, A. Goldmann, and R. R. Edelman. High-speed black blood imaging of vessel stenosis in the presence of pulsatile flow. J Magn Reson Imaging, vol. 2, pp. 437-41, 1992.

[91] E. M. Haacke, D. Li, and S. Kaushikkar. Cardiac MR imaging: principles and techniques. Top Magn Reson Imaging, vol. 7, pp. 200-17, 1995.

[92] H. Sakuma, K. Takeda, and C. B. Higgins. Fast magnetic resonance imaging of the heart. Eur J Radiol, vol. 29, pp. 101-13, 1999.

[93] K. Butts, S. J. Riederer, R. L. Ehman, R. M. Thompson, and C. R. Jack. Interleaved echo planar imaging on a standard MRI system. Magn Reson Med, vol. 31, pp. 67-72, 1994.

[94] F. Hennel and J. F. Nedelec. Interleaved asymmetric echo-planar imaging. Magn Reson Med, vol. 34, pp. 520-4, 1995.

[95] F. H. Epstein, S. D. Wolff, and A. E. Arai. Segmented k-space fast cardiac imaging using an echo-train readout. Magn Reson Med, vol. 41, pp. 609-13, 1999.

[96] S. B. Reeder, E. Atalar, A. Z. Faranesh, and E. R. McVeigh. Multi-echo segmented k-space imaging: an optimized hybrid sequence for ultrafast cardiac imaging. Magn Reson Med, vol. 41, pp. 375-85, 1999.

[97] H. J. Lamb, J. Doornbos, E. A. van der Velde, M. C. Kruit, J. H. Reiber, and A. de Roos. Echo planar MRI of the heart on a standard system: validation of measurements of left ventricular function and mass. J Comput Assist Tomogr, vol. 20, pp. 942-9, 1996.

[98] D. A. Leung, J. F. Debatin, S. Wildermuth, G. C. McKinnon, and G. K. von Schulthess. Cardiac imaging: comparison of two-shot echo-planar imaging with fast segmented K-space and conventional gradient-echo cine acquisitions. J Magn Reson Imaging, vol. 5, pp. 684-8, 1995.

[99] D. R. Wetter, G. C. McKinnon, J. F. Debatin, and G. K. von Schulthess. Cardiac echo-planar MR imaging: comparison of single- and multiple-shot techniques. Radiology, vol. 194, pp. 765-70, 1995.

[100] P. Mansfield. Multi planar image formation using NMR spin echoes. J Phys C, vol. 10, pp. L55-L58, 1977.

[101] C. P. Davis, G. C. McKinnon, J. F. Debatin, S. Duewell, and G. K. von Schulthess. Single-shot versus interleaved echo-planar MR imaging: application to visualization of cardiac valve leaflets. J Magn Reson Imaging, vol. 5, pp. 107-12, 1995.

[102] M. Markl and J. Hennig. Cardiac Multi-Phase k-Space Segmented Echo Planar Imaging with Black Blood Preparation for Fast Velocity Mapping of Myocardial Motion. presented at Magnetic Resonance in Cardiovascular Research, 4th international symposium, Würzburg, Germany, 1998.

[103] M. Doyle, E. G. Walsh, G. G. Blackwell, and G. M. Pohost. Block regional interpolation scheme for k-space (BRISK): a rapid cardiac imaging technique. Magn Reson Med, vol. 33, pp. 163-70, 1995.

[104] M. Doyle, E. G. Walsh, R. E. Foster, and G. M. Pohost. Rapid cardiac imaging with turbo BRISK. Magn Reson Med, vol. 37, pp. 410-7, 1997.

[105] T. K. Foo, M. A. Bernstein, A. M. Aisen, R. J. Hernandez, B. D. Collick, and T. Bernstein. Improved ejection fraction and flow velocity estimates with use of view sharing and uniform repetition time excitation with fast cardiac techniques. Radiology, vol. 195, pp. 471-8, 1995.

Chapter 10

Myocardial Spatiotemporal Tracking

Yudong Zhu
GE Corporate Research and Development,
Schenectady, New York

Norbert J. Pelc
Stanford University,
Palo Alto, California

10.1 Introduction

The past two decades of magnetic resonance imaging (MRI) research witnessed the development of noninvasive technologies that are capable of both motion quantification and spatiotemporal resolution. Representative examples include the MR tagging [1-5] and the phase contrast MR velocity mapping techniques [6-10]. Among clinical applications that have been established, or are being developed, use of the technologies for evaluating cardiac motion may be one that is most rewarding, yet exceedingly challenging.

The function of a human heart as a pump is characterized by its deforming motion in space and time. While myocardial status may be most fundamentally understood at a microscopic or biochemical level, its diseased state is often revealed by appreciable alterations of wall motion patterns. It is known, for example, that regional contractile abnormality is correlated with ischemia in the myocardium [11,12]. With its potential value in the diagnosis and management of ischemic heart disease and conduction abnormalities, this finding has motivated the development of techniques to differentiate abnormal wall contraction patterns from normal ones. The MR techniques noted above promise the ability to evaluate cardiac motion and to assess the effects of cardiovascular disease and therapeutic interventions. The complexity of the task however challenges further technological development on both the data acquisition and image post-processing fronts.

A.A. Amini and J.L. Prince (eds.),
Measurement of Cardiac Deformations from MRI: Physical and Mathematical Models, 257–288.

10.1.1 Imaging Cardiac Motion

A variety of imaging techniques have been developed and tested for qualitative or quantitative evaluation of myocardial motion. Radiologic imaging of the blood pool within the chambers (projection format, with radiopaque contrast agents or radionuclides) can indirectly depict the motion of the endocardial surface [13-15]. Echocardiography [16-18], computerized x-ray tomography (CT) [19,20] and conventional magnetic resonance imaging [21-24] can delineate both the endocardial and epicardial surface motion (contrast agents required in the CT case). The heart wall border motion captured by these noninvasive techniques enables qualitative examinations of cardiac motion and function, and to some extent, allows quantitative evaluations of the heart as a whole with such measures as chamber volumes, myocardial mass and cardiac output. These techniques however, are very limited in their ability to accurately follow and further quantify the motion/contraction of individual myocardial samples throughout the cardiac cycle [25,1,3,26]. This is because the motion of the heart wall is much more than a simple radial deformation. In fact, the heart translates, rotates, twists and shortens as it contracts and relaxes [27]. Without trackable fiducial marks inside the myocardium, knowledge of changing of the wall borders alone is not sufficient for unambiguously resolving the complex myocardial deformation.

Cardiac disorders such as coronary heart disease are frequently characterized by localized abnormalities in the wall. Reflecting the need for accurate measurement of regional motion and contractility, techniques have been developed that track natural or artificial landmarks. For example, regional endocardial trajectories have been derived by identifying endocardial landmarks [28], and motion of regions on the epicardial surface have been quantified through locating the bifurcation points of coronary arteries [29-31]. Since these landmarks may not be present near all regions of interest and do not go beyond the heart wall surfaces, the associated techniques still fall short in general cases, e.g., the study of intramural contraction. High quality measurements at points within the myocardium are possible by invasive techniques that use surgically placed landmarks or probes. Examples include distance measurement between implanted pulse transit sonomicrometry crystal pairs [32-34], ultrasonic echo measurement of inserted sutures [35] and fluoroscopic tracking of implanted metallic markers [36,27,37-39]. Accurate yet invasive techniques like these are responsible for much of today's knowledge about myocardial dynamics and still are the gold standards for quantitative analysis of myocardial motion. Their clinical applicability however, is limited because of the highly invasive nature of the required surgical process. Practical limitations on the number of markers and possible mechanical alteration of regional tissue also lessen the techniques' appeal.

Recent advances in magnetic resonance imaging, particularly the development of the MR tagging technique [1-5] and the phase contrast velocity mapping technique [6-10] have enabled regional myocardial motion and deformation to be quantified noninvasively. MR tagging is a marker technique. With this technique, a large number of magnetic landmarks can be noninvasively generated inside the myocardium through spatially selective perturbation of the local tissue magnetization; imaging after a short time delay will show the perturbed regions as low signal fiducial marks depicting the underlying tissue motion (Chapter 2). The phase contrast technique measures the velocity field by encoding the velocity into the phase of the local transverse magnetization, allowing individual tissue samples to be tracked. Compared to MR tagging, the phase contrast technique does not have the limitation of tag fading due to T_1 recovery and is capable of achieving greater sampling density of the motion field. Disadvantages are that the phase measurements tend to be more susceptible to imaging artifacts and at the present time, a longer scan time is needed to map 3D motion. Due to the noninvasive nature of the measurement process and the constantly improving quality of the image data, both techniques demonstrate great potential as tools for evaluating cardiac function. This chapter will primarily focus on illustrating the principle of phase contrast velocity mapping and describing an effective post-processing technique that further maps displacement and strain from the velocity data. As will be described however, the processing technique is also able to use displacement data from MR tagging.

10.1.2 Mapping Velocity With Phase Contrast MRI

An MR image (planar or volumetric) reconstructed from the acquired magnetic resonance signal portrays the spatial distribution of the transverse magnetization of spins (Chapter 9) — each image element, having both magnitude and phase, represents the average transverse magnetization vector of a corresponding neighborhood in space. While the direction (phase) information of the transverse magnetization is ignored in typical MRI exams, it has been known for decades that in the presence of a magnetic field gradient, transverse magnetization of moving spins accrue different phases than those of the static spins [40]. Van Dijk [6] originally proposed and demonstrated the potential use of MRI phase images for cardiac motion study. Nayler et al [7] first combined phase contrast with cine MRI and obtained time-resolved velocity images. Pelc et al [8] introduced interleaved velocity encoding and further developed cine phase contrast MRI. Today, phase contrast MRI represents a family of imaging techniques that measure and/or map the motion-induced phase shifts for the goal of quantifying motion.

Let $M(\cdot)$ represent, in complex terms, the distribution of the transverse magnetization at the time of the signal echo ($\tau = TE$). Consider a moving volume element whose trajectory is $(x(\tau), y(\tau), z(\tau))$ and whose position at $\tau = TE$ is (x, y, z). Its contribution to the signal received during the spatial encoding and data acquisition window (τ_1, τ_2) (assumed to be narrow such that relaxation and motion effects are of secondary significance), can be expressed as

$$M(x,y,z)e^{-j\omega_0(\tau-TE)}e^{-j\gamma\int_{\tau_1}^{\tau}(G_x(\mu)x+G_y(\mu)y+G_z(\mu)z)d\mu}dx\,dy\,dz\,, \qquad (10.1)$$

where ω_0 denotes the Larmor frequency and the G's describe the linear gradient field. For convenience we will express (10.1) as $\overline{M}(x, y, z)$. We may also find the following shorthand,

$$\overline{G}(\mu, x, y, z) = (G_x(\mu)x + G_y(\mu)y + G_z(\mu))d\mu\,,$$

useful. Now, the expression for the total signal is then a volume integral of the contributions from all the excited elements:

$$s_r(\tau) = \iiint \overline{M}(x, y, z)\,. \tag{10.2}$$

$\mathbf{M}(x, y, z)$ can be mapped with the spatial encoding principle as discussed before (see Chapter 9). Conventional dynamic MR imaging focuses on the magnitude of the reconstructed image which portrays the strength of the transverse magnetization at the time of image acquisition. The phase contrast technique further utilizes the phase of the reconstructed image. Particularly, the technique encodes velocity information into the phase by playing out extra gradients during a velocity encoding period

$(0, \tau_v)$ that is placed between the excitation and τ_1. Assume $(0, \tau_v)$ is so short that during the period the motion of the volume element is well described by its initial position (x_0, y_0, z_0) and average velocity (v_x, v_y, v_z): $x(\tau) = x_0 + v_x\tau$, $y(\tau) = y_0 + v_y\tau$, and $z(\tau) = z_0 + v_z\tau$. Then $\mathbf{M}(x, y, z)$ is related to $\mathbf{M}_0(x_0, y_0, z_0)$, the transverse magnetization right after the RF excitation, by

$$\mathbf{M}(x, y, z) = \mathbf{M}_0(x_0, y_0, z_0)e^{-TE/T_2}e^{-j\omega_0 TE}e^{j\phi}\,, \tag{10.3}$$

where the extra phase accrued

$$\phi = -\gamma \int_0^{\tau_v} \overline{G}(\mu, x_0 + v_x\mu, y_0 + v_y\mu, z_0 + v_z\mu)\,, \tag{10.4}$$

represents effects of gradients played during $(0, \tau_v)$.

Let a reference signal be defined as one acquired with all gradients turned off in $(0, \tau_v)$ (thus $\phi = 0$). The image reconstructed from it has an approximate complex value $\mathbf{M}_0(x_0, y_0, z_0)e^{-TE/T_2}e^{-j\omega_0 TE}$ at (x, y, z). Suppose in a separate acquisition, $G_x(\tau)$ is turned on during $(0, \tau_v)$ and its waveform is controlled so that

$$\int_0^{\tau_v} G_x(\mu)d\mu = 0 \quad \text{and} \quad \int_0^{\tau_v} G_x(\mu)\mu d\mu = \alpha_1 \neq 0\,. \tag{10.5}$$

The phase expression (10.4) then becomes $\phi = -\gamma\alpha_1 v_x$. Reconstruction based on this signal yields an image with value at (x, y, z) being approximately equal to

$\mathbf{M}_0(x_0, y_0, z_0)e^{-TE/T_2}e^{-j\omega_0 TE}e^{-j\gamma\alpha_1 v_x}$. While the images from both acquisitions show the same magnitude, their phase difference at (x, y, z) is $\Delta\phi = \gamma\alpha_1 v_x$.

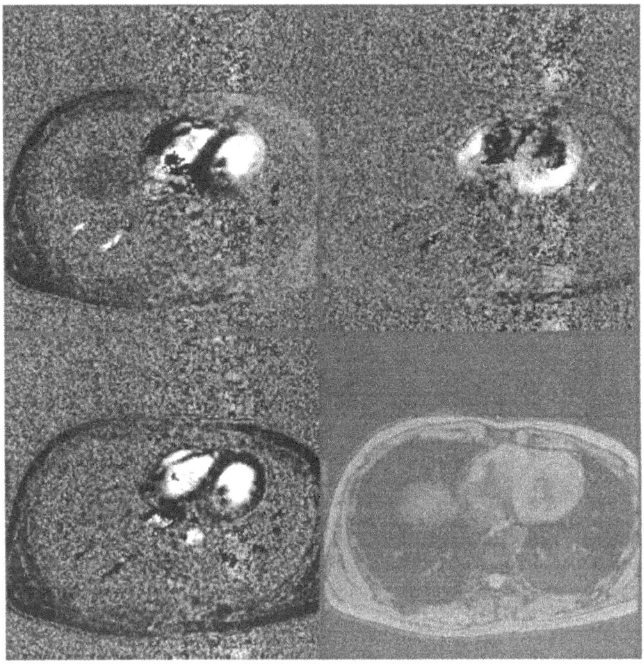

Figure 10.1: Sample images from cine phase contrast acquisition: v_x (top left), v_y (top right), v_z (bottom left), and magnitude (bottom right) images at a certain point in the cardiac cycle are shown.

One can therefore calculate v_x as $v_x = (v_{\text{enc}}/\pi)\Delta\phi$, where v_{enc} denotes the velocity that produces a phase shift of π radians (commonly used to represent velocity encoding strength). Thus, the two magnitude images will reflect the element's transverse magnetization strength at the acquisition time and the phase difference image will show its velocity x-component at the velocity encoding time. Maps of velocity y- and z-components can be similarly produced by velocity encoding with G_y and G_z, respectively. An acquisition of a reference signal is needed in practice, as phase accumulation due to sources other than velocity, such as B_0 field inhomogeneities and RF effects, may be present but can be subtracted by contrasting each velocity-encoded signal with the reference.

The value of an image element reflects both the transverse magnetization strength and velocity at about the same moment. Repeating the "excitation + velocity encoding + acquisition" at multiple time instants generates images depicting the object configuration and velocity distribution at corresponding phases of the object motion. Cine PC MR imaging technique [8] is a practical implementation of this strategy. Figure 10.1 shows some sample CINE PC images.

Let the velocity field associated with an object that undergoes cyclic motion be denoted by $\mathbf{v}(\mathbf{r}, t)$ (for given $\mathbf{r}$ and t, it is the velocity of a material point occupying position $\mathbf{r}$ at time t). At multiple phases of the object motion, Cine PC MR imaging measures this periodic velocity field with respect to a fixed laboratory frame and provides image frames each containing velocity samples at a set of fixed points in space (i.e., a spatial description of the kinematics). With measurement noise, the sampling can be expressed as

$$\mathbf{v}_{i,j,k,n} = \mathbf{v}(i\Delta x, j\Delta y, k\Delta z, n\Delta t) + \boldsymbol{\epsilon}_{i,j,k,n}\,, \tag{10.6}$$

where i, j, k, and n are sample indices, Δx, Δy, Δz, and Δt are sampling intervals, and $\boldsymbol{\epsilon}$ denotes the noise. This simplified yet useful view of the cine PC MR imaging is reasonable since many imaging imperfections, such as spatially dependent phase offsets due to eddy current effect and temporal low-pass filtering due to cine interpolation effect, can be rectified [41].

10.1.3 Analyzing Motion

Differentiating normal and diseased states in a myocardial region based on analyzing its motion and deformation pattern may be realized by computing from image data such local indices as strain rate tensor [9,10], strain tensor [5,26,42,43], as well as radial thickening, circumferential shortening, and longitudinal shortening [8,44-47,41]. A material description of regional deformation in terms of one or more indices listed above answers the basic question of how a certain myocardial sample moves and deforms. As a result, an integrated evaluation can be made of both the instantaneous tissue contractile state and its evolution over an extended period of time.

Central to this analysis are the fundamental tasks of tracking material points and measuring stretching/contraction. With the MR tagging technique, following the establishment of a number of fiducial markers in the myocardium through spatially selective excitation (usually applied at about end diastole), a sequence of image frames is acquired that captures the time-varying configuration of the tags as they deform along with the myocardium. In a post processing stage, establishment of marker correspondence between image frames provides samples of the displacement field.

With the PC velocity imaging technique, the phase shift of spins due to their motion through magnetic field gradients is used to generate a sequence of velocity-encoded images covering a heart cycle. Temporal integration of the measured velocity field samples then yields trajectory estimates of material points. To further quantify regional stretching/contraction, both techniques rely on measuring the difference in motion between neighboring material points, which essentially amounts to estimating the spatial derivatives of the displacement field. Reconstructing the displacement and strain fields based on the displacement samples from MR tagging or the velocity samples from PC MRI is generally made more difficult by the complex nature of the heart wall motion in the spatiotemporal domain. This section reviews issues mainly concerning PC MR data processing. Aspects of MR tagging data analysis are addressed in Chapters 2-8.

As described earlier, PC MR imaging depicts a periodically-varying velocity field with respect to a fixed laboratory frame, providing data samples with finite temporal and spatial resolutions. Deriving a material description of the motion and deformation (including trajectories of material points, segmental stretching and contraction, and Lagrangian strain field) from this spatial (Eulerian) description requires, either explicitly or implicitly, both temporal modeling and spatial modeling of the data. This is because a) integration of material velocity samples in time requires modeling of the waveform between data samples, b) when a material point's velocity is retrieved from the measured data for temporal integration, one generally needs an estimation scheme since velocity fields measured are Eulerian and data samples are only available at fixed grid locations, and c) spatial/temporal differentiation (for extracting parameters indicative of regional stretching or contraction) must assume a model for the variation between data samples.

To deal with nonrigidity, local methods [45-47,41,48,43] track motion and compute deformation by modeling the spatiotemporal variation of the motion field of only a small region. The "forward-backward" tracking method [47] for example, numerically integrates a myocardial sample's velocity measurements with respect to time, assuming the temporal variation of the velocity waveform is linear in sampling intervals. A weighted sum of trajectories obtained by integrating forward and backward in time effectively minimizes the noise and eddy current effects, which generally induce errors that propagate and increase along either integration direction. With local methods, applying the computation repeatedly with the region centered at various locations within the myocardium can provide myocardial displacement and strain field estimates. To ensure accuracy however, the size of the region must be kept small due to possible high order heterogeneity of the motion field as well as constraints imposed by the myocardial geometry (particularly in the radial direction). As a result, the reproducibility of the computed displacement may be limited, and that of the strain quantification may be particularly low since estimating spatial derivatives is highly sensitive to noise. A further limitation of local methods is that the modeling lacks cohesiveness — a regional model centered at one location and the same model centered at a neighboring location generally will not reconcile with each other in the overlapped supporting area.

Intuitively, compared to generally noise-sensitive local approaches, a global computation using the velocity samples from a large portion of the myocardium and all time frames can be more reproducible, and can also be more efficient in estimating the whole-body strain field. Further, a global model-based computational method yields a cohesive and structured view of the motion, which facilitates interpreting as well quantifying the displacement and strain fields. Modeling of the nonrigid motion of an extended region in this case has to address the complex geometry of the ventricular myocardium and the rich temporal characteristics of the dynamics. Use of large analytical shapes that have few configuration parameters (e.g., cylinders and ellipsoids), generally only leads to gross approximations of the ventricular geometry, and local refinement is often necessary to improve modeling accuracy

[49,50]. Use of linear, or other low-order polynomial temporal integration models [45-48], may give rise to various degrees of error in capturing the temporal characteristics of the dynamics [41].

Standard finite element methods approximate the spatial variation of a field with piecewise smooth functions [51]. They have been traditionally used as simulation tools to provide numerical solutions to partial differential equations. Application of finite element modeling to studying nonrigid motion has recently been explored, such as physically-based elastic models [49,52], and interpolation/smoothing approaches [42,53]. The main focus of the remainder of this chapter is a nonrigid motion tracking method (DMESH) [54-56], which uses a dynamic finite element mesh model to simultaneously capture a fields temporal behavior as well as its spatial variation. With the parameters of the mesh model obtained from fitting the velocity samples of an extended region at all time frames, the displacement field can be analytically constructed, as can other quantities that are spatial/temporal derivatives of the displacement field. The model expresses the complex deforming motion in space and time with time-varying basic elements, which represents an extension to the standard finite element concept. The model provides a flexible tradeoff between accuracy and reproducibility with controllable built-in spatiotemporal smoothing (determined by the fineness of the defined mesh and the richness of the included Fourier temporal harmonics), which enables cohesive and precise mapping of the displacement and strain fields with little compromise in accuracy. The model and the method can be further extended to analyze cyclic motion using, or incorporating, other motion information, such as MR tagging data (displacement information), and optic flow data (apparent motion information inferred from spatiotemporal intensity variation in the images).

10.2 DMESH Motion/Strain Mapping

Estimating (material descriptions of) the motion and deformation fields is a problem of reconstructing temporal functions based on measured velocity data. In the temporal domain, the sampling theorem asserts that one can at best accurately estimate spectral components of these functions with frequencies not exceeding half the data sampling frequency. The present approach models each element's periodic temporal variation using Fourier harmonics of up to half the sampling frequency, which achieves the highest accuracy supported by the data. Complete spatiotemporal modeling of the continuum kinematics in the present approach is accomplished by using a group of elements that interconnect in space and whose deforming motion are each characterized by Fourier harmonics. This allows optimization of the balance between analysis accuracy and reproducibility, as adjustment of the fineness of the local mesh tessellation and the number of Fourier harmonics facilitates smooth and controllable transition from a coarse (but highly reproducible) modeling at one end, to a fine one (approaching perfect spatiotemporal representation but at the cost of poorer reproducibility) at the other.

10.2.1 The Spatiotemporal Finite Element Model

For a periodically moving and deforming object, we consider a mesh whose node points are attached to a set of material points of the underlying region of interest such that the mesh moves and deforms along with the material region. With non-overlapping time-varying basic mesh elements, such as triangular or quadrilateral elements in 2-D and tetrahedral or hexahedral elements in 3-D, the mesh constitutes a partition of the region (see Figure 10.2 for a 2D example). Depending on the shape functions used in the element domain and the modeling in the temporal domain, the dynamic mesh configuration approximates the material kinematics with various degrees of accuracy.

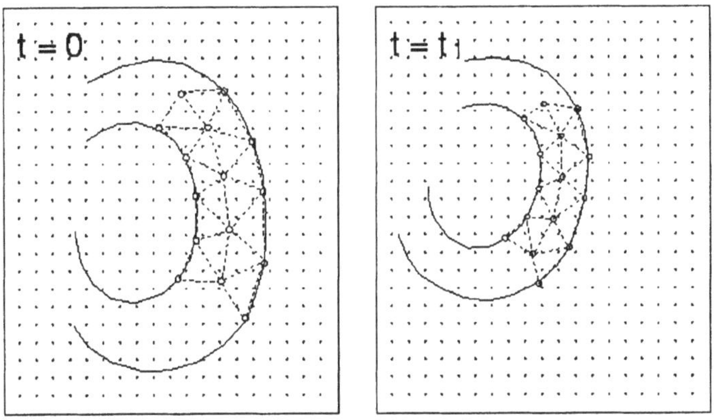

Figure 10.2: A moving and deforming object and an example spatiotemporal finite element mesh model. (From Zhu and Pelc, ref [56], Copyright 1999 IEEE.)

Specifically, the partitioning mesh is initialized by selecting a set of nodal points at a reference state ($t = 0$). The spatiotemporal trajectories of these points, along with the finite element shape functions, specify the mesh configuration at subsequent time instants and define the moving and deforming domain of each element. With the concept of isoparametric element [51], the element-wise kinematics of the supporting local material region is modeled spatially as in the following. At any time t for any material point in the eth element:

$$\mathbf{x}^e(\boldsymbol{\xi}, t) = \sum_{a=1}^{n_{en}} N_a(\boldsymbol{\xi})\mathbf{x}^e(\boldsymbol{\xi}_a, t), \tag{10.7}$$

$$\mathbf{v}^e(\boldsymbol{\xi}, t) = \sum_{a=1}^{n_{en}} N_a(\boldsymbol{\xi})\mathbf{v}^e(\boldsymbol{\xi}_a, t). \tag{10.8}$$

In the above equations, a is the local node index, n_{en} is the number of nodes in the eth mesh element, $\boldsymbol{\xi}$ are the local coordinates of the material point, and $\boldsymbol{\xi}_a$ and

N_a are, respectively, the local coordinates and shape function associated with the ath node. $\mathbf{x}^e(\boldsymbol{\xi}, t)$ and $\mathbf{v}^e(\boldsymbol{\xi}, t)$ represent, respectively, the trajectory and velocity of the material point, and $\mathbf{x}^e(\boldsymbol{\xi}_a, t)$ and $\mathbf{v}^e(\boldsymbol{\xi}_a, t)$ represent, respectively, the trajectory and velocity of the ath node of the eth element. Equation (10.7) states the form of the mapping from the eth element's current local coordinate system to the fixed lab coordinate system, and Equation (10.8), derived from differentiating both sides of Equation (10.7) is the spatial model of the velocity field within the element's supporting region. The shape functions are typically chosen to be Lagrange polynomials. The implementation of triangular elements for 2-D problems and tetrahedral elements for 3-D problems, both with piecewise linear shape functions (first order Lagrange polynomials), will be described in later sections.

Periodicity of motion and deformation allows the ath node's spatiotemporal trajectory to be expressed in terms of its Fourier harmonics:

$$\mathbf{x}^e(\boldsymbol{\xi}_a, t) = \sum_{k=-M}^{M} \mathbf{g}_a^e(k) e^{j2\pi k f_0 t} . \tag{10.9}$$

Differentiation of Equation (10.9) yields the frequency component representation of the node's material velocity:

$$\mathbf{v}^e(\boldsymbol{\xi}_a, t) = \sum_{k=-M, k\neq 0}^{M} (j2\pi k f_0) \mathbf{g}_a^e(k) e^{j2\pi k f_0 t} . \tag{10.10}$$

In Equations (10.9) and (10.10), $f_0 = 1/T_0$ (T_0 = motion period) is the fundamental frequency, k is the index for the harmonics, and M is the highest value of k. This component of the present spatiotemporal model stems directly from Fourier tracking — a method developed for computing the trajectory of material points based on velocity field measurements [57,41,43,58]. The key idea of Fourier tracking is to integrate velocity samples through fitting Fourier harmonics (with FFT or least squares); this eliminates undesirable low-pass filtering effects inherent in algorithms that use constant, linear or polynomial temporal models [45-48] and achieves the highest accuracy supported by the data samples.

Equations (10.7) through (10.10) constitute the statement of the present spatiotemporal finite element mesh model. Combining Equations (10.8) and (10.10) leads to:

$$\mathbf{v}^e(\boldsymbol{\xi}, t) = \sum_{a=1}^{n_{en}} \left(N_a(\boldsymbol{\xi}) \sum_{k=-M, k\neq 0}^{M} (j2\pi k f_0) \mathbf{g}_a^e(k) e^{j2\pi k f_0 t} \right) , \tag{10.11}$$

indicating that the present spatiotemporal finite element mesh model has the $\mathbf{g}_a^e(k)$'s, the Fourier coefficients of the preselected node points' trajectories, as its parameters.

10.2.2 The DMESH Tracking Algorithm

Given spatial and temporal samples of the velocity fields, we can apply the mesh model and quantify the deforming motion using the algorithm presented below. Since the mapping Equation (10.7) and the modeling Equation (10.11) require knowledge of mesh configuration estimates at all time instants in advance, the algorithm must be iterative. A set of selected node points defines the initial mesh configuration. Independent tracking of these points with the Fourier tracking method [41] initializes the mesh configuration estimates at subsequent time instants. Then, fitting the velocity data to the spatiotemporal finite element mesh model yields refined Fourier coefficient estimates of the nodal points' trajectories, as well as the updated mesh configuration estimates at all time instants. Specifically,

- For each time instant $n\Delta t$, with the configuration estimate from the previous iteration, we identify every contributing data grid point and its associated element domain, evaluate the point's corresponding $\boldsymbol{\xi}$ and $N_a(\boldsymbol{\xi})$ values, and obtain an equation of form (10.11) (or its equivalent real version). Consider, for example, a 2-D implementation using triangular elements and linear shape functions (i.e., $N_1(\xi_1, \xi_2) = \xi_1$, $N_2(\xi_1, \xi_2) = \xi_2$, and $N_3(\xi_1, \xi_2) = 1 - \xi_1 - \xi_2$). Suppose we have a velocity measurement $\mathbf{v}$ at location $\mathbf{x}$ and time $n\Delta t$, and we find the location $\mathbf{x}$ to be inside the eth element of the mesh configuration at this time. This data point then contributes a vector equation (2 scalar linear equations) that constrains the Fourier coefficients of the trajectories of the eth element's node points:

$$\sum_{k=-M, k\neq 0}^{M} j2\pi k f_0 e^{j2\pi k f_0 n\Delta t}(\xi_1 \mathbf{g}_1^e(k) + \xi_2 \mathbf{g}_2^e(k) + (1 - \xi_1 - \xi_2)\mathbf{g}_3^e(k)) = \mathbf{v}\,, \tag{10.12}$$

where the components of $\boldsymbol{\xi}$ are evaluated beforehand by solving Equation (10.7) and M is chosen to be,

$$\left(\frac{\text{total number of data time frames}}{2}\right) - 1\,.$$

- Going through all elements and all time instants, (using the equation assembling technique from the finite element analysis theory) we systematically collect a set of linear equations: $\mathbf{A}\mathbf{g} = \mathbf{b}$, where $\mathbf{A}$ is the matrix that contains the coefficients of the equations (and thus depends on data point positions relative to the mesh configuration computed from the previous iteration, as well as the shape functions and the number of Fourier harmonics implemented), $\mathbf{g}$ is the vector that contains the unknown $\mathbf{g}_a^e(k)$'s (the Fourier coefficients of the nodal points' trajectories), and $\mathbf{b}$ is the data vector that collects velocity measurements.

- A least squares fit yields updated $\mathbf{g}_a^e(k)$'s ($k \neq 0$). The $\mathbf{g}_a^e(0)$'s can then be determined from Equation (10.9) using the initial conditions:

$$\mathbf{g}_a^e(0) + \sum_{k=-M,k\neq 0}^{M} \mathbf{g}_a^e(k) = \mathbf{x}^e(\boldsymbol{\xi}_a, 0) \,. \tag{10.13}$$

This fitting+updating step is repeated until the coefficient estimates converge, or until a prespecified number of iterations has been performed. The model and the mesh configuration estimates at all time instants can then be used to derive other motion and deformation quantities associated with the region of interest, such as the displacement field, the deformation gradient field and the strain field. The trajectory of any material point (with initial coordinate $\mathbf{X}$) within the region of interest, for example, is computed as:

$$\hat{\mathbf{x}}(\mathbf{X}, t) = \hat{\mathbf{x}}^e(\boldsymbol{\xi}, t) = \sum_{a=1}^{n_{en}} N_a(\boldsymbol{\xi})\hat{\mathbf{x}}^e(\boldsymbol{\xi}_a, t) \,, \tag{10.14}$$

where e identifies the element within which the material point is initially located, and $\boldsymbol{\xi}$ denotes the point's local coordinates in that element. The deformation gradient tensor $\mathbf{F}$ in the neighborhood of the material point is computed as

$$\hat{\mathbf{F}}_{i,J}(\mathbf{X}, t) = \frac{\partial \hat{x}_i}{\partial X_J} = \sum_{a=1}^{n_{en}} \hat{x}_i^e(\boldsymbol{\xi}_a, t) \left(\sum_{j=1}^{n_{sd}} \frac{\partial N_a}{\partial \xi_j} \frac{\partial \xi_j}{\partial X_J} \right) \,, \tag{10.15}$$

where n_{sd} denotes the number of spatial dimensions (e.g., n_{sd}=2 for 2-D problems). Expression (11.15) can be efficiently evaluated for the triangular or tetrahedral linear elements, using analytically derived partial derivative expressions. It is to be noted that each time-varying component of the estimated motion trajectory and deformation gradient tensor turns out to be a linear combination of the Fourier coefficients of the nodal points' trajectories. Organizing the estimated values of the component at all time instants into a vector form, we may express the vector as $\hat{\mathbf{y}} = \mathbf{D}\mathbf{g}$, where $\mathbf{D}$ is a matrix that collects, in the right order, the corresponding combination coefficients.

10.2.3 Reproducibility Analysis

Reproducibility of the computed motion and deformation, as measured by the corresponding covariance matrices, can be analyzed after each computation. Assuming that the noise in the velocity component measurements are uncorrelated with mean zero and identical variance σ_v^2, and that the perturbation to $\mathbf{A}^T\mathbf{A}$ caused by the noise in the mesh configuration estimates is negligible, we can readily show that

$$\text{Cov}(\mathbf{g}) = \sigma_v^2(\mathbf{A}^T\mathbf{A})^{-1} \,, \tag{10.16}$$

where the superscript T denotes matrix transpose (conjugate transpose, if complex rather than real equations are assembled). Being a linear combination of the Fourier coefficients,

$$\mathrm{Cov}(\hat{\mathbf{y}}) = \sigma_v^2 \mathbf{D}(\mathbf{A}^T\mathbf{A})^{-1}\mathbf{D}^T . \tag{10.17}$$

The measurement noise variance σ_v^2 may be estimated from the fitting residual (the estimate is unbiased for a fitting model of high accuracy):

$$\hat{\sigma}_v^2 = \frac{\text{RSS}}{\text{degrees of freedom for residue}} , \tag{10.18}$$

where RSS is the residual sum of squares, and the *degrees of freedom* is the difference between the number of rows and the number of columns in $\mathbf{A}$. Using this estimate of σ_v^2 in Equations (10.16) and (10.17), we obtain a prediction for the estimated quantities' reproducibility as part of the motion/strain mapping process.

A formal proof, confirming the expectation that a global computation tends to yield more reproducible results than a local approach, has been given previously [56]. It showed that, in general, extending an initial mesh model by incorporating additional elements (which are coupled to the original elements and are sufficiently supported by corresponding data) results in increased reproducibility of the motion and deformation estimates for the original elements. It additionally showed that, with the support of more data (due to more available measurements, e.g., displacement measurements), motion analysis using the same mesh modeling is generally at least as precise as that without the new data.

10.2.4 Lagrangian Strain Field Computation

The mutually orthogonal principal components of the Lagrangian finite strain tensor $\mathbf{E}$ (defined as $\mathbf{E} = (\mathbf{F}^T\mathbf{F} - \mathbf{I})/2$) fully characterize how a local segment with arbitrary initial state changes in size and shape, and are thus appropriate for use as indices of the regional deformation. However, as it essentially relies on measuring the difference in motion between neighboring material points (estimating spatial derivatives), quantifying the strain field is inherently more noise-sensitive than reconstructing the displacement field. Additionally, use of low order polynomial shape functions may not constrain the spatial derivatives to be continuous across element boundaries [51]. Smoothing of the strain field estimation that is directly computed from $\hat{\mathbf{E}} = (\hat{\mathbf{F}}^T\hat{\mathbf{F}} - \mathbf{I})/2$ may therefore be desirable.

Assuming element-wise homogeneous strain, the present spatiotemporal model implementation uses linear shape functions. A straightforward reconstruction of the strain field according to $\hat{\mathbf{E}} = (\hat{\mathbf{F}}^T\hat{\mathbf{F}} - \mathbf{I})/2$, where $\hat{\mathbf{F}}$ denotes the deformation gradient computed using Equation (10.15), generally leads to discontinuities at element boundaries. To improve the overall quality of the continuous strain field estimation, we introduce smoothing [51] by solving the following optimization problem for each component of the strain tensor

$$\min \int_{\Omega} \left(\tilde{E} - \hat{E}\right)^2 d\Omega \,, \tag{10.19}$$

where $\hat{E}$ denotes a component of the element-wise constant strain field estimation (from $\hat{\mathbf{E}} = (\hat{\mathbf{F}}^T\hat{\mathbf{F}} - \mathbf{I})/2$) and the minimization is taken over all continuous and element-wise linear functions $\tilde{E}$. This formulation translates into solving linear equations assembled using techniques from the finite element analysis theory. The result is a continuous strain field estimate whose element-wise spatial variation is constrained to be linear.

10.2.5 Extended Use of DMESH Tracking

While DMESH is well suited for processing the velocity data measured using PC MR scans, it can also be used for processing velocity information from other sources such as optic flow and Doppler ultrasound. This flexibility is largely due to the controllable model configuration (e.g. definition of initial mesh geometry and tessellation, use of finite element shape functions, and inclusion of Fourier harmonics) and the fact that the velocity modeling Equation (10.11) does not require the data to be uniformly sampled in space or time.

Some imaging techniques allow displacement information to be extracted. The displacement information, for example, can be inferred from temporal correspondence established through matching unique geometric patterns in images at different times, e.g., surgically implanted markers [36,39], bifurcation points of coronary arteries [29,30], and curvature-based features on myocardial boundaries [59,60]. With the MR tagging technique which noninvasively creates a large number of fiducial markers that move along with the underlying tissue, the displacement information can be extracted from the images with good spatial coverage and particularly high fidelity [5,50]. DMESH is adaptable to processing displacement information through displacement field modeling:

$$\Delta \mathbf{x}^e(\boldsymbol{\xi}, t) = \sum_{a=1}^{n_{en}} \left(N_a(\boldsymbol{\xi}) \sum_{k=-M}^{M} \mathbf{g}_a^e(k)(e^{j2\pi k f_0 t} - 1) \right) . \tag{10.20}$$

For analyzing MR tagging data in particular, lines detected from tagged images typically generate, for each tag point, the component of its displacement vector that is orthogonal to its corresponding initial tag plane. Based on such displacement information, the component-wise form of Equation (10.20) can be readily used for reconstructing the displacement field.

In cases where data from multiple measurement processes are available, the concept of improving analysis quality by taking advantage of all the information naturally arises. By incorporating both velocity modeling and displacement modeling, the DMESH method provides a unique framework that integrates information from various sources. A (weighted) least squares solution to a set of equations of form (10.11) or (10.20) for example, may represent an optimal integration of velocity data (from velocity imaging or optic flow) and displacement data (from correspondence established from trackable intensity features).

10.3 Experiments

The analysis software used in all the studies described below was written in Matlab (MathWorks, Natick, MA) and executed on Sun workstations (Sun Microsystems, Palo Alto, CA). Analysis time varies with the size of matrix **A**, and certainly depends on the processor speed and amount of memory available. In the volumetric simulation study described below for example, each iteration required 6.5 minutes to assemble **A** (about 77,100×2,500 in size) and 8.5 minutes to solve $\mathbf{Ag} = \mathbf{b}$ on a Sun Ultra2 workstation (300MHz dual-processor, 256MB RAM). With the heart data analysis case on the other hand, each iteration required 1.0 minute to assemble **A** (about 26,400×1,500 in size) and 0.5 minutes to find the least squares solution.

10.3.1 Computer simulation studies

The DMESH tracking method was evaluated with computer synthesized data of an object undergoing nonuniform deformation. The object consisted of a nonrotating outer cylindrical shell ($R_0 = 47.6$ mm), a periodically rotating inner cylinder ($R_i = 18.4$ mm), and deforming material between the two (Figure 10.3). The rotation of the inner cylinder $\theta(t)$ was specified as a waveform with period $T_0 = 0.96$ s and peak-to-peak excursion of 41 degrees. At radius R within the deforming material the rotation was $\theta_R(t) = \theta(t)(R_0^{-2} - R^{-2})/(R_0^{-2} - R_i^{-2})$ [61]. The object remained still along the z direction in 2D simulation studies, but translated and deformed along the z direction in 3D simulation studies: $z(Z,t) = 1.5\sin(2\pi t/T_0) + (0.86 + 0.14\cos(2\pi t/T_0))Z$, where Z is the position in the z direction at $t = 0$.

In a first simulation study, single transaxial slice data with 1.2×1.2 mm^2 resolution, 16 time frames covering the 0.96 s period, and $v_{\text{enc}} = 15$ cm/s was used to validate the tracking method and verify the error analysis. A set of nodal points was preselected to define an initial mesh configuration covering part of the deforming annular region (Figure 10.3). The mesh was composed of a single element (filled triangle) in case A (to examine local modeling) and all four elements in case B (to investigate potential benefits of extended modeling). In each case, the algorithm described in 11.2.2 was used to compute the Fourier coefficients of the nodal points' trajectories. For each mesh element and each time instant, the center point position $\boldsymbol{x}_c$, the deformation gradient tensor $\boldsymbol{F}$ and the strain tensor $\boldsymbol{E}$, were then derived from the model and compared to the true values. The method's performance in the two cases was evaluated with noisy data sets as well as a noiseless one.

For noisy data with an apparent SNR of 45 (white Gaussian noise of standard

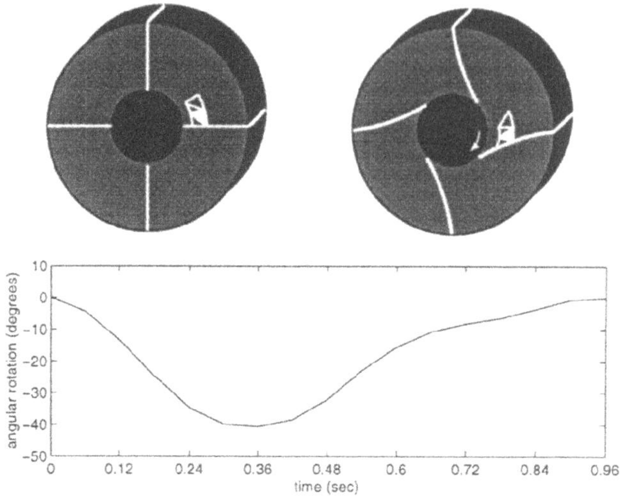

Figure 10.3: The simulated deforming object at two time instants and the angular rotation of the inner cylinder. (From Zhu and Pelc, ref [56], Copyright 1999 IEEE.)

deviation 0.15 cm/s was added to both the v_x and v_y components of the velocity data), a total of 1000 experiments were performed. Figures 10.4 and 10.5 show the measured means and standard deviations of the computed quantities (center point position and deformation gradient) of the filled triangle in both cases: single mesh element (local) modeling of this region (case A) and extended mesh element modeling in which the other three elements were also included in the analysis (case B). In both cases, the estimates from the noiseless data and the averages of the estimates from the noisy data were in excellent agreement with the true values (Figure 10.4). The theoretically predicted and experimentally measured standard deviations also agreed well (Figure 10.5). Figures 10.4 and 10.5 further show that the extended mesh modeling resulted in lower standard deviation but comparably high accuracy. This is consistent with the theoretical prediction. Under the present situation, adding neighboring elements to the analysis reduced the standard deviations of the computed quantities within the filled triangle by a factor of up to 2. The good agreement and the conclusions held true when the study was repeated at SNR=15, corresponding to a noise-induced standard deviation in the velocity data of 0.45 cm/s.

To further examine the performance of the method in displacement and strain field quantification, in a second study, a much extended mesh was applied to analyze a single transaxial slice (with the same data resolutions as above and an SNR of 45). In the reference state ($t = 0$), user-selected node points defined an initial mesh covering the inner portion of the annular region where the material deforms with great amplitude. The node points were individually tracked to initialize the mesh configuration estimates at subsequent time instants. Iteratively

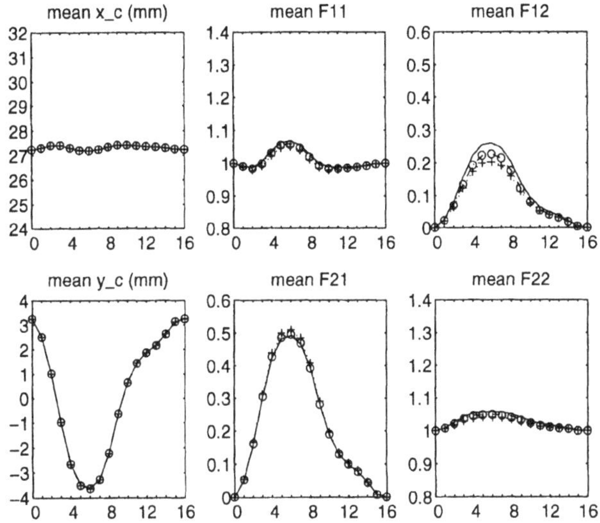

Figure 10.4: Mean of the computed center point position (x_c and y_c) and deformation gradient (F_{ij}) as functions of time frame — solid line: true value, circle: single-element mesh, cross: extended mesh. As a comparison, same quantities computed using noiseless data are also shown — dashdot line: single-element mesh, dotted line: extended mesh. (From Zhu and Pelc, ref [56], Copyright 1999 IEEE.)

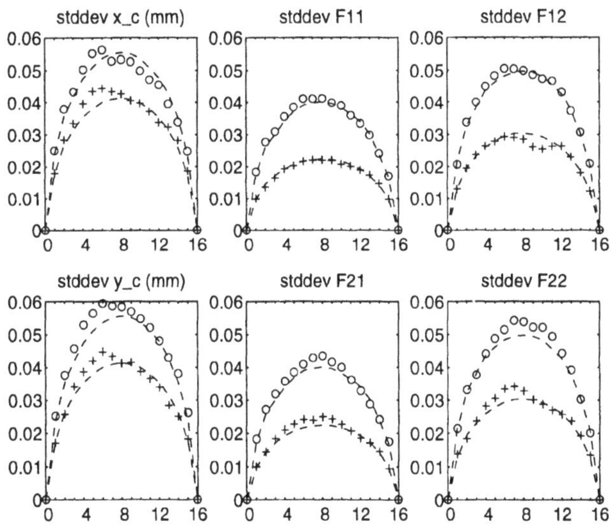

Figure 10.5: Standard deviation of the computed center point position (x_c and y_c) and deformation gradient (F_{ij}) as functions of time frame — dashed line: theoretical prediction, circle: single-element mesh, cross: extended mesh. (From Zhu and Pelc, ref [56], Copyright 1999 IEEE.)

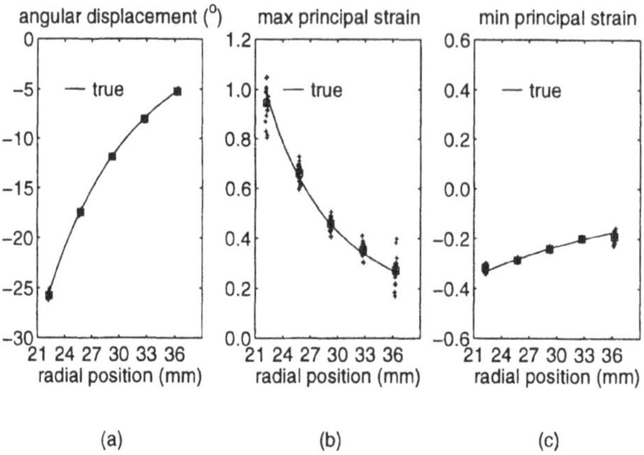

Figure 10.6: The computed fields at multiple radial and angular positions were examined. (a), (b) and (c) show respectively, computed angular displacement, maximum principal strain and minimum principal strain at time frame 7 (about maximum deformation) as a function of radial position. Each + symbol corresponds to one material point and each square symbol represents the average of the results of the points at the same radial position. (From Zhu and Pelc, ref [56], Copyright 1999 IEEE.)

fitting the velocity data to the spatiotemporal finite element mesh model led to refined estimates of the mesh configuration. The displacement field and (element-wise constant) strain field $\hat{\mathbf{E}}$ were then derived. Solving the minimization problem Equation (10.19) subsequently provided a continuous strain field estimate for each time instant. The computed fields at multiple radial and angular positions were examined. Figure 10.6 (a), (b) and (c) show, respectively, computed angular displacement, maximum principal strain and minimum principal strain at time frame 7 (near maximum deformation) as a function of radial position. As the comparison with the true values demonstrated, the computed displacements were very accurate and precise, and the strain quantification approach that included the smoothing process was capable of reconstructing the strain field with high accuracy and good reproducibility.

A third study evaluated a 3-D implementation. A total of 9 transaxial slices simulated a volumetric data set with a $1.2\times1.2\times2.4$ mm^3 resolution. The temporal resolution and SNR were kept the same as above. An initial mesh covering about a quarter of the annular volume was prescribed, and then analyzed following the same steps as in the second study. Results from the 3D implementation of the method and volumetric data from the third simulation study were also in good agreement with the true values. By displaying various strain levels as shades of gray, Figure 10.7 shows the reconstructed maximum principal strain field evaluated on the surface of the estimated mesh configuration at time frame 7. Such display of the deformation state of the underlying material region is easily inter-

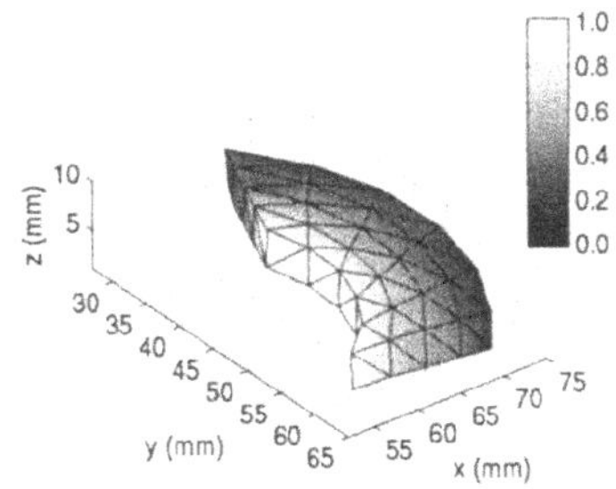

Figure 10.7: 3D simulation: reconstructed maximum principal strain field evaluated on the surface of the estimated mesh configuration is shown as shades of grey (time frame 7). (From Zhu and Pelc, ref [56], Copyright 1999 IEEE.)

preted visually. Since the present method reconstructs the time-varying strain field over the whole volume of interest, volumetric rendering of the functional index with interactive user guidance and cine display is possible, and is expected to be more intuitive and informative than numerical or other graphical formats.

10.3.2 *In vitro* and *in vivo* studies

A phantom [62] with an identical geometry to the object described above was imaged to evaluate the analysis method in actual experimental studies. The outer and inner cylinders were made of acrylic (R_i=18.4 mm, R_o=47.6 mm). The deformable material in between was a silicone gel (Silgard, Primerless Dielectric Gel 527, Dow Corning, Midland, MI), mixed as one part catalyst to one part resin. The motion of the inner cylinder was computer controlled with a period of 0.96 s and a simulated physiological velocity and displacement. For tracking performance evaluation, 12 beads were embedded inside the gel (identifiable in magnitude images with appropriate slice prescription). Velocity data for a single axial slice were collected using a 1.5T MRI system (Signa Horizon, GE Medical Systems, Milwaukee, WI), with a quadrature head coil and a phase contrast spoiled GRE cine sequence. The peak-to-peak angular excursion of the inner cylinder was 41°. Other acquisition parameters were *TR*/*TE*=18/7 ms, 30 cm FOV, 30° flip angle, 7 mm slice thickness, $v_{\text{enc}} = 20$ cm/s, 256×256 acquisition matrix and 2 NEX. The acquired data were processed in the same way as in the 2-D simulation study. Figure 10.8 shows magnitude image frames 3, 7, 11, and 15 (out of 16) during a whole motion cycle, with the tracked mesh configuration at corresponding time instants each displayed as an overlay on the associated image. The location of the fiducial markers embedded in the deforming material are visible as regions of reduced signal. Good agreement is seen between the actual motion as evidenced by the beads and the computed motion as portrayed by the overlaid mesh. With the estimated time-varying displacement field (material description), the spatiotemporal trajectory of

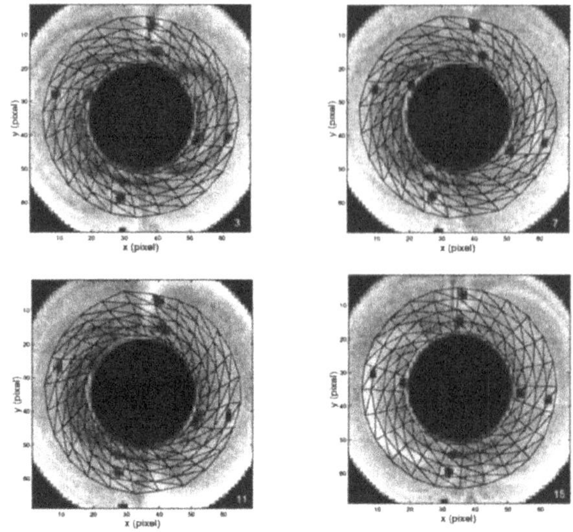

Figure 10.8: Magnitude image frames 3, 7, 11, and 15 of the phantom during a whole motion cycle. The time-varying mesh configuration is computed and the result at each corresponding time instant is shown as an overlay on the associated magnitude image. (From Zhu and Pelc, ref [56], Copyright 1999 IEEE.)

any material point initially located within the tracked material region can be readily computed. Figure 10.9 shows computed trajectories (with the initial locations marked as circles) for 20 evenly spaced material points along each of eight user-defined line segments.

Cine PC data were acquired of a patient with an idiopathic hypertrophic subaortic stenosis to test the method *in vivo*. A midventricular transaxial slice was imaged using a body coil. The cine PC sequence had *TR*/*TE*=30/8.9 ms, 32 cm FOV, 30° flip angle, 10 mm slice thickness, $v_{\text{enc}} = 20$ cm/s, 256×256 matrix, 2 NEX, cardiac synchronization using the ECG signal, and respiratory compensation. The total acquisition time was about 8 minutes. An initial mesh covering much of the left ventricular wall on this slice was prescribed and analyzed. Figure 10.10 (image frames 3, 7, 11, and 15 out of 16) shows the estimated principal strain distribution in a manner similar to that used in Figure 10.7. The result suggests the presence of a nonuniform contraction pattern in the circumferential direction near end systole.

As another *in vivo* application, cyclic motion of the biceps was examined. Parameters similar to those above were used to image a sagittal plane of a human volunteers upper arm while the subject was performing a repeated biceps curl exercise at a rate of 35 cycles/min. The data collection was synchronized to the motion cycle by an optical transducer. Twenty four temporal frames were acquired. An initial mesh covering part of the biceps was defined and analyzed. Figure 10.11 (image frames 2, 6, 10, 14, 18 and 22 out of 24) shows the estimated principal

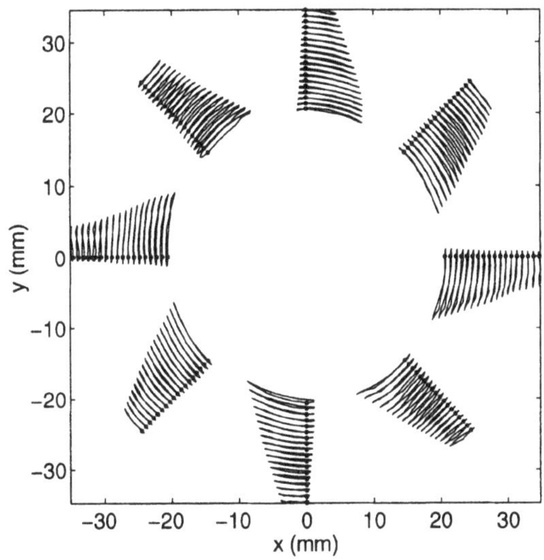

Figure 10.9: Material description of the computed displacement field evaluated on eight user-defined line segments: resultant trajectories (with the initial locations marked as circles) for 20 evenly spaced material points along each of the line segments are shown. (From Zhu and Pelc, ref [56], Copyright 1999 IEEE.)

strain distribution and reveals some features of the muscle deformation. Most noticeable appears to be a significant heterogeneity along the fiber direction at about the mid-point into the cycle.

10.3.3 Combined use of displacement and velocity data

A computer simulation study was carried out to investigate the extendibility and value of the DMESH method for analyzing data that contains both velocity and displacement information. The setting was similar to that of case B in the first simulation study of DMESH (see Section 11.3.1). The only difference was that tagging data was additionally simulated and the DMESH tracking algorithm was used to reconstruct the displacement and strain fields with both velocity and tagging data taken into account. The simulated tagging data represented a typical data set acquired with SPAMM [3]: for the first three quarters of the motion period (time frames 1 through 12 out of 16 frames that evenly cover the whole period) two sets of tag lines were detectable in the images with one set roughly horizontal and the other vertical. The two sets of tag lines were the intersections of the imaging plane with the tag surfaces which were initially parallel planes in horizontal and vertical directions, respectively. The initial spacing between adjacent parallel tag planes was 5 mm. The spacing between adjacent detected tag points along each tag line was around 1.2 mm. Noise was added to the detected tag positions such that the

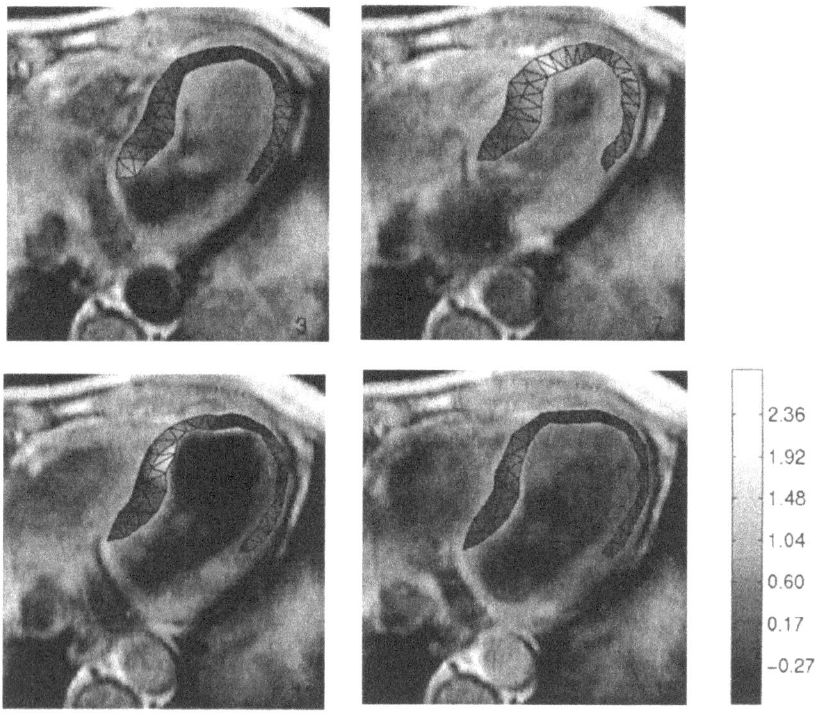

Figure 10.10: Left ventricular wall: reconstructed maximum principal strain field across the estimated mesh configuration is represented as shades of gray and overlaid on the magnitude images (time frames 3, 7, 11 and 15 out of 16). (From Zhu and Pelc, ref [56], Copyright 1999 IEEE.)

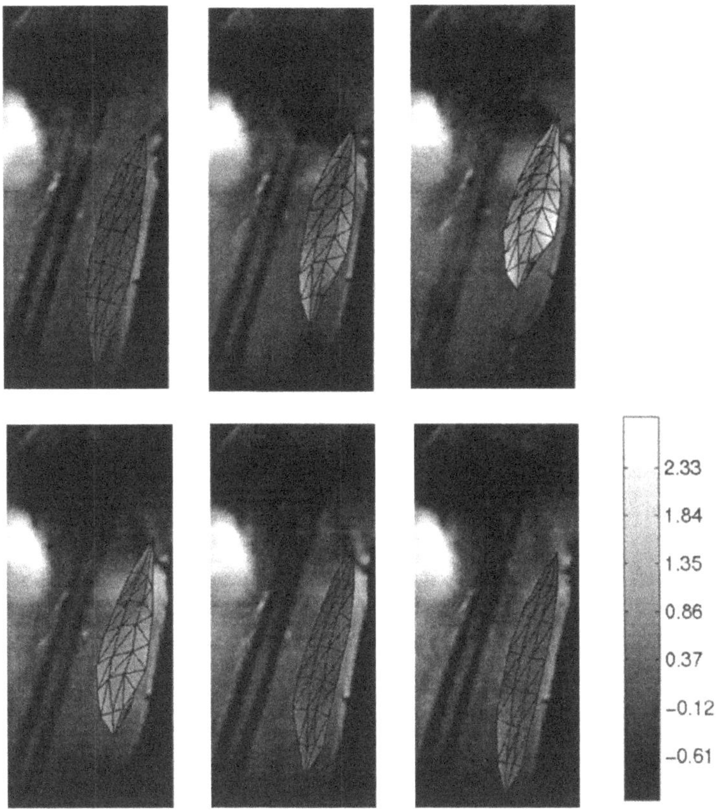

Figure 10.11: Biceps: reconstructed maximum principal strain field across the estimated mesh configuration is represented as shades of gray and overlaid on the magnitude images (time frames 2, 6, 10, 14, 18 and 22 out of 24). (From Zhu and Pelc, ref [56], Copyright 1999 IEEE.)

standard deviation in the measured vertical or horizontal displacement of each tag point was 0.12 mm.

The DMESH algorithm was used to analyze the same 4-element mesh as in case B of Section 11.3.1. The tagging data contributed additional equations that were based on the displacement modeling (Equation (10.20) in its component-wise form). A weighted least squares solution to the whole set of equations (velocity from PC and displacement from tagging) provided estimations of the Fourier coefficients of the nodal points' trajectories. For each mesh element and each time instant, the center point position $\boldsymbol{x}_c$, the deformation gradient tensor $\boldsymbol{F}$, and the strain tensor $\boldsymbol{E}$ were derived from the model and the coefficients. These were compared to the true values. A total of 1000 experiments were performed to measure the mean and standard deviation of the quantities. The averages of the estimated quantities (center point position and deformation gradient) indicate that the results are of the same level of accuracy as that of case B of Section 11.3.1. In Figure 10.12, the standard deviation of the estimated quantities within the filled triangle element in the present case is shown, along with results from case B of Section 11.3.1 (included as a comparison). The figure suggests good agreement between the theoretically predicted and experimentally measured standard deviations, and shows that incorporating the displacement information resulted in lower standard deviations. Note that the improvements are most noticeable in the time frames where displacement data are available. The improvement in reproducibility is again consistent with the theoretical prediction.

10.4 Discussion

At the core of the DMESH method is the dynamic mesh model, which expresses complex deforming motion with time-varying finite elements and provides a flexible trade-off between accuracy and reproducibility through built-in spatiotemporal smoothing. Compared to methods that use local models, analyzing a single element with DMESH and analyzing a similarly-sized region with a local method (e.g., [43]) have about the same reproducibility. With DMESH however, extending the finite element mesh by adding more elements offers enhanced reproducibility, while at the same time, due to the element-wise parameterization, high estimation accuracy that is comparable to that of the local method can still be obtained. Further, simultaneously taking into account all measurements from the analyzed region enables DMESH to extract a cohesive view of the object motion, which is difficult to achieve with a local method.

Assuming the input data is reasonably accurate, motion tracking and strain quantification accuracy is then primarily determined by the mesh element sizes specified, the shape functions used and the Fourier harmonics included. In theory, as the finite element mesh is further and further refined, the displacement field associated with the object's motion and its spatial derivatives approach constant values over each element domain, ensuring that the spatial variation of the motion can

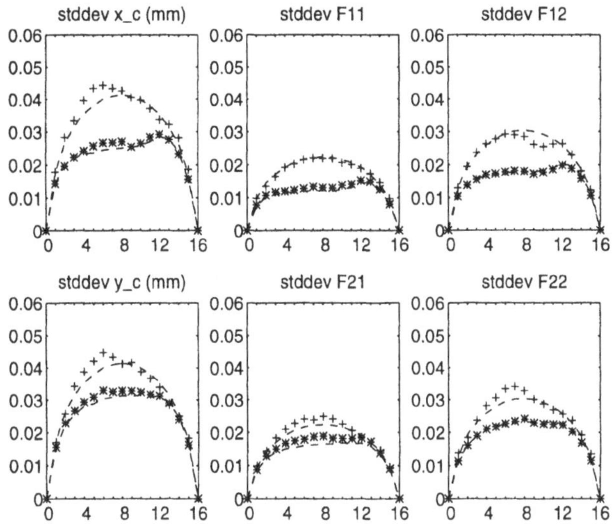

Figure 10.12: Standard deviation of the computed center point position (x_c and y_c) and deformation gradient (F_{ij}) as functions of time frame — dashed line: theoretical prediction, cross: with velocity samples only, star: with both velocity and displacement samples. (From Zhu and Pelc, ref [56], Copyright 1999 IEEE.)

be represented with sufficient accuracy. Alternatively, increasing the order of the polynomial shape functions while retaining the same mesh element dimensions will also improve model accuracy. However, due to the finite spatial resolution of the data, one cannot arbitrarily refine the mesh or increase the order of the shape functions without rendering the problem ill-posed. As the determination of the model parameters is not sufficiently supported by the data, the matrix **A** becomes singular. The situation is similar with the temporal modeling. Higher accuracy in the temporal domain is achievable by including more Fourier harmonics, with a limit that the highest harmonic frequency must not exceed half the temporal sampling frequency.

Of equal importance, we note that as we refine the spatial/temporal modeling for higher accuracy, the reproducibility of the estimates tends to get worse (prior to reaching the ill-posedness extreme). This tradeoff between accuracy and reproducibility is intrinsic to a modeling process, but with the DMESH method a good balance is achievable. In the spatial domain, the tradeoff can be handled by appropriately adjusting the initial mesh definition, making the elements' sizes match the expected local deformation heterogeneity. In the temporal domain, smoothing can be introduced by incorporating low-pass filtering (attaching appropriate weights to the exponentials in Equations (10.11) and (10.20)) [41]. Guidance from the computed covariance matrix could be helpful when adjusting the initial mesh definition and the filtering weights. Alternatively, one can introduce regularization into the modeling to restore well-posedness or improve reproducibility, which may be particularly effective when data is under-sampled or nonuniformly-sampled.

The DMESH method may be extended to analyze motion information from various sources. In the particular case where both velocity and displacement information is encoded with a hybrid tagging-PC technique, a computer simulation demonstrated that an improved performance was achievable by an extended version of the DMESH method that uses both velocity and displacement measurements. Processing of the velocity data requires temporal integration. Propagation of velocity measurement noise through this integration causes uncertainty in the tracking and deformation quantification results which is characterized by a curve that typically peaks at the middle of the motion cycle [56]. When analyzing the displacement data, temporal integration is not necessary. The effect of displacement measurement noise is characterized by a curve that is usually much flatter during the time the tags are detectable. Incorporating displacement data into the analysis thus not only improves the overall reproducibility but also tends to flatten the uncertainty curve (Figure 10.12). Furthermore, the combination of PC velocity data and tagging displacement data may represent a denser sampling of the motion field and thus have the potential to support higher order element-wise modeling for improving quantification accuracy.

On the data acquisition front, current state of the art imaging capabilities, certainly with PC imaging but even with MR tagging, still fall short of providing high quality time-resolved volumetric data in a clinically acceptable scan time. The volume coverage as a result, is routinely compromised. The presented *in vivo* data were obtained with single slice acquisitions, and thus the DMESH tracking had to ignore the through-plane motion component. In the presence of nontrivial 3-D motion and deformation, such a 2-D approach may cause significant errors in the motion field reconstruction [63] and may lead to unusually high strain estimates at some locations. We expect 3-D DMESH analysis will avoid this problem and provide accurate and precise *in vivo* measurements. With the current activity toward developing more rapid and efficient readout and spatial encoding methods (e.g., [64,65]), we anticipate the emergence of a significantly faster MR imaging technology which makes clinical examinations of 3-D motion/deformation a reality.

Acknowledgments

The authors thank Drs. M. Drangova and J.O. Fredrickson for assisting in the phantom experiments, and Drs. R.J. Herfkens, G. Pappas and J.E. Drace for providing human subject data. Much of the presented work received grant sponsorships from NIH, GE Medical Systems, Phil N. Allen Trust and the Lucas Foundation.

References

[1] E. Zerhouni, D. Parish, W. Rogers, A. Yang, and E. Shapiro. Human heart: tagging with MR imaging – a method for noninvasive assessment of myocardial motion. Radiology 169: 59-63 (1988).

[2] L. Axel and L. Dougherty. MR imaging of motion with spatial modulation of magnetization. Radiology 172: 349-350 (1989).

[3] L. Axel and L. Dougherty. Heart wall motion: improved method of spatial modulation of magnetization for MR imaging. Radiology 172: 349-350 (1989).

[4] L. Axel. Three-dimensional MR imaging of heart wall motion. Radiology 173: 233 (1989)

[5] E. R. McVeigh and E. Zerhouni. Noninvasive measurement of transmural gradients in myocardial strain with MR imaging. Radiology 180: 677-683 (1991)

[6] P. Van Dijk. Direct cardiac NMR imaging of heart wall and blood flow velocity. Journal Computer Assisted Tomography 8: 429-436 (1984).

[7] G. L. Nayler, D. N. Firmin, and D. B. Longmore. Blood flow imaging by cine magnetic resonance. Journal of Computer Assisted Tomography 10:715-722 (1986).

[8] N. J. Pelc, R. J. Herfkens, A. Shimakawa, and D. R. Enzmann. Phase Contrast Cine Magnetic Resonance Imaging. Magnetic Resonance Quarterly 7: 229-254 (1991).

[9] V. J. Wedeen. Magnetic resonance imaging of myocardial kinematics. Technique to detect, localize, and quantify the strain rates of active human myocardium. Magn. Reson. Med. 27: 52-67 (1992).

[10] N. J. Pelc, R. J. Herfkens, and L. R. Pelc. 3D analysis of myocardial motion and deformation with phase contrast cine MRI. Proc. SMRM. 18 (1992).

[11] M. V. Herman and R. Gorlin. Implications of left ventricular asynergy. American Journal of Cardiology, 23:538-547, (1969).

[12] W. A. Baxley and T. J. Reeves. Abnormal regional myocardial performance in coronary artery disease. Progress in Cardiovascular Diseases, 13:405-421, (1971).

[13] M. V. Herman, R. A. Heinle, M. D. Klein, and R. Gorlin. Localized disorders in myocardial contraction. New England Journal of Medicine 227:222-232 (1967).

[14] J. S. Borer, S. L. Bacharach, M. V. Green, K. M. Kent, S. E. Epstein, and G. S. Johnston. Real-time radionuclide cineangiography in the noninvasive evaluation of global and regional left ventricular function at rest and during exercise in patients with coronary-artery disease. New England Journal of Medicine 296:839-844 (1977).

[15] J. Tillisch, R. Brunken, R. Marshall, M. Schwaiger, M. Mandelkern, M. Phelps, and H. Schelbert. Reversibility of cardiac wall-motion abnormalities predicted by positron tomography. New England Journal of Medicine 314:884-888 (1986).

[16] A. N. Lieberman, J. L. Weiss, B. I. Judgutt, and et al. Two-dimensional echocardiography and infarct size: relationship of regional wall motion and thickening to the extent of myocardial infarction in the dog. Circulation 63:739-746 (1981).

[17] J. F. Ren, M. N. Kotler, A. H. Hakki, I. P. Panidis, G. S. Mintz, and J. Ross. Quantification of regional left ventricular function by two-dimensional echocardiography. 1. Pattern of contraction of the normal ventricle. American Heart Journal 110:552-560 (1985).

[18] P. E. Assmann, C. J. Slager, S. G. Van der Borden, J. G. P. Tijssen, J. A. Oomen, and J. R. Roelandt. Comparison of models for quantitative left ventricular wall motion analysis from two-dimensional echocardiograms during acute myocardial infarction. American Journal of Cardiology 71:1262-1269 (1993).

[19] R. F. Mattrey and C. B. Higgins. Detection of regional myocardial dysfunction during ischemia with computerized tomography: documentation and physiologic basis. Investigative Radiology 17:329-335 (1982).

[20] D. Farmer, M. J. Lipton, C. B. Higgins, H. Ringertz, P. B. Dean, R. Sievers, and D. P. Boyd. *In vivo* assessment of left ventricular wall and chamber dynamics during transient myocardial ischemia using cine computed tomography. American Journal of Cardiology 55:560-565 (1985).

[21] M. R. Fisher, G. K. von Schulthess, and C. B. Higgins. Multiphasic cardiac magnetic resonance imaging: normal regional left ventricular wall thickening. American Journal of Roentgenology 145:27-40 (1985).

[22] C. B. Higgins, W. Holt, P. Pflugfelder, and U. Sechtem. Functional evaluation of the heart with magnetic resonance imaging. Magnetic Resonance in Medicine 6:121-139 (1988).

[23] H. Sakuma, N. Fujita, T. K. F. Foo G. R. Caputo, S. J. Nelson, J. Hartiala, A. Shimakawa, and C. B. Higgins. Evaluation of left ventricular volume and mass with breath-hold cine MR imaging. Radiology 188:377-380 (1993).

[24] E. R. Holman, H. W. Vliegen, R. J. van der Geest, J. H. C. Reiber, P. R. M. van Dijkman, A. van der Laarse, A. de Roos, and E. E. van der Wall. Quantitative analysis of regional left ventricular function after myocardial infarction in the pig assessed with cine magnetic resonance imaging. Magnetic Resonance in Medicine 34:161-169 (1995).

[25] H. L. Falsetti, M. L. Marcus, R. E. Kerber, and D. J. Skorton. Quantification of myocardial ischemia and infarction by left ventricular imaging. Circulation 63: 747-751 (1981).

[26] L. Axel, R. C. Goncalves, and D. Bloomgarden. Regional heart wall motion: two-dimensional analysis and functional imaging with MR imaging. Radiology 183: 745-750 (1992).

[27] N. B. Ingels, G. T. Daughters, E. B. Stinson, and E. L. Alderman. Measurements of midwall dynamics in intact man by radiography of surgically implanted markers. Circulation 52:859-867 (1975).

[28] C. J. Slager, T. E. H. Hooghoudt, P. W. Serruys, J. C. H. Schuurbiers, J. H. C. Reiber, G. T. Meester, P. D. Verdouw, and P. G. Hugenholtz. Quantitative assessment of regional left ventricular motion using endocardial landmarks. Journal of the American College of Cardiology 7:317-326 (1986).

[29] H. C. Kim, B. G. Min, M. M. Lee, J. D. Seo, Y. W. Lee, and M. C. Han. Estimation of local cardiac wall deformation and regional wall stress from biplane coronary cineangiograms. IEEE Trans. Biomed. Eng. 32:503-511 (1985).

[30] C. W. Chen and T. S. Huang. Epicardial motion and deformation estimation from coronary artery bifurcation points. Proc. of 3rd International Conference on Computer Vision, pp. 456-459 (1990).

[31] A. A. Young. Epicardial deformation from coronary cineangiograms. In L. Glass, P. Hunter, A. McCulloch, eds., Theory of Heart: biomechanics, biophysics, and nonlinear dynamics of cardiac function New York, Springer-Verlag, pp. 175-207 (1991).

[32] J. S. Rankin, P. A. McHale, C. E. Arentzen, D. Ling, J. C. Greenfield, and R. W. Anderson. The three-dimensional dynamic geometry of the left ventricle in the conscious dog. Circulation Research 39:304-313 (1976).

[33] P. Theroux, J. J. Ross, D. Franklin, J. Covell, C. Bloor, and S. Sasayama. Regional myocardial function and dimensions early and late after myocardial infarction in the unanesthetized dog. Circulation Research 40:158-165, (1977).

[34] F. J. Villarreal, L. K. Waldman and W. Y. W. Lew. Technique for measuring regional two-dimensional finite strains in canine left ventricle. Circulation Research 62:711-721 (1988).

[35] J. H. Myers, M. C. Stirling, M. Choy, A. J. Buda, and K. P. Gallagher. Direct measurement of inner and outer wall thickening dynamics with epicardial echocardiography. Circulation 74:164-172 (1986).

[36] D. C. Harrison, A. Goldblatt, E. Braunwald, G. Glick, and D. T. Mason. Studies on cardiac dimensions in intact unanesthetized man. Circulation Research, 13:448-467 (1963).

[37] R. W. Brower, H. J. ten Katen, and G. T. Meester. Direct method for determining regional myocardial shortening after bypass surgery from radiopaque markers in man. American Journal of Cardiology 41:1222-1229 (1978).

[38] N. B. Ingels, G. T. Daughters, E. B. Stinson, and E. L. Alderman. Evaluation of methods for quantitating left ventricular segmental wall motion in man using myocardial markers as a standard. Circulation 61:966-972 (1980).

[39] G. Daughters, W. Sanders, D. Miller, A. Schwarzkopf, C. Mead, and N. Ingels. A comparison of two analytical systems for 3-D reconstruction from biplane videoradiograms. Computers in Cardiology, 15:79-82 (1989).

[40] E. L. Hahn. Detection of sea-water motion by nuclear precession. Journal of Geophysical Research 65:776-777 (1960).

[41] Y. Zhu, M. Drangova, and N. J. Pelc. Fourier tracking of myocardial motion using cine PC data. Magn. Reson. Med. 35: 471-480 (1996).

[42] A. A. Young and L. Axel. Three-dimensional motion and deformation of the heart wall: estimation with spatial modulation of magnetization – a model-based approach. Radiology 185:241-247 (1992).

[43] Y. Zhu, M. Drangova and N. J. Pelc. Estimation of deformation gradient and strain from cine-PC velocity data. IEEE Transactions on Medical Imaging vol. 16, no. 6, pp. 840-851 (1997).

[44] N. R. Clark, N. Reichek, P. Bergey, E. A. Hoffman, D. Brownson, L. Palmon, and L. Axel. Circumferential Myocardial Shortening in the Normal Human Left Ventricle. Circulation 84: 67-74 (1991).

[45] R. J. Herfkens, N. J. Pelc, L. R. Pelc, and J. R. Sayre. Right ventricular strain measured by phase contrast MRI. Proc. SMRM. 163 (1991).

[46] R. T. Constable, K. M. Rath, A. J. Sinusas, and J. C. Gore. Development and evaluation of tracking algorithms for cardiac wall motion analysis using phase velocity MR mapping. Magn. Reson. Med. 32: 33-42 (1994).

[47] N. J. Pelc, M. Drangova, L. R. Pelc, Y. Zhu, D. Noll, B. Bowman, and R. J. Herfkens. Tracking of cyclical motion using phase contrast cine MRI velocity data. JMRI 5:339-345 (1995).

[48] A. Lingamneni, P. A. Hardy, K. Powell, N. J. Pelc, and R. D. White. Validation of cine phase-contrast MR imaging for motion analysis. JMRI 5: 331-338 (1995).

[49] D. Terzopoulos and D. Metaxas. Dynamic 3D models with local and global deformations: deformable superquadrics. PAMI, vol. 13, no. 7, pp. 703-714 (1991).

[50] W. G. O'Dell, C. C. Moore, W. C. Hunter, E. A. Zerhouni, and E. R. McVeigh. Displacement field fitting for calculating 3D myocardial deformations from tagged MR images. Radiology 195:829-835 (1995).

[51] T. J. R. Hughes. The Finite Element Method: Linear Static and Dynamic Finite Element Analysis. Prentice-Hall (1987).

[52] A. Pentland and B. Horowitz. Recovery of nonrigid motion and structure. PAMI, vol. 13, no. 7, pp. 730-742 (1991).

[53] F. G. Meyer, R. T. Constable, A. J. Sinusas, and J. S. Duncan. Tracking Myocardial Deformation Using Phase Contrast MR Velocity Fields: A Stochastic Approach. IEEE Trans. Med. Imaging vol. 15, no. 4: 453-465 (1996).

[54] Y. Zhu and N. J. Pelc. Myocardial function analysis using a spatiotemporal finite element mesh model and cine-PC velocity data. Proc. of the 5th meeting of the ISMRM, p. 464 (1997).

[55] Y. Zhu and N. J. Pelc. A spatiotemporal finite element mesh model of cyclical deforming motion and its application in myocardial motion analysis using phase contrast MR images. Proc. IEEE International Conference on Image Processing, vol II, pp. 117-120 (1997).

[56] Y. Zhu and N. J. Pelc. A spatiotemporal model of cyclic kinematics and its application to analyzing nonrigid motion with MR velocity images. IEEE Transactions on Medical Imaging vol. 18, no. 7, pp. 557-569 (1999).

[57] Y. Zhu, M. Drangova, and N. J. Pelc. Fourier tracking of myocardial motion using cine PC data. Proc. of the 2nd meeting of the Society of Magnetic Resonance, p. 1477 (1994).

[58] M. Drangova, Y. Zhu, B. S. Bowman, and N. J. Pelc. *In vitro* verification of myocardial-motion tracking from phase-contrast velocity data. Magnetic Resonance Imaging, 16:863-870 (1998).

[59] A. Amini and J. Duncan. Pointwise tracking of left-ventricular motion in 3-D. Proc. IEEE Workshop on Visual Motion, pp. 294-298 (1991).

[60] S. K. Mishra and D. B. Goldgof. Motion analysis and modeling of epicardial surfaces from point and line correspondences. Proc. IEEE Workshop on Visual Motion, pp. 300-305 (1991).

[61] A. A. Young, L. Axel, L. Dougherty, D. K. Bogen, and C. S. Parenteau. Validation of Tagging with MR Imaging to Estimate Material Deformation. Radiology 188:101-108 (1993).

[62] M. Drangova, B. Bowman, and N. J. Pelc. Physiologic motion phantom for MRI applications. JMRI 6:513-518 (1996).

[63] Y. Zhu and N. J. Pelc. Three-dimensional motion tracking with volumetric phase contrast MR velocity imaging. Journal of Magnetic Resonance Imaging, 9:111-118 (1999).

[64] D. N. Firmin, P. D. Gatehouse, G. Z. Yang, P. Jhooti, and J. Keegan. A 7-dimensional echo-planar flow imaging technique using a novel k-space sampling scheme with velocity compensation. Proc. of the 5th meeting of the ISMRM, p. 118 (1997).

[65] D. K. Sodickson and W. J. Manning. Simultaneous acquisition of spatial harmonics (SMASH): fast imaging with radiofrequency coil arrays. Magn. Reson. Med. 38: 591-603 (1997).

[66] Y. Zhu. Quantifying cyclic motion and deformation with magnetic resonance velocity images. Ph.D. Dissertation, Department of Electrical Engineering, Stanford University, Palo Alto, California, 1998.

Chapter 11

Computational Platforms for Integrated Cardiac Image Analysis

Xenophon Papademetris
Department of Diagnostic Radiology,
Yale University School of Medicine,
New Haven, Connecticut 06520-8042
papad@noodle.med.yale.edu

Albert J. Sinusas
Section of Cardiovascular Medicine, Department of Internal Medicine,
Yale University School of Medicine,
New Haven, Connecticut 06520-8042

James S. Duncan
Department of Diagnostic Radiology, Department of Electrical Engineering,
Yale University School of Medicine,
New Haven, Connecticut 06520-8042

11.1 Introduction

Ischemic heart disease is a major clinical problem. Myocardial injury caused by ischemic heart disease is often regional, and causes regional alterations in the deformation patterns in the left ventricle (LV). It is the fundamental goal of many forms of cardiac imaging and image analysis to measure the regional function of the LV in an effort to isolate the location and extent of ischemic or infarcted myocardium.

There has been a lot of work in medical image analysis to estimate 3D cardiac deformation non-invasively from image data, as this book demonstrates. (See also a recent review article [31]). In the case of magnetic resonance imaging, the image data utilized are typically acquired in 16–20 frames consisting of 10–16 slices each. Alternative sources of image data are 3D echocardiography, and 3D cine-CT. Most

A.A. Amini and J.L. Prince (eds.),
Measurement of Cardiac Deformations from MRI: Physical and Mathematical Models, 289–313.

researchers have focused almost exclusively on the motion and deformation of the left ventricle. More recently, however, some preliminary work on right ventricular deformation has also appeared in the literature [17], and in Chapter 5 of this book.

The primary emphasis of this chapter is on the development of a methodology for the estimation of cardiac image deformation from a any one of a variety of image modalities, and especially the important aspect of properly modeling the myocardium in order to ensure reliable and robust estimation of this deformation. Modeling is needed as the image-derived displacement estimates generated from a number of methods (to be described in section 2) have the following characteristics:

- They are *sparse*. Displacements and/or velocities are only available at certain points and not the whole of the myocardium.
- They are *noise-corrupted*. This is an inherent problem in all medical image analysis methods, although the level of noise is very method dependent.
- They may contain only *partial* information. Even where displacements and/or velocities are available, only a certain component of the displacement vector may be known.

The selection of an appropriate model and an appropriate modeling framework are of great importance for the estimation of complete and smooth displacement fields which in turn will allow us to estimate the complete cardiac deformation that is typically expressed in terms of myocardial strains. (Strain is defined in section 11.3.1; see also Chapter 1).

The rest of this chapter reads as follows. In section 2 we briefly describe various methods for the estimation of displacements. With the exception of the shape-tracking method, all of these techniques have been described in more detail in the previous chapters (see Chapters 3–5). In section 3, we describe in more detail the process of modeling the left ventricle and creating an estimation framework that represents an approach for integrating image derived information and estimating the complete displacement field. In section 4, we present some experimental results from the application of this methodology. Some possible future research directions are presented in section 5.

11.2 Obtaining Estimates of Cardiac Displacements

11.2.1 Methods Relying on Magnetic Resonance Tagging

In magnetic resonance tagging, grid lines at certain positions can be generated at one point in the cardiac cycle and their deformation tracked over a portion of the cycle using gated acquisition techniques. The development of the cardiac tagging approach to the measurement of myocardial strain has been vigorously pursued by two groups in particular: the University of Pennsylvania [3] and Johns Hopkins [27], who are the original developers of the tagging ideas.

Much of these groups' current efforts are focused on how to create dense fields of measurements in 3D by putting together several orthogonal tagging grid acquisitions. Their approaches certainly show promise, because of the inherent capability of including discernible patterns that deform with the tissue, but currently have the following limitations:

i.) It is difficult to track the tags over the *complete* LV cycle due to decay of the tags with time.

ii.) Multiple acquisitions are required to assemble 3D information.

iii.) It is still non-trivial to assemble the detected tags into a robust 3D analysis/display.

All of these problems are being aggressively pursued by the two primary groups mentioned above, as well as at a few other institutions (e.g. Amini [1]).

In general, there seem to be three different approaches to estimating initial displacement data from magnetic resonance tagging as follows:

- Tagging in multiple intersecting planes and using the tag intersections as tokens for tracking [1,25,48].
- Tagging in multiple intersecting planes and then for each tagging plane estimating the magnitude of the motion perpendicular to the plane. This generates a sense of partial displacements (i.e. the component parallel to the tag lines is missing) to be combined later [8,17,21].
- Attempting to model the tag fading over time using a model for the Bloch equations and using a variable brightness optical flow approach to extract the displacements [16,39].

The details of these methods are explored in Chapters 4-8 of this book.

11.2.2 Methods Relying on Phase Contrast MRI

Several investigators have employed changes in phase due to motion of tissue within a fixed voxel or volume of interest to assist in estimating instantaneous, localized velocities, and ultimately cardiac motion and deformation. While the basic ideas were first suggested by van Dijk [46] and Nayler [29], it was Pelc and his team [36–38] that first bridged the technique to conventional cine MR imaging and permitted the tracking of myocardial motion throughout the cardiac cycle (see also Chapters 9 & 10 of this book). In general there seem to be the following two common approaches to extracting useful information from phase contrast images:

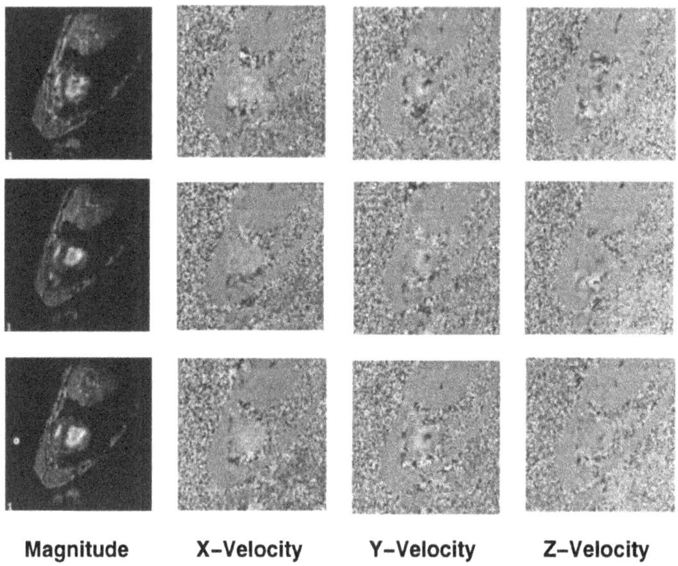

Figure 11.1: Three-slice thick volumetric dataset obtained using magnetic resonance phase contrast images. The left column shows the magnitude images for the three slices and the other columns show the components of the velocity in the X, Y and Z directions respectively. From Shi et al [41]

- Processing the data directly to estimate strain rate tensors [37, 47].
- Integrating the velocities over time, via some form of tracking mechanism to estimate displacements [7, 18, 28, 49].

We also note that Shi [41] combined the phase-contrast velocities with shape-based displacements [42] within an integrated framework based on continuum mechanics.

11.2.3 Computer-Vision Based Methods

Quantifying the deformation of the LV could be seen as a two-step process: first establishing correspondence between certain points on the LV at time t and time $t+1$; and second, using these correspondences as guides, to solve for a complete mapping the of the LV between any two time frames. This problem could be posed for the entire myocardium or just portions of it, such as the endocardial surface alone.

One common approach to establishing correspondence is to track shape-related features on the LV over time as reported by Duncan [10], Amini [2], Kambhamettu [24], Cohen [6], McEachen [26] and Shi [42]. The preliminary displacement estimates here are, in general, generated using the following steps:

1. First extract the endocardial and epicardial surfaces from the images.

2. Then calculate the quantity that is used as the shape feature from these surfaces. These tend to be the curvatures; either the principal curvatures [42] or the Gaussian curvature [24].

3. Track points on the surfaces from one frame to the next by minimizing a metric such as bending energy or difference in curvature.

Then the displacement field is smoothed (as was the case with previous methods) to produce the final output displacements. A validation study of shape-based tracking by comparing trajectories with implanted markers was reported by Shi [42], which found that the accuracy of tracking was within the resolution of the image voxel sizes. Another interesting approach by Tagare [44] poses the mapping problem in 2D as a bimorphism between two curves, thus eliminating the basic asymmetry in the tracking process. This, last idea, has not been extended to 3D yet.

In general, all of the methods here depend on an accurate segmentation of the LV surfaces, but have the advantage of being imaging-modality-independent. They have been used on MR, CT [42], and 3D ultrasound [34]. The dependency on obtaining an accurate segmentation, however, remains a significant issue, as there are still no fully automated, robust, and efficient LV surface segmentation methods. The accuracy of the LV segmentation needed for these methods to be successful is obviously greater than in the case of methods using MR tagging. This is because the surfaces themselves provide the features as opposed to being bounding surfaces within which to search for intersections.

11.2.4 The Shape-Based Tracking Approach

In this section we describe the curvature tracking approach as this was implemented in the work of Shi [42] and subsequently extended by Papademetris [34]. Displacement data generated using this technique are used to form most of the results presented later in this chapter.

Curvature Computation

Before proceeding to describe the curvature tracking technique, we define what is meant by the principal curvatures. Given any point p on a differentiable surface we can find a local parameterization x parameterized along vectors u and v. We also define the outward normal of the surface at this point to be N. (In practice, we fit a bi-quadratic surface patch to the neighborhood of p and then use this surface to define the local parameterization (u, v) close to point p [42].)

We then proceed to define the following quantities at point $p = (u_0, v_0)$:

$$\begin{aligned}
E(u_0, v_0) &= < \mathbf{x}_u, \mathbf{x}_u >, & (11.1)\\
F(u_0, v_0) &= < \mathbf{x}_u, \mathbf{x}_v >, & (11.2)\\
G(u_0, v_0) &= < \mathbf{x}_v, \mathbf{x}_v >, & (11.3)\\
e(u_0, v_0) &= - < N_u, \mathbf{x}_u > = < N, \mathbf{x}_{uu} >, & (11.4)\\
f(u_0, v_0) &= - < N_v, \mathbf{x}_u > = < N, \mathbf{x}_{uv} > = - < N_u, \mathbf{x}_v >, & (11.5)\\
g(u_0, v_0) &= - < N_v, \mathbf{x}_v > = < N, \mathbf{x}_{vv} >, & (11.6)
\end{aligned}$$

where $\mathbf{x}_u$ signifies the derivative of $\mathbf{x}$ with respect to u.

These quantities which appear in the definition of the first and second fundamental forms of the surface [9] enable us to define the the *Weingarten Mapping Matrix* as follows:

$$[\beta] = -\begin{pmatrix} e & f \\ f & g \end{pmatrix}\begin{pmatrix} E & F \\ F & G \end{pmatrix}^{-1}. \tag{11.7}$$

This is also known as the shape operator matrix of the surface. This matrix determines surface shape by relating the intrinsic geometry of the surface to the Euclidean (extrinsic) geometry of the embedding space. The *Gaussian curvature* of a surface can be defined from the Weingarten mapping matrix as its determinant:

$$K = det[\beta] = \frac{eg - f^2}{EG - F^2}. \tag{11.8}$$

Meanwhile, the *mean curvature* of a surface is similarly defined as half of the trace of the Weingarten mapping matrix:

$$H = \frac{tr[\beta]}{2} = \frac{eG - 2fF + gE}{2(EG - F^2)}. \tag{11.9}$$

We also define the principal curvatures which are the eigenvalues of the Weingarten mapping matrix, with their directions along the two eigenvectors. They are can be calculated in terms of the Gaussian and mean curvatures as:

$$\begin{aligned}
\kappa_1 &= H + \sqrt{H^2 - K}, & (11.10)\\
\kappa_2 &= H - \sqrt{H^2 - K}. & (11.11)
\end{aligned}$$

The Shape-Tracking Algorithm

The first step in this algorithm is to estimate for all points on the first surface their symmetric nearest neighbor [33]. Next, for any given point p_1 on a surface s_1 at time t_1 and which has a corresponding point p_2 on surface s_2 at time t_2 as a result of the symmetric nearest neighbor estimation step, we construct a plausible

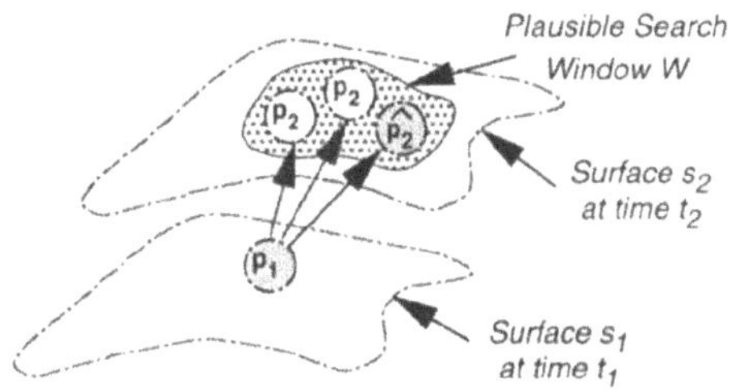

Figure 11.2: Example of the shape-tracking approach. The goal here is to map the original surface to the final surface. For a point p_1 on the original surface a window W of plausible matching points on the final surface is first generated. Then the point p_2 in W which has the most similar shape-properties to p_1 is selected as the candidate match point. The distance function for shape-similarity is typically based on the curvature(s).

search window W on s_2. This search window W consists of all the points on s_2 that have a connectivity distance less than a threshold t from p_2 on s_2; i.e. $p_w \in W$ iff $d_c(p_2, p_w) < t$, where the connectivity distance is defined in terms of the surface triangulation.

Next, a search is performed within this plausible region W on the deformed surface s_2 and the point $\hat{p}_2$ which has the local shape properties closest to those p_1 is selected. The shape properties here are captured in terms of the principal curvatures κ_1 and κ_2.

This is illustrated in figure 11.2. The distance measure used is the bending energy required to bend a curved plate or surface patch to a newly deformed state. This is labeled as d_{be} and is defined as [40]:

$$d_{be}(p1, p2) = \left(\frac{(\kappa_1(p_1) - \kappa_1(p_2))^2 + (\kappa_2(p_1) - \kappa_2(p_2))^2}{2} \right). \tag{11.12}$$

The displacement estimate vector for each point p_1, u_1^m is given by

$$u_1^m = \hat{p}_2 - p_1 \quad , \quad \hat{p}_2 = \arg\min_{p_2 \in W} \left[d_{be}(p1, p2) \right].$$

Confidence Measures

The bending energy measures for all the points inside the search region W are recorded as the basis to measure the *goodness* and *uniqueness* of the matching choices. The value of the minimum bending energy in the search region between the matched points indicates the goodness of the match. Denoting this value as m_g, we have the following measure for match goodness:

$$m_g(p_1) = -d_{be}(p_1, \hat{p}_2)\,. \tag{11.13}$$

On the other hand, it is desirable that the chosen matching point be a unique choice among the candidate points within the search window. Ideally, the bending energy value of the chosen point should be much smaller than the values of the rest of the points. If we denote the mean values of the bending energy measures of all the points inside window W except the chosen point as $\bar{d}_{be}$ and the standard deviation as σ^d_{be}, we define the uniqueness measure as:

$$m_u(p_1) = \frac{d_{be}(p_1, \hat{p}_2)}{\bar{d}_{be} - \sigma^d_{be}}\,. \tag{11.14}$$

This uniqueness measure has a high value if the bending energy of the chosen point is small compared to some smaller value (mean minus standard deviation) of the remaining bending energy measures. Combining these two measures together, we arrive at one *confidence measure* $c^m(p_1)$ for the matched point $\hat{p}_2$ of point p_1:

$$c^m(p_1) = \frac{1}{k_{1,g} + k_{2,g} m_g(p_1)} \times \frac{1}{k_{1,u} + k_{2,u} m_u(p_1)}\,, \tag{11.15}$$

where $k_{1,g}, k_{2,g}, k_{1,u}$, and $k_{2,u}$ are scaling constants for normalization purposes. We normalize the confidences to lie in the range 0 to 1.

Modeling the Initial Displacement Estimates

Given a set of displacement vector measurements u^m and confidence measures c^m, we model these estimates probabilistically by assuming that the noise in the individual measurements is normally distributed with zero mean and a variance $\sigma^2 = \frac{1}{c^m}$. In addition, we assume that the measurements are uncorrelated. This essentially models the measurement $u^m = u + n$ where n is the noise. Given these assumptions we can write the measurement probability for each point as:

$$p(u^m|u) = \frac{1}{\sqrt{2\pi\sigma^2}} e^{\frac{-(u-u^m)^2}{2\sigma^2}}\,. \tag{11.16}$$

11.3 Modeling used for Interpolation and Smoothing

The estimation of accurate myocardial deformation requires a dense, smooth, and complete displacement field. This is because the deformation is typically captured in terms of the strain, which is a function of the derivatives of the displacement field. The process of taking derivatives is very noise-sensitive and this is what makes this problem so challenging as compared to other measurement tasks. For example estimating the volume of the LV is an integral measure, and is therefore less sensitive to noise.

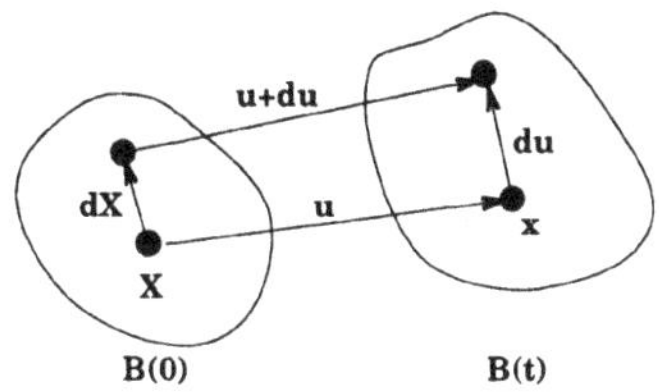

Figure 11.3: Definition of displacement

The methodology to be described in this section presupposes two underlying assumptions. The first is that the properties of the cardiac displacement field are best captured in terms of the mechanical properties of the tissue itself, as these have been described by work in biomechanics (see the article collections [22,30] as well as Chapter 1 of this book), introducing appropriate simplifications/linearizations as dictated by computational requirements. The second assumption is that we will proceed to model the image noise in the displacement estimates probabilistically. This general procedure is followed in many digital signal/image processing applications. By adopting these two assumptions we create a growth path for handling more complicated and difficult situations.

There are two primary alternative approaches which deserve mention here. The first is the so-called 'physics-based' vision paradigm (e.g Metaxas and Terzopoulos [45]). In this case the object is modeled using a mechanical model and data is applied using 'data-forces'. The limitation of this approach is that it tries to model the image noise in terms of forces, which makes incorporation of probabilistic noise models into such a framework problematic. The second approach is the general regularization framework (e.g. Horn and Schunk [20].) In this case the object is modeled as having a smooth displacement field by penalizing the derivatives of the displacement field. It can be shown (see [31, 33]) that this often is equivalent to a mechanical model that has a number of undesirable properties, such as lack of invariance to coordinate transformations.

The major goal of this section is to describe how to *consistently* incorporate knowledge of the mechanical properties of the left ventricle within an image analysis problem and to understand some of the underlying problems inherent in such an approach. To do so we first define the concepts of strain and a strain energy function, which are needed to define the material model. Then we demonstrate the relationship between such a material model and probabilistic models known as Markov random fields (MRF). Then we discuss issues related to unit reconciliation, and the presence of bias in the output estimates.

11.3.1 The Strain Tensor

In this section we follow the presentations in Spencer [43, chapter 6] and Hunter [23]. Consider a body $B(0)$ which after time t moves and deforms to body $B(t)$.

A material particle initially located at some position X on $B(0)$ moves to a new position x on $B(t)$. If we further assume that material cannot appear or disappear there will be an one-to-one correspondence between X and x, so we can always write the path of the particle as:

$$x = x(X, t)\,. \tag{11.17}$$

We can also define the displacement vector for this particle as

$$u(t) = x(t) - X\,. \tag{11.18}$$

This relationship is invertible, so that given x and t we can find X. Now consider two neighboring particles located at X and $X + dX$ on $B(0)$. In a new configuration $B(t)$, using 11.17 we can write:

$$dx = \frac{\partial x}{\partial X} dX\,. \tag{11.19}$$

The Jacobian matrix $F(t) = \partial x(t)/\partial X$ is called *the deformation gradient matrix.* We note that by definition $F(0) = I$, $u(0) = 0$. Using this, we can rewrite (11.17) more fully as:

$$\begin{aligned} dx(t) &= F(t)dX\,, \\ F_{ij} &= \frac{\partial x_i}{\partial X_j}\,, \\ &= \frac{\partial u_i}{\partial X_j} + \delta_{ij}\,, \end{aligned} \tag{11.20}$$

where δ_{ij} is equal to zero unless $i = j$.

The mapping defined by equations (11.17) through (11.20) has two components: a rigid motion component and a change in the shape or deformation of the object. For the purposes of capturing the material behavior we need to extract from F the component that is a function of the rigid motion and the component that is a function of the deformation.

Infinitesimal Deformations

If the deformations and the rotations are small, we use the approximation [43, section 6.6]:

$$\frac{\partial u}{\partial x} \approx \frac{\partial u}{\partial X}\,. \tag{11.21}$$

From here we can re-write $F = RU$ as:

$$F = RU = (I + \omega)(I + \epsilon) \approx I + \omega + \epsilon . \tag{11.22}$$

Here ω is the small rotation tensor and is antisymmetric. ϵ is the small(infinitesimal) strain tensor and is symmetric. Ignoring second order terms, we define ω and ϵ as:

$$\omega = \frac{1}{2}(F - F^t), \tag{11.23}$$

$$= \begin{bmatrix} 0 & \frac{1}{2}\left(\frac{\partial u_1}{\partial x_2} - \frac{\partial u_2}{\partial x_1}\right) & \frac{1}{2}\left(\frac{\partial u_1}{\partial x_3} - \frac{\partial u_3}{\partial x_1}\right) \\ \frac{1}{2}\left(\frac{\partial u_2}{\partial x_1} - \frac{\partial u_1}{\partial x_2}\right) & 0 & \frac{1}{2}\left(\frac{\partial u_2}{\partial x_3} - \frac{\partial u_3}{\partial x_2}\right) \\ \frac{1}{2}\left(\frac{\partial u_3}{\partial x_1} - \frac{\partial u_1}{\partial x_3}\right) & \frac{1}{2}\left(\frac{\partial u_3}{\partial x_2} - \frac{\partial u_2}{\partial x_3}\right) & 0 \end{bmatrix},$$

$$\epsilon = \frac{1}{2}(F + F^t) - I, \tag{11.24}$$

$$= \begin{bmatrix} \frac{\partial u_1}{\partial x_1} & \frac{1}{2}\left(\frac{\partial u_1}{\partial x_2} + \frac{\partial u_2}{\partial x_1}\right) & \frac{1}{2}\left(\frac{\partial u_1}{\partial x_3} + \frac{\partial u_3}{\partial x_1}\right) \\ \frac{1}{2}\left(\frac{\partial u_2}{\partial x_1} + \frac{\partial u_1}{\partial x_2}\right) & \frac{\partial u_2}{\partial x_2} & \frac{1}{2}\left(\frac{\partial u_2}{\partial x_3} + \frac{\partial u_3}{\partial x_2}\right) \\ \frac{1}{2}\left(\frac{\partial u_3}{\partial x_1} + \frac{\partial u_1}{\partial x_3}\right) & \frac{1}{2}\left(\frac{\partial u_3}{\partial x_2} + \frac{\partial u_2}{\partial x_3}\right) & \frac{\partial u_3}{\partial x_3} \end{bmatrix}. \tag{11.25}$$

Often, taking advantage of the symmetries these tensors are written in vector form as:

$$e = [\epsilon_{11}, \epsilon_{22}, \epsilon_{33}, \epsilon_{12}, \epsilon_{13}, \epsilon_{23}]^t, \theta = [0, 0, 0, \omega_{12}, \omega_{13}, \omega_{23}]^t,$$

This e is the classical definition for strain in infinitesimal linear elasticity [43].

Finite Deformations

The infinitesimal deformation measures are applicable only for very small deformations and rotations. In the case of soft-tissue deformation and specifically the left ventricle, these are not applicable. In this case we can define the *Lagrangian (or Green) strain* tensor E as:

$$E = \frac{1}{2}\left(F^t F - I\right). \tag{11.26}$$

The components of E become equal to zero when there is no deformation, and in the case of small deformations and rotations reduce to the strain tensor of classical infinitesimal elasticity theory, and provide a proper definition for the strain tensor in the case of larger deformations. We can also write this, in component form, as:

$$E_{ij} = \frac{1}{2}\left(\sum_k \frac{\partial x_k}{\partial X_i}\frac{\partial x_k}{\partial X_j} - \delta_{ij}\right) = \frac{1}{2}\left(\frac{\partial u_i}{\partial X_j} + \frac{\partial u_j}{\partial X_i} + \sum_k \frac{\partial u_k}{\partial X_i}\frac{\partial u_k}{\partial X_j}\right). \tag{11.27}$$

11.3.2 Material Models

So far we have restricted our description to the geometry of the deformation. In this section we extend this to account for what happens when a material deforms, and relate the deformation to the change in the internal structure of the material. Before proceeding to give examples of possible material models, we first note that there are some theoretical guidelines that must be observed [12]. The most important ones for this work are:

1. *The axiom of objectivity* – this requires the material model to be invariant with respect to rigid motion or the spatial frame of reference.

2. *The axiom of material invariance* – this implies certain symmetry conditions dependent on the type of anisotropy of the material, and implicitly reduces the number of free parameters.

The first axiom can be satisfied by postulating an internal or strain energy function that depends on the gradient deformation matrix F only through Green strain tensor E, or in small deformation cases, the infinitesimal strain tensor ϵ. The strain energy function serves as the material model.

Violation of the fist axiom leads to the following problem. Consider an internal energy that is not invariant to a global rotation. Assume also that work is needed to rotate the object clockwise. From conservation of energy principles, this energy will be returned when the object is turned counter-clockwise. We can keep turning the object counter-clockwise to get more and more energy and in this way we have created a *perpetual motion machine* and violated the second law of thermodynamics. Such an energy function is inadmissible as a material model.

Linear Elastic Energy Functions

In this section e will be used to denote the vector form of either the Green strain tensor E or the infinitesimal strain tensor ϵ as appropriate. The simplest useful continuum model in solid mechanics is the linear elastic one which is of the form:

$$W = \frac{1}{2}e^t C e, \tag{11.28}$$

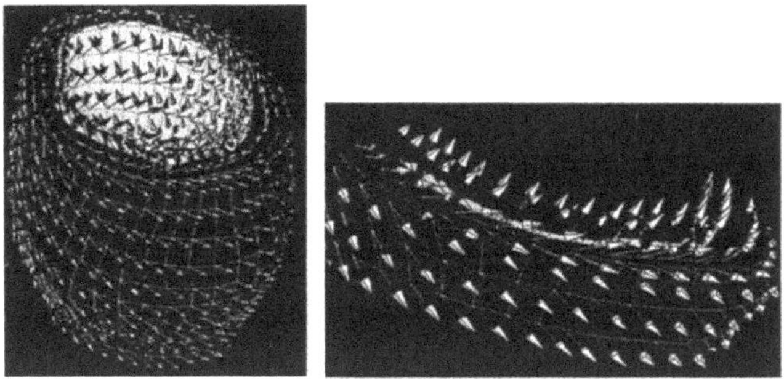

Figure 11.4: Fiber direction in the left ventricle as defined in Guccione et al [15]. Note on the small section shown on the right the transition of fiber angle from approximately -45 degrees (from the horizontal) on the epicardium to +90 degrees on the endocardium. More details can be found in Chapter 1 of this book.

where C is a 6×6 matrix and defines the material properties of the deforming body. The simplest model is the isotropic linear elastic model used elsewhere in the image analysis literature [11, 17]. In this case the matrix C takes the form:

$$C^{-1} = \frac{1}{E}\begin{bmatrix} 1 & -\nu & -\nu & 0 & 0 & 0 \\ -\nu & 1 & -\nu & 0 & 0 & 0 \\ -\nu & -\nu & 1 & 0 & 0 & 0 \\ 0 & 0 & 0 & 2(1+\nu) & 0 & 0 \\ 0 & 0 & 0 & 0 & 2(1+\nu) & 0 \\ 0 & 0 & 0 & 0 & 0 & 2(1+\nu) \end{bmatrix}, \qquad (11.29)$$

where E is the Young's modulus, which is a measure of the stiffness of the material, and ν is the Poisson's ratio, which is a measure of incompressibility.

In this work, the left ventricle of the heart is specifically modeled as a transversely elastic material to account for the preferential stiffness in the direction of the muscle fibers in the myocardium [15]. This is an extension of the isotropic linear elastic model which allows for one of the three material axis to have a different stiffness from the other two. In this case the matrix C takes the form:

$$C^{-1} = \begin{bmatrix} \frac{1}{E_p} & \frac{-\nu_p}{E_p} & \frac{-\nu_{fp}}{E_f} & 0 & 0 & 0 \\ \frac{-\nu_p}{E_p} & \frac{1}{E_p} & \frac{-\nu_{fp}}{E_f} & 0 & 0 & 0 \\ \frac{-\nu_{fp}E_f}{E_p} & \frac{-\nu_{fp}E_f}{E_p} & \frac{1}{E_f} & 0 & 0 & 0 \\ 0 & 0 & 0 & \frac{2(1+\nu_p)}{E_p} & 0 & 0 \\ 0 & 0 & 0 & 0 & \frac{1}{G_f} & 0 \\ 0 & 0 & 0 & 0 & 0 & \frac{1}{G_f} \end{bmatrix}, \qquad (11.30)$$

where E_f is the fiber stiffness, E_p is cross-fiber stiffness and ν_{fp}, ν_p are the corresponding Poisson's ratios and G_f is the shear modulus across fibers. ($G_f \approx E_f/(2(1 + \nu_{fp}))$. If $E_f = E_p$ and $\nu_p = \nu_{fp}$ this model reduces to the more common isotropic linear elastic model.

Non-Linear Energy Functions

Linear models do not capture the progressive hardening of many materials (especially soft tissue) when it is stretched. In the case of linear elastic models the effective stiffness is a constant with respect to the strain whereas in practice the stiffness increases as the strain increases. The reader is referred to Chapter 1 for more details.

A Probabilistic Interpretation of Material Models

As previously demonstrated by Geman and Geman [14] and applied to medical image analysis problems in [5, 13] there is a correspondence between an internal energy function and a Gibbs probability density function. If the mechanical model is described in terms of an internal energy function $W(C, u)$, where C represents the material properties and u the displacement field, then we can write an equivalent prior probability density function $p(u)$ of the Gibbs form [14]:

$$p(u) = k_1 \exp(-W(C, u)) \,, \tag{11.31}$$

where k_1 is a normalization constant.

Furthermore, we note that the Markov random field (MRF) then can be thought of as the probabilistic analog of the continuum mechanical model. There are two interesting similarities: (i) both can be defined using energy functions, and (ii) the energy functions at any given point have local support, i.e. they are functions only of the values at that point and its immediate neighbors. In the case of the MRF model, point (ii) comes from the fact that the the Gibbs probability density function is often defined on first and/or second order cliques which are very local neighborhoods of the point. So if the displacement field is modeled as a MRF, the probability of the displacement of a given point p effectively only depends on the displacement of its neighbors. In the case of the mechanical model described using a strain energy function, the value of the internal energy function, (which via exponentiation in (11.31) becomes the probability density function), at a given point depends only on the local strains. These local strains are only dependent on the displacements of the neighbors of the point and not on the displacements of the whole volume.

The expression of the mechanical model as a MRF allows us to solve the problem within a Bayesian estimation framework. This has the advantage of allowing us to model the noise in the displacement estimates probabilistically while still maintaining the description of the model in the language of continuum mechanics.

11.3.3 A Bayesian Estimation Framework

We now derive a probabilistic interpretation of the energy minimization framework. This is an abridged version of [33]. In this setup, we aim to estimate the output displacements u from a set of measurements u^m. We further assume that we are given the measurement probability density function $p(u^m|u)$, which also corresponds to the noise model for the measurements, and the prior probability density function for u, $p(u)$. We now pose this within a Bayesian *a-posteriori* estimation problem. Within this framework, the solution $\hat{u}$ is the u that maximizes the posterior probability density $p(u|u^m)$. Using Bayes' rule we can write the posterior probability as:

$$\hat{u} = \arg\max_u p(u|u^m)\,, \quad p(u|u^m) = \frac{p(u^m|u)p(u)}{p(u^m)}\,. \tag{11.32}$$

Note that $p(u^m)$ is a constant once the measurements have been made, and can therefore be ignored in the maximization process. We can now rewrite the above expression by taking logarithms to arrive at:

$$\hat{u} = \arg\max_u \left(\log p(u) + \log p(u^m|u)\right). \tag{11.33}$$

As discussed earlier, given a strain energy function $W(C, u)$, we can write an equivalent prior probability density function $p(u)$ [see (11.32)] of the Gibbs form [14]):

$$\begin{aligned} p(u) &= k_1 \exp(-W(C, u)), \\ \log(p(u)) &= \log(k_1) - W(\alpha, u, x), \end{aligned} \tag{11.34}$$

where k_1 is a normalization constant.

Next we define the noise $n = u - u^m$. Then we can model the noise probabilistically, using a multinomial Gaussian distribution, as:

$$\begin{aligned} p(n) &= k_2 \exp\left(\frac{-n^t\Sigma^{-1}n}{2}\right), \\ \log p(n) &= \log k_2 - \frac{1}{2}n^t\Sigma^{-1}n\,, \end{aligned} \tag{11.35}$$

where k_2 is also a normalization constant and Σ is the covariance matrix which in this case can be assumed to be diagonal. The mean of the noise is assumed to be equal to zero. Substituting for n in the this expression we get:

$$\log p(u^m|u) = \log k_2 - \frac{1}{2}(u^m - u)^t\Sigma^{-1}(u^m - u). \tag{11.36}$$

The Problem of Unit Reconciliation

The fact that the model stiffness is measured in different units than the image-derived noise variance in the displacement estimates causes a problem which call 'the problem of unit reconciliation.' This is best explained by means of an example.

Using $W = \frac{1}{2}e(u)^t Ce(u)$, which is the linear elastic model defined in equation (11.28) and the noise model defined in equation (11.35), we re-write equation (11.33) (ignoring the constant terms k_1 and k_2) as:

$$\hat{u} = \arg\max_u \; - \left(\frac{1}{2}e(u)^t Ce(u) + \frac{1}{2}(u^m - u)^t \Sigma^{-1}(u^m - u)\right). \qquad (11.37)$$

The modeling terms in this expression are C and Σ. C defines the mechanical model and Σ^{-1} the noise/data covariance. We can write both of these matrices in the following general form (using the $n \times n$ matrix M to be either C or Σ^{-1}) as:

$$M = \begin{bmatrix} M_{11} & \dots & M_{1n} \\ \vdots & & \vdots \\ M_{n1} & \dots & M_{nn} \end{bmatrix} = M_{max}\left[\bar{M}\right],$$

$$\left[\bar{M}\right] = \begin{bmatrix} \frac{M_{11}}{M_{max}} & \dots & \frac{M_{1n}}{M_{max}} \\ \vdots & & \vdots \\ \frac{M_{n1}}{M_{max}} & \dots & \frac{M_{nn}}{M_{max}} \end{bmatrix}, \qquad (11.38)$$

where M_{max} is the maximum value of M. In the case of the material matrix C, C_{max} would be the highest value of the stiffness or the Young's Modulus, whereas in the case of the covariance matrix Σ^{-1}, Σ^{-1}_{max} would be the smallest variance, or the highest confidence in any of the measurements. We can now rewrite equation (11.37) as:

$$\hat{u} = \arg\max_u \; - \left(C_{max}e(u)^t[\bar{C}]e(u) + \Sigma^{-1}_{max}(u^m - u)^t[\bar{\Sigma}^{-1}](u^m - u)\right),$$

$$\hat{u} = \arg\max_u \; - \Big(\underbrace{e(u)^t[\bar{C}]e(u)}_{\text{dimensionless}} + \frac{\Sigma^{-1}_{max}}{C_{max}}\underbrace{(u^m - u)^t[\bar{\Sigma}^{-1}](u^m - u)}_{\text{dimensionless}}\Big). \qquad (11.39)$$

At this point, it is clear that the absolute values of C_{max} and Σ^{-1}_{max} enter into the functional only through their ratio $\frac{\Sigma^{-1}_{max}}{C_{max}}$. Given that the rest of the expressions in equation (11.39) are dimensionless (i.e. are pure numbers and have no units,) for equation (11.39) to add up from a dimensionality viewpoint we need to convert this ratio $\frac{\Sigma_{max}^{-1}}{C_{max}}$ in order to also make it dimensionless.[1] This is done by multiplying by a scaling constant k_{sc} of the appropriate units, i.e,

$$\frac{\Sigma_{max}^{-1}}{C_{max}} \longmapsto \frac{k_{sc}\Sigma_{max}^{-1}}{C_{max}}. \tag{11.40}$$

From a dimensionality viewpoint the value of the scaling constant k_{sc} is completely arbitrary. This value can be interpreted as defining in some sense the ratio of the relative confidences in the data *as a whole* and the model *as a whole*.

The Problem of Bias

The material models described up to this point are *passive* models. They assume that the tissue deform under the influence of external effects. Further, if one looks at the internal energy functions (i.e. $W = \frac{1}{2}e^tCe$) these penalize all deformations. Essentially the internal energy functions act like a prior probability density function with zero mean and a covariance-like structure defined by the material properties matrix C. Hence, the expectation in using such a model is that the material *will not* deform! When such a model is used to model the deformation of a deforming body such as the left ventricle it results in the underestimation of the deformation as it biases the whole estimation towards zero.

In this work, this problem is dealt with using two complementary strategies. First the deformation is estimated in a frame-by-frame approach which keeps it small, and hence reduces the effect of the bias. Second, we apply bias correction by mapping all points that were on the endo- and epi-cardial surfaces of the heart at time t to lie on the (pre-segmented) endo and epi-cardial surfaces at time $t+1$, using the symmetric nearest neighbor method (briefly described in section 11.2.4.)

11.4 Experimental Results

In this section we present results from the application of this integrated biomechanics-based image analysis methodology presented in the last section to magnetic resonance images. We further note that this methodology has also been applied successfully to 3D Ultrasound Images [34] and ultrafast CT images [33].

The images were segmented interactively and the surfaces sampled to 0.5 voxel resolution, at which point curvatures were calculated and the shape-tracking algorithm was used to generate initial displacement estimates. The heart wall was divided into 1000 – 1500 hexahedral elements (depending on the exact geometry of the heart) and the transversely-isotropic linear elastic model was used to regularize the displacements. The fiber stiffness was set to be 3.5 times greater than the cross-fiber stiffness [15]. The Poisson's ratios were both set to 0.4 to model

1 - C_{max} is measured in Pascals and Σ_{max} in voxels. Hence their ratio will not be dimensionless.

approximate incompressibility. The bias problem was dealt with by adopting a frame-by-frame approach and by forcing the nodes which lie on the endocardial and epicardial surfaces at time t to lie on the segmented surfaces at the time $t+1$. The scaling constant k_{sc} was set adaptively to be as large as possible (which pushes the optimum towards the data side) subject to solution convergence. In this way we make the following assumption: the best solution is the one which adheres as much as possible to initial estimate of the displacement field but still results in a connected solid. Convergence fails when the Jacobian of the deformation field[1] becomes singular. In this case we lower the value of this weight to produce a smoother displacement field.

A commercial finite element solver ABAQUS [19] was used to solve the resulting equations. The computational time after the segmentation was of the order of 3-4 hours/dog (depending on the heart rate and hence the number of image frames) on a Silicon Graphics Octane with an R10000 195 MHz processor and 128 MB RAM. An example of the strain output for the full cardiac cycle is shown in figure 11.5. Note here, that in the case of circumferential strain (top) for example, the heart shortens during the first half of the cycle (End Diastole to End Systole) resulting in positive circumferential strain and it returns to its original shape at the end of the cycle resulting close to zero circumferential strain.

We also note that the algorithm was validated by comparing its strain estimates to those obtained using implanted markers (in the case of cine-MRI data) and sonomicrometers (in the case of 3D Echocardiography) [35].

11.4.1 Pre and post-occlusion comparison

In figure 11.6, we show results from one canine study in which two sets of images were acquired. The first set of images was acquired under baseline conditions and the second set of images was acquired after occlusion of the left anterior descending artery (LAD). This occlusion caused an area of dysfunction where there was reduced blood flow, and in broad terms simulated the effect of a 'heart attack'.

To understand the results two key points must be kept in mind. (i) Unlike a balloon, a heart acts like a pump and it contracts under increasing pressure. Because the tissue in the heart wall is close to incompressible, this contraction results in an increased thickening of the wall and a shortening of the heart around its circumference. These effects are captured using the radial and circumferential strain components, which can be thought of as percentage changes in length in their specific directions. (ii) In the case of loss of regional blood flow in the myocardial wall, that part of the wall 'switches' to 'balloon' mode, as it no longer is capable of actively contracting. In this case the tissue bulges out instead of contracting with an associated decrease in thickness and an increase in the circumferential length. In figure 11.6 this change is clearly shown for both radial and circumferential strains.

---

1 - The Jacobian of the deformation is the matrix F defined in equation (11.20)

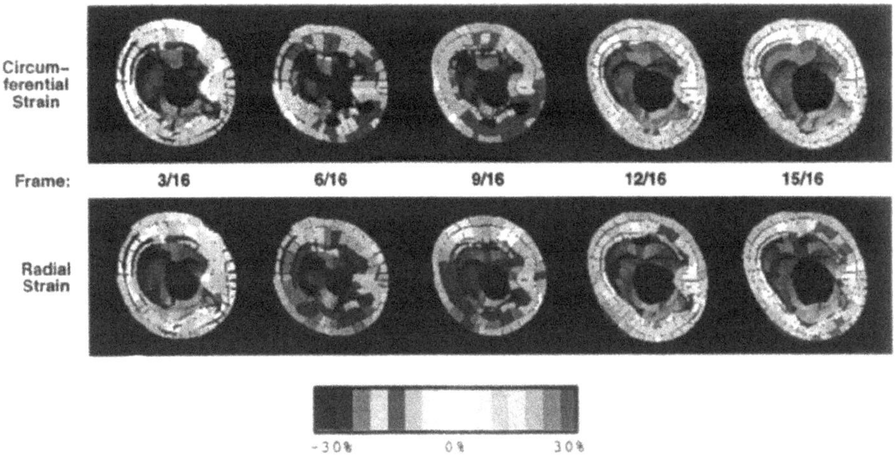

Figure 11.5: Strain Development in Baseline Canine LV derived from cine-MRI. In this figure we show results from every third frame for circumferential (top) and radial (bottom) strain development in a normal canine LV. See color Plate 9.

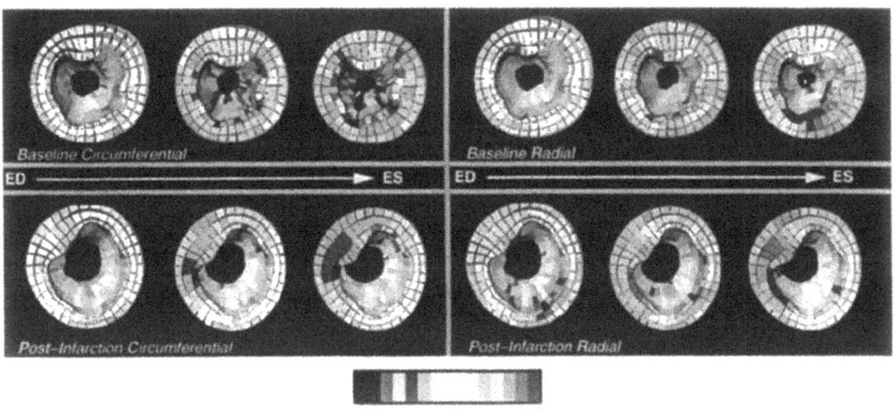

Figure 11.6: Strain Development in Post-Infarction (and vs. Baseline) Canine LV derived from cine-MRI. Left side: mid-ventricle cut-away views through the 3D reconstructed volume show the strain patterns that develop at 1/3, 2/3 and 3/3 of the time between ED and ES. The leftmost displays illustrate the circumferential (CC) strains (normal ED-ES shortening is in the blue-green region). The displays just to the right show the radial (RR) strains (normal ED-ES thickening in yellow-red region). See color Plate 10.

The area of dysfunction (or infarct region) is in the lower left of the ventricle.

11.4.2 Shape-Based Estimates vs MR Tagging

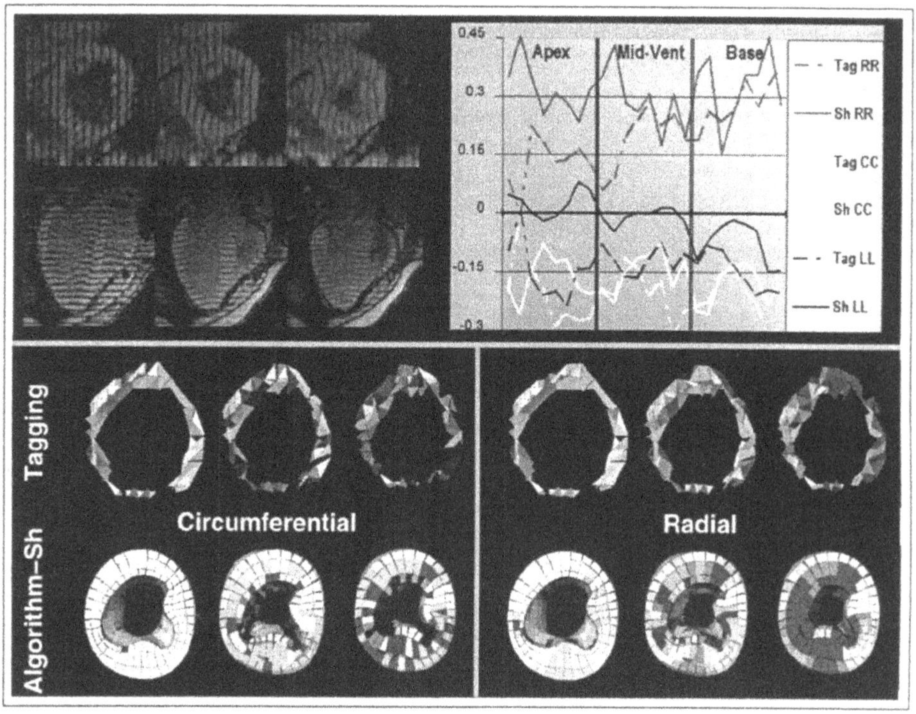

Figure 11.7: MR Tagging-derived strains vs. strains from cine-MRI, derived using our algorithm using shape-based displacements. Top-left: Image slices shown with MR line tags in 2 (out of 3) orthogonal views at three time points. Bottom-left: MR tagging-derived (upper) and our-algorithm-derived (lower) circumferential strains at times 1/3, 2/3 and 3/3 from ED to ES. Refer to color scale in figure 11.6. Bottom-right: MR tagging-derived (upper) and our -algorithm-derived (lower) radial strains at same times. For MR tag displays, tetrahedra connect only the tracked points. Top-right: Comparison of circumferential (CC,yellow), radial (RR,red) and longitudinal (LL,blue) ED-ES strains in a helical path from apex to base of LV derived using MR-tagging (Tag, dotted lines) and our-algorithm (Sh, solid lines). See color Plate 11.

In another experiment we illustrate the application of this methodology using shape -based displacements as compared to the results of the magnetic resonance tagging-based method of Kerwin [25]. The image data set is from a normal human volunteer and was provided to us by Dr Jerry Prince, of John Hopkins University. The resulting comparison is shown in Figure 11.7.

11.5 Future Research Directions

The rational for the use of biomechanical models in the recovery of soft tissue deformation from medical images, is that they capture something of the real material properties of the object. If the object though, as in the case of the left ventricle, is deforming actively a passive model such as those discussed earlier in this chapter has severe bias problems.

We can try to deal with the effects of the bias problems in a number of ways as discussed in the previous section, but none of these methods can provide the following properties:

1. Have a prior model for the deformation which preferentially penalizes some deformations but not others.
2. Ability to model the deformation from start to finish and at any time in the process penalize the deformation from the original state.

Regarding the first point, most elastic models will penalize deviations from rigid motion, that is all deformations. Models based on the thin-plate spline [4] penalize any deviations from an affine deformation. This would be a good choice if we knew that the true deformation was on average affine, but this is not very likely in arbitrary soft tissue deformation.

The second point would allow the imposition of constraints such as fiber hardening or locking. In the case of the left ventricle (and generally where elastomers are concerned) a material will become rigid in certain directions after a certain amount of deformation. Any attempt to deform it further in this direction will result in a twisting motion as the deformation has to be captured in a direction other than the one that has locked.

The Active Model Paradigm One possible correction for the elastic models is the adjustment of the model for non-zero bias. Consider the following generalization of the standard linear elastic model, which we will label the *active elastic model*:

$$W = \frac{1}{2}(e - e^a)^t C(e - e^a) \tag{11.41}$$

This is equivalent to having a non-zero mean prior probability density for the deformation. The strain e is divided into two parts: the part e^a which is energy free, and the part $e - e^a$ which is penalized. If this model were used, we would be assuming that the expected value of the deformation would be close to e^a and not to zero as is currently done. This has the advantage over the thin-plate spline model (which also penalizes only part of the deformation) of being able to map the part of the active deformation directly in terms of local strains. Some preliminary results using this model can be found in [32].

Acknowledgments

The authors would like to thank Dr R. Todd Constable of the Department of Diagnostic Radiology, Yale University School of Medicine for acquiring the MR images.

References

[1] A. A. Amini, Y. Chen, R. W. Curwen, V. Manu, and J. Sun. Coupled B-snake grids and constrained thin-plate splines for analysis of 2D tissue deformations from tagged MRI.

[2] A. A. Amini and J. S. Duncan. Bending and stretching models for LV wall motion analysis from curves and surfaces. Image and Vision Computing, 10(6):418–430, 1992.

[3] L. Axel. Physics and technology of cardiovascular MR imaging. Cardiology Clinics, 16(2):125–133, 1998.

[4] F. L. Bookstein. Principal warps: Thin-plate splines and the decomposition of deformations. IEEE Transactions on Pattern Analysis and Machine Intelligence, 11(6):567–585, 1989.

[5] G. E. Christensen, R. D. Rabbitt, and M. I. Miller. 3D brain mapping using deformable neuroanatomy. Physics in Medicine and Biology, 39:609–618, 1994.

[6] I. Cohen, N. Ayache, and P. Sulger. Tracking points on deformable objects using curvature information. Lecture Notes in Computer Science-ECCV92, pages 458–466. Springer Verlag, 1992.

[7] T. Constable, K. Rath, A. Sinusas, and J. Gore. Development and evaluation of tracking algorithms for cardiac wall motion analysis using phase velocity MR imaging. Magn. Reson. Med., 32:33–42, 1994.

[8] T. S. Denney Jr and J. L. Prince. Reconstruction of 3-D left ventricular motion from planar tagged cardiac MR images: An estimation theoretic approach. IEEE Transactions on Medical Imaging, 14(4):625–635, December 1995.

[9] M. P. do Carmo. Differential Geometry of Curves and Surfaces. Prentice-Hall, New Jersey, 1976.

[10] J. S. Duncan, R. L. Owen, L. H. Staib, and P. Anandan. Measurement of non-rigid motion using contour shape descriptors. In Computer Vision and Pattern Recognition, pages 318–324, Lahanai,Maui, HI, June 1991. IEEE.

[11] J. S. Duncan, P. Shi, R. T. Constable, and A. Sinusas. Physical and geometrical modeling for image-based recovery of left ventricular deformation. Progress in Biophysics and Molecular Biology, 69(2-3):333–351,1998.

[12] A. C. Eringen. Mechanics of Continua. Krieger, New York, NY, 1980.

[13] J. C. Gee, D. R. Haynor, L. Le Briquer, and R. K. Bajcsy. Advances in elastic matching theory and its implementation. In CVRMed-MRCAS, pages 63–72, Grenoble, France, March 1997.

[14] D. Geman and S. Geman. Stochastic relaxation, Gibbs distribution and Bayesian restoration of images. IEEE Transactions on Pattern Analysis and Machine Intelligence, 6:721–741, 1984.

[15] J. M. Guccione and A. D. McCulloch. Finite element modeling of ventricular mechanics. In P. J. Hunter, A. McCulloch, and P. Nielsen, editors, Theory of Heart, pages 122–144. Springer-Verlag, Berlin, 1991.

[16] S. N. Gupta and J. L. Prince. On variable brightness optical flow for tagged MRI. In Information Processing in Medical Imaging, pages 323–334, June 1995.

[17] E. Haber, D. N. Metaxas, and L. Axel. Motion analysis of the right ventricle from MRI images. In Medical Image Computing and Computer Aided Intervention (MICCAI), pages 177–188, Cambridge, MA, October 1998.

[18] R. Herfkens, N. Pelc, L. Pelc, and J. Sayre. Right ventricular strain measured by phase contrast MRI. In Proceedings of the 10th Annual SMRM, page 163, San Francisco, 1991.

[19] Inc. Hibbit, Karlsson & Sorencen. Abaqus Version 5. 7. Rhode Island, USA, 1997.

[20] B. K. P. Horn and B. G. Schunk. Determining optical flow. Artificial Intelligence, 17:185–203, 1981.

[21] J. Huang, D. Abendschein, V. G. Dávila-Román, and A. A. Amini. Spatiotemporal tracking of myocardial deformations with a 4-D B-spline model from tagged MRI. IEEE Transactions on Medical Imaging 18(10):957–972, October 1999.

[22] P. J. Hunter, A. McCulloch, and P. Nielsen, editors. Theory of heart. Springer-Verlag, Berlin, 1991.

[23] P. J. Hunter, M. P. Nash, and G. B. Sands. Computational electromechanics of the heart. In A. V. Panfilov and A. V. Holden, editors, Computational Biology of the Heart, pages 346–407. John Wiley &Sons, 1997.

[24] C. Kambhamettu and D. Goldgof. Curvature-based approach to point correspondence recovery in conformal nonrigid motion. CVGIP: Image Understanding, 60(1):26–43, July 1994.

[25] W. S. Kerwin and J. L. Prince. Cardiac material markers from tagged MR images. Medical Image Analysis, 2(4):339–353, 1998.

[26] J. McEachen, A. Nehorai, and J. Duncan. A recursive filter for temporal analysis of cardiac function. In IEEE Workshop on Biomedical Image Analysis, pages 124–133, Seattle, June 1994.

[27] E. R. McVeigh. Regional myocardial function. Cardiology Clinics, 16(2):189–206, 1998.

[28] F. G. Meyer, R. T. Constable, A. J. Sinusas, and J. S. Duncan. Tracking myocardial deformation using phase contrast MR velocity fields: A stochastic approach. IEEE Transactions on Medical Imaging, 15(4), August 1996.

[29] G. Nayler, N. Firmin, and D. Longmore. Blood flow imaging by cine magnetic resonance. J. Comp. Assist. Tomog., 10:715–722, 1986.

[30] A. V. Panfilov and A. V. Holden, editors. Computational Biology of the Heart. John Wiley &Sons, 1997.

[31] X. Papademetris and J. S. Duncan. Cardiac image analysis: Motion and deformation. In J. M. Fitzpatrick and M. Sonka, editors, SPIE Handbook on Medical Imaging - Volume III: Medical Image Processing and Analysis. SPIE, 2000.

[32] X. Papademetris, E. T. Onat, A. J. Sinusas, D. P. Dione, R. T. Constable, and J. S. Duncan. The active elastic model. To appear in Information Processing in Medical Imaging, 2001.

[33] X. Papademetris, Estimation of 3D left ventricular deformation from medical images using biomechanical models, Ph. D. dissertation, Yale University, New Haven CT. (URL = http:// noodle.med.yale.edu/ thesis) (May 2000).

[34] X. Papademetris, A. J. Sinusas, D. P. Dione, and J. S. Duncan. Estimation 3D left ventricular deformation from echocardiography. Medical Image Analysis, 5(1):17–28, 2001.

[35] X. Papademetris, A. J. Sinusas, D. P. Dione, and J. S. Duncan R. T. Constable. Estimating 3D strain from 4D cine-MRI and echocardiography: In-vivo validation. In Medical Image Computing and Computer Aided Intervention (MICCAI), pages 678-686, Pittsburgh, U.S.A., October 2000.

[36] N. Pelc, R. Herfkens, A. Shimakawa, and D. Enzmann. Phase contrast cine magnetic resonance imaging. Magn. Res. Quart., 7(4):229–254, 1991.

[37] N. J. Pelc. Myocardial motion analysis with phase contrast cine MRI. In Proceedings of the 10th Annual SMRM, page 17, San Francisco, 1991.

[38] N. J. Pelc, R. Herfkens, and L. Pelc. 3D analysis of myocardial motion and deformation with phase contrast cine MRI. In Proceedings of the 11th Annual SMRM, page 18, Berlin, 1992.

[39] J. L. Prince and E. R. McVeigh. Motion estimation from tagged MR image sequences. IEEE Transactions on Medical Imaging, 11:238–249, June 1992.

[40] P. Shi. Image Analysis of 3D Cardiac Motion Using Physical and Geometrical Models. Ph. D. dissertation, Yale University, New Haven CT, May 1996.

[41] P. Shi, A. J. Sinusas, R. T. Constable, and J. S. Duncan. Volumetric deformation analysis using mechanics–based data fusion: Applications in cardiac motion recovery. International Journal of Computer Vision, 35(1):65–85, November 1999.

[42] P. Shi, A. J. Sinusas, R. T. Constable, E. Ritman, and J. S. Duncan. Point-tracked quantitative analysis of left ventricular motion from 3D image sequences. IEEE Transactions on Medical Imaging, 19(1):36–50, January 2000.

[43] A. Spencer. Continuum Mechanics. Longman, London, 1980.

[44] H. D. Tagare. Non-rigid curve correspondence for estimating heart motion. In Information Processing in Medical Imaging, pages 489–494, Vermont, USA, June 1997.

[45] D. Terzopoulos and D. Metaxas. Dynamic 3D models with local and global deformation: Deformable superquadrics. IEEE Transactions on Pattern Analysis and Machine Intelligence, 13(17), 1991.

[46] P. van Dijk. Direct cardiac NMR imaging of heart wall and blood flow velocity. J. Comp. Assist. Tomog., 8:429–436, 1984.

[47] V. Wedeen. Magnetic resonance imaging of myocardial kinematics: Technique to detect, localize and quantify the strain rates of active human myocardium. Magn. Reson. Med., 27:52–67, 1992.

[48] A. A. Young, D. L. Kraitchman, L. Dougherty, and L. Axel. Tracking and finite element analysis of stripe deformation in magnetic resonance tagging. IEEE Transactions on Medical Imaging, 14(3):413–421, September 1995.

[49] Y. Zhu, M. Drangova, and N. J. Pelc. Estimation of deformation gradient and strain from cine-PC velocity data. IEEE Transactions on Medical Imaging, 16(6):840–851, 1997.

Index

A

active contour, 152, 159
atria, 94
  anatomy, 94
  echocardiography of, 94
  FGRE MR imaging, 98
  fibrillation, 94
  FSE MR imaging, 98
  left atrial motion, 106
  left atrial shape, 106
  motion field, 104, 107
  MRI, 91, 95, 96
  pathologies, 94, 95
  right atrial motion, 106
  surface fitting, 102
  surface registration, 104
    iterative closest point (ICP), 104
  variability in motion field, 112

B

B-snake, 185
  coupled grids, 188
    optimization, 190
  dynamic programming, 185
B-solid, 185
B-spline, 186
  advantages of, 186
  coupled grids, 188
    optimization, 190
  curves, 188
  definition, 186
  discrete sampled, 187
  properties, 187
  recursive definition, 186
  representation for deformation field, 193
  representation for tag planes, 206–209
  three-dimensional motion field, 97, 185
  uniform, 186
biplane radiography, 8
black blood image,
  see cardiac MRI

C

cardiac MRI, 18, 91, 257,
  see also HARP MRI,
  see also phase-contrast MRI,
  see also SPAMM,
  see also tagged MRI
  3D ventricular geometry, 2
  adenosine stress, 9
  black blood image, 163
  diffusion imaging, 2
  diffusion MRI, 2, 3, 22
    fiber architecture, 2, 3
  dobutamine stress, 9, 19
  ejection fraction, 183
  imaging protocol, 18
  in estimation of stress and strain, 2
  interferometric techniques, 219
  phase-contrast MRI, 219, 220, 258
  true FISP, 18
  vs. conventional methods, 17–18, 257–258
  vs. invasive methods, 17, 258
  white blood images, 166
cardiac simulator, 196
  error norms for validation with, 200
    angular error, 200
    length error, 200
    Relative RMS (RRMS), 200
  ground truth deformation field, 196
  k-parameters, 196
  myocardial beads from, 211
  prolate spheroids, 196
  tagged images, 196
Cholesky factorization, 195
CINE-HARP (CHARP), 120, 127
  HARP targeting, 128
  HARP tracking

- backward, 129
- elongation, 130
- forward, 129
- *Lagrangian* strain, 130
  - circumferential, 130
  - deformation gradient tensor, 131
  - in a paced canine LV, 131–133
  - radial, 130–131
- optical flow, 120, 134
- strain rate maps, 137
  - in a paced canine LV, 138
- velocity fields, 134

congestive heart failure, 1
coordinate system
- left ventricle, 40
- prolate spheroidal, 2

coronary artery
- disease, 169
- left anterior descending, 9

D

deformable contours, 2, 185, 188
deformable model, 64, 185, 188
- B-spline, 188
- dynamics, 65

deformation gradient tensor, 203, 298
- in infinitesimal deformation, 298

diffusion coefficient, 3
diffusion tensor, 2
dobutamine, 9, 23

F

finite elements, 7, 37–56, 64, 264
- ABAQUS, 306
- basis functions, 8, 39
- DMESH, 263, 264
  - computer simulation, 271
  - covariance of trajectories, 268
  - deformation gradient tensor, 268
  - factors affecting accuracy, 280
  - fitting, 268
  - *in-vitro* studies, 275
  - *in-vivo* studies, 275
  - local *vs.* global analysis, 268–269
  - material point trajectory, 265–268
  - material point velocity, 265
  - mesh initialization, 265–266
  - multiple information sources, 270
  - reproducibility, 268
  - run-time, 270
  - smoothing the strains, 270
  - strain accuracy, 272
  - tracking accuracy, 271
- geometric fits, 43
- in ventricular mechanics, 8–10
- shape functions, 85
- strain calculation, 86

full width at half maximum, 154, 165

G

Gaussian random vector, 154
graphical user interface, 176

H

HARmonic Phase MRI,
- **see** HARP MRI

HARP MRI,
- **see also** CINE-HARP and Single-shot HARP
- *Eulerian vs. Lagrangian* strains, 146
- harmonic image, 119, 122
  - magnitude image, 119, 122
  - phase image, 119, 122
- harmonic peaks, 122
- harmonic phase, 123
  - derivatives of, 127
  - material property, 123
  - slope, 125
- phase-demodulation, 126
- phase-wrapping, 123–126
- small-bandwidth, 123

heart, 92,
- **see also** atria,

see also left ventricle,
see also right ventricle
anatomy, 2
biventricular model, 61, 79
chambers, 92
relations between, 92
volumes, 95
coupled RV-LV model, 65
fiber orientation, 2
MRI of atria, 91
MRI of the whole heart, 91
MRI of ventricles, 91
pathology, 9
rotation, 79
strain, 1
stress, 1
hypertrophic cardiomyopathy, 3

I

implanted radiopaque markers, 8
iterated conditional modes, 167

L

Law of *LaPlace*, 7
least squares, 44
left ventricle, 59
geometry, 2, 40, 53
modes, 53
prolate spheroidal coordinate system, 40
remodeling, 27
ACE inhibitors, 27
strain, 42,
see also myocardial strain
suction, 22
twist, 21
untwisting, 22
likelihood function, 178
longitudinal relaxation, 154

M

magnetic field gradients
bipolar, 221, 222
motion compensation, 221
switching, 221
Markov Random Field (MRF), 302
displacement estimation, 302–304
for material modeling, 302
Gibbs distribution, 302
problem of bias, 306
maximum a posteriori, 152
maximum-likelihood, 152
MR elastography, 10
MRI, 259,
see also cardiac MRI,
see also MR elastography,
see also phase-contrast MRI,
see also tagged MRI
magnitude image, 259
noise, 154
phase image, 259
signal phase, 245
velocity encoding, 259
myocardial beads, 204
computation of, 207
for cardiac simulator data, 211
in a normal volunteer, 212
in a patient with old MI, 214
validations of, 213
myocardial contractility, 24
in ischemic heart disease, 24
myocardial fiber architecture, 3
myocardial hybernation, 10
myocardial infarction, 1
myocardial ischemia, 1
myocardial material properties, 7
myocardial mechanics, 1, 2
determinants of, 2, 10
related to (patho)physiology, 2
role of tagged MRI, 2
myocardial segment shortening, 20, 24
circumferential shortening, 20
in normal humans, 22
cross-fiber shortening, 21
fiber shortening, 21
in infarction, 27
with dobutamine stress, 24
myocardial strain,

see also strain
circumferential strains, 21
coefficient of variation, 105
in normal humans, 105
definition, 4
fiber *vs.* cross-fiber strains, 22, 24
from triangular elements, 21
homogenous analysis, 8
in a paced canine LV, 131–133, 138, 143–145, 147
in a patient with old MI, 201, 202, 204
in a pig with acute MI, 204, 205
in border zone, 10
in FE model validations, 9
in ischemia, 21
in MI patients, 27
in normal humans, 105
nonhomogeneous analysis, 8
trade offs, 8
orthogonal coordinates, 4
principal axis in systole, 5
principal strains, 4, 21
radial strains, 21
sensitivity to noise, 297
shear strains, 4
tetrahedral measurements, 8
torsional shear
in diastole, 6
in systole, 5
myocardial stress, 3
3D model of, 7
in hypertrophy, 1
Law of *LaPlace*, 7
nine components of, 3, 4
non-homogeneous nature, 7
orthogonal coordinates, 4
principal stresses, 4
shear stress, 4
myocardial stunning, 10
myocardial velocities,
see also phase-contrast MRI,
see also velocity fields **under** CINE-HARP
in healthy volunteers, 234–236
in infarcted patients, 237
in infarction, 243
r, ϕ decomposition, 232
rotational *vs.* radial, 243
rotational twist, 237
systolic range, 243
transmural gradients, 236
myocardial viability, 9, 25
dobutamine MRI, 9, 24, 27
myocardium
detection, 161
material parameters, 9
perfusion, 10
shortening, 5
stunned *vs* hibernating, 10
viability, 9

P

papillary muscles, 7
phase-contrast MRI, 219–246, 260,
see also finite elements **under** DMES
see also myocardial velocities
3D velocity acquisition, 221, 222
black blood preperation, 224
sandwich pulse, 224
breath-hold acquisition, 223, 229
cine imaging, 260
data acquisition time, 229
gradient echo, 223
gradient echo *vs.* echo-planar, 228
imaging artifacts, 224
k-space sampling, 230
MR-angiography, 220
parametric images, 233
phase-contrast, 7
reference scan, 221, 222
segmented acquisition, 224
segmented echo-planar acquisition, 226
SMASH and SENSE, 244
v_{enc}, 223

velocity aliasing, 221, 222
velocity encoding, 221, 222, 260
gradients, 260
strength, v_{enc}, 261
velocity sensitive scan, 221, 222
view sharing, 230
vs. TI-201 SPECT in infarct, 242
vs. tagged MRI, 244
phase-shift, 220, 259, 261, 262
field-inhomogeneity, 261
motion-induced, 220, 259
other sources, 221, 222
Poisson's ratio, 301

R

regularization, 9, 46, 192
Tikhonov, 44
right ventricle, 48, 59, 93
anatomy, 93
circumferential strains, 105, 110
contour segmentation, 62
contraction pattern, 93
free wall, 48
function, 94
geometry, 2, 49
hypertrophy, 74, 79
invasive imaging, 94
motion parameters, 72
MRI, 95
RVH,
see also right ventricle **under** hypertrophy

S

Shape-Based Tracking, 293–295
bending energy, 295
confidence measures, 295
surface curvatures for, 293
first and second fundamental form, 294
Gaussian curvature, 294
mean curvature, 294
principal curvature, 294
Weingarten Mapping, 294
Single-shot HARP (SHARP), 120, 139
contraction angle, 145
in a paced canine, 145
Eulerian strain, 140–141
circumferential, 141
in a paced canine LV, 143, 144, 147
principal strains, 142
radial, 141
tag-line visualization, 139
unit elongation, 141
snake, 159
snake algorithm,
see active contour
SPAMM, 18, 60, 184,
see also tagged MRI
coupled B-snake grid, 188
deformable model for, 65
external forces, 67
internal forces, 70
stiffness, 70
deformation field from, 190
approximating subspace, 193
computation time, 203
constrained thin-plate reconstruction, 192
constraints for computing, 192
effect of B-spline order, 202
effect of weights, 202
in a patient with old MI, 200
in a pig with acute MI, 203
shifted B-spline representation, 193
validation with cardiac simulator, 196
tag grid lines, 184
tag planes, 184
strain, 4–10, 262
Cauchy-Green strain tensor, 42
deformation gradient tensor, 42
energy function, 300
isotropic linear elastic, 301
non-linear, 302
transversely clastic, 301

Eulerian, 203, 263
Green, 299
in finite deformation, 299
in infinitesimal deformation, 298
Lagrangian, 72, 263, 299
principal axes, 5
principle strain, 73
shear, 6, 43
strain rate, 7, 137, 262
stress, 3–9
sum-of-squared-differences (SSD), 189

T

tag center, 156
tag detection, 151, 188
tag intersection, 191
tag line
detection, 161, 188
tag lines, 152–163
tag pattern
phase modulation due to motion, 125
tag profile, 153
tag tracking, 151, 188
tagged MRI, 8, 17, 37, 65, 151,
see also cardiac MRI,
see also HARP MRI,
see also SPAMM
2D *vs.* 3D, 21, 205
apparent motion, 125
Fourier spectra in, 119
Fourier Transform, 120
model tags, 43, 45, 49
of dilated cardiomyopathy, 30
of hypertrophic cardiomyopathy, 29
of LVH, 28
of pericardial constriction, 30
of right ventricle, 95
of right ventricular hypertrophy, 30
tag surfaces, 67, 206–209
vs. invasive methods, 8
vs. phase-contrast MRI, 258
vs. sonomicrometry, 20
tagging,
see tagged MRI
thin-plate splines, 192
torsion, 4
trabeculae, 7

W

white blood images,
see cardiac MRI

Y

Young's modulus, 301

www.ingramcontent.com/pod-product-compliance
Lightning Source LLC
LaVergne TN
LVHW051049210926
848486LV00001B/54

9781402002229